Notice

This volume attempts to provide a useful guide to surgical intensive care. The manual does not attempt to define in exhaustive detail a particular patient's requirements for therapy, nor to prejudge for a particular physician the therapeutic regimen he or she may deem necessary in regard to that patient. The Committee does not claim that methods or approaches other than those presented in this volume may not be equally successful in the management of surgical patients.

MANUAL OF
SURGICAL
INTENSIVE
CARE

BY THE COMMITTEE ON
PRE AND POSTOPERATIVE CARE

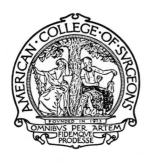

AMERICAN
COLLEGE
OF
SURGEONS

Editorial Subcommittee

JOHN M. KINNEY, M.D., *Chairman*
HENRIK H. BENDIXEN, M.D.
SAMUEL R. POWERS, JR., M.D.

W. B. SAUNDERS COMPANY • PHILADELPHIA • LONDON • TORONTO

W. B. Saunders Company: West Washington Square
Philadelphia, PA 19105

1 St. Anne's Road
Eastbourne, East Sussex BN21 3UN, England

1 Goldthorne Avenue
Toronto, Ontario M8Z 5T9, Canada

Library of Congress Cataloging in Publication Data

American College of Surgeons. Committee on Pre and
Postoperative Care.

Manual of surgical intensive care.

1. Therapeutics, Surgical.   2. Critical care medicine.
    3. Intensive care units.   I. Title. [DNLM: 1. Intensive
care units.   2. Preoperative care.   3. Postoperative care.
    WX218 A512m]

RD51.A45 1976   617   76–51009

ISBN 0–7216–1180–X

American College of Surgeons   ISBN   0-7216-1180-X

Last digit is the print number: 9   8   7   6   5   4   3   2

COMMITTEE ON
PRE AND POSTOPERATIVE CARE

*JOHN A. COLLINS, Chairman, *Stanford*
*STANLEY J. DUDRICK, Vice Chairman, *Houston*

Active Members

J. WESLEY ALEXANDER,
Cincinnati

ARTHUR E. BAUE,
New Haven

*CHARLES R. BAXTER,
Dallas

CHARLES E. BRACKETT,
Kansas City

LARRY C. CAREY,
Columbus, Ohio

CHARLES J. CARRICO,
Seattle

JOSEPH M. CIVETTA,
Miami

P. WILLIAM CURRERI,
New York

JAMES H. DUKE, JR.,
Houston

JOHN H. DUFF,
London, Canada

RUBEN F. GITTES,
Boston

LAZAR J. GREENFIELD,
Richmond

FRANK E. GUMP,
New York

E. JOHN HINCHEY,
Montreal

JOHN W. MADDEN,
Tucson

JOHN A. MANNICK,
Boston

WILLIAM W. MONAFO, JR.,
St. Louis

GERALD S. MOSS,
Chicago

JOHN M. PALMER,
Sacramento

*SAMUEL R. POWERS, JR.,
Albany

*MARC I. ROWE,
Miami

GEORGE F. SHELDON,
San Francisco

ROGER T. SHERMAN,
Tampa

JOHN J. SKILLMAN,
Boston

ROBY C. THOMPSON, JR.,
Minneapolis

HASTINGS K. WRIGHT,
New Haven

*Executive Committee

Senior Members

Contributors

HENRIK H. BENDIXEN, M.D. Professor and Chairman, Department of Anesthesiology, College of Physicians and Surgeons, Columbia University. Chief of the Anesthesiology Service, Presbyterian Hospital, New York.

HARVEY R. BERNARD, M.D., F.A.C.S. Professor of Surgery, Albany Medical College of Union University, Albany, New York.

LAWRENCE B. BONE, M.D. Clinical Instructor in Surgery, State University of New York at Buffalo. Chief Resident in Surgery, E. J. Meyer Memorial Hospital and Veterans Administration Hospital, Buffalo, New York.

JOHN R. BORDER, M.D., F.A.C.S. Professor of Surgery, State University of New York at Buffalo. Director of the Trauma Service and Attending in Surgery, E. J. Meyer Memorial Hospital, Buffalo, New York.

JOHN E. BRIMM, M.D. Postdoctoral Fellow, Department of Pathology, University of California, San Diego.

JOSEPH M. CIVETTA, M.D., F.A.C.S. Professor of Surgery, Anesthesiology, Medicine and Pathology, University of Miami School of Medicine. Director, Surgical Intensive Care, Jackson Memorial Hospital, Miami, Florida.

JOHN A. COLLINS, M.D., F.A.C.S. Professor of Surgery and Chairman of the Department of Surgery, Stanford University School of Medicine, Stanford, California.

J. FRANCIS DAMMANN, JR., M.D. Professor of Pediatric Cardiology and Biomedical Engineering, University of Virginia, Charlottesville.

S. RAYMOND GAMBINO, M.D. Professor of Pathology, College of Physicians and Surgeons, Columbia University. Director of the Clinical Chemistry Service, Presbyterian Hospital, New York.

AKE GRENVIK, M.D. Professor of Anesthesiology and Critical Care Medicine, and Director of Critical Care Medicine, University of Pittsburgh School of Medicine. Medical Director, Intensive Care Unit, Presbyterian-University Hospital, Pittsburgh, Pennsylvania.

FRANK E. GUMP, M.D., F.A.C.S. Professor of Surgery, College of Physicians and Surgeons, Columbia University. Attending Surgeon, Presbyterian Hospital, New York.

JOHN M. KINNEY, M.D., F.A.C.S. Professor of Surgery, College of Physicians and Surgeons, Columbia University, New York.

DONALD S. KORNFELD, M.D. Professor of Clinical Psychiatry, College of Physicians and Surgeons, Columbia University. Attending Psychiatrist, New York Psychiatric Institute, New York.

HAROLD LAUFMAN, M.D., F.A.C.S. Professor of Surgery, Albert Einstein College of Medicine. Director, Institute for Surgical Studies, and Attending Surgeon, Montefiore Hospital and Medical Center, Bronx, New York.

STANLEY M. LEVENSON, M.D., F.A.C.S. Professor of Surgery, Albert Einstein College of Medicine. Director, Surgical ICU-Burn Unit, Bronx Municipal Hospital Center, Bronx, New York.

RICHARD M. PETERS, M.D., F.A.C.S. Professor of Surgery and Bioengineering, University of California, San Diego. Head, Division of Thoracic Surgery, University Hospital, San Diego, California.

HENNING PONTOPPIDAN, M.D. Professor of Anaesthesia, Harvard Medical School. Chief, Respiratory Unit and Respiratory Care Department, Massachusetts General Hospital, Boston.

SAMUEL R. POWERS, Jr., M.D., D.Sc.(Med.), F.A.C.S. Professor of Surgery, Albany Medical College. Attending Surgeon-in-Chief, Albany Medical Center Hospital, Albany, New York.

BASIL A. PRUITT, Jr., M.D., COL MC, F.A.C.S. Commander and Director, U.S. Army Institute of Surgical Research, Brooke Army Medical Center, Ft. Sam Houston, Texas.

MICHAEL A. RIE, M.D. Instructor in Anesthesia, Harvard Medical School. Assistant in Anesthesia and Assistant in Medicine, Massachusetts General Hospital, Boston.

PETER SAFAR, M.D. Professor and Chairman, Department of Anesthesiology, University of Pittsburgh School of Medicine. Director, Department of Anesthesiology, Presbyterian-University Hospital, Pittsburgh, Pennsylvania.

RAJIINDAR SINGH, M.D. Assistant Professor of Cardiology, Chicago Medical School. Chief of Cardiology, Veterans Administration Hospital, North Chicago, Illinois.

WILLIAM M. STAHL, Jr., M.D., F.A.C.S. Professor of Surgery, New York University School of Medicine. Attending Staff, University Hospital, Bellevue Hospital and Manhattan Veterans Administration Hospital, New York.

GARY W. WELCH, M.D., Ph.D. Assistant Professor, Department of Anesthesiology, University of Massachusetts Medical School, Worcester.

CARL W. WALTER, M.D., F.A.C.S. Clinical Professor of Surgery Emeritus, Harvard Medical School. Surgeon Emeritus, Peter Bent Brigham Hospital, Boston.

Preface

This volume is divided into three general sections: Development of Surgical Intensive Care, General Aspects of Surgical Intensive Care and Management of Specific Conditions. The chapters vary in length and several have been given extra space because they represent subjects of central importance (such as the management of ventilatory failure) or special difficulty not commonly faced by all surgeons (such as management of the major burn patient). There is no single discipline of medicine where the conventional training qualifies a person to manage all of the different kinds of challenges which may be met in a busy intensive care unit for surgical patients. The editors, representing two disciplines, surgery and anesthesiology, have included a chapter on the psychological aspects of an ICU, the legal problems of the ICU, and a separate chapter on the problems of the clinical laboratory in relation to the ICU. These widely varying areas of competence have become important in providing modern intensive care.

For the optimum care of their patients, informed surgeons will have more and more to accept some responsibility for the quality of intensive care in their hospital. Routine operative procedures have become more complex and are more frequently applied to the treatment of the very young, the very old and the poor-risk patient with preoperative complications. Modern intensive care is an important determinant of survival for such patients. In addition, it is often necessary for informed surgeons to apply appropriate pressure to surmount the local roadblocks to development of modern intensive care in their institutions. For this reason, a chapter has been included in this book dealing with the location and design of an intensive care unit.

The intensive care unit has been called the "hospital's hospital" for many different reasons. An ICU segregates and concentrates all of the assets of an institution for care of the critically ill. A poorly designed or carelessly operated ICU may segregate and concentrate liabilities of care, such as medication errors, infection exposure, electrical hazards and psychological trauma. Certain important features of ICU design may easily be omitted unless the surgical staff are aware of their importance and hence speak out in their defense.

Intensive care on an individual basis dates back to the first concerned physician struggling with the care of a critically ill patient. But the field of intensive care, as a formal discipline, has developed since World War II. It is a young and rapidly growing field without clearly defined boundaries and facing increasingly complex problems. Many of these current problems are related to the rapid growth of the intensive care concept. Our ability to apply advanced intensive care is exceeding our limits of money and manpower to provide such care. Therefore, we find ourselves not only striving for the optimum care for every patient but also forced to become selective in the allocation of the resources which are available for intensive care.

The ideal person to direct the day-to-day activities of a surgical ICU is not automatically someone trained in one or another specialty, but rather is the individual who is most effective in mobilizing the resources of a given institution to meet the problems of a particular patient in an effective and integrated manner. The chapter on Therapeutic Conflicts in the Intensive Care Unit highlights some of the areas where the optimum treatment of one organ system is at the expense of another. Modern intensive care demands rapid and effective communication at every level in order to achieve the greatest benefit with the least risk for the particular combination of problems presented by any one patient.

It is fitting that this book has been prepared under the auspices of the American College of Surgeons. Just as the definition of intensive care is changing rapidly and evolving in complexity, so is the responsibility of the surgeon. The concept of modern intensive care represents an unusual opportunity to demonstrate the principles set forth in the fellowship pledge of that College:

"... I pledge myself to pursue the practice of surgery with scientific honesty and to place the welfare of my patients above all else; to advance constantly in knowledge; and to render willing help to my colleagues, regard their professional interest, and seek their counsel when in doubt as to my own judgment."

JOHN M. KINNEY, M.D., *Chairman*
HENRIK H. BENDIXEN, M.D.
SAMUEL R. POWERS, JR., M.D.
Editorial Subcommittee

Contents

Part I:

DEVELOPMENT OF SURGICAL INTENSIVE CARE

Part II:

GENERAL ASPECTS OF SURGICAL INTENSIVE CARE

Part III:

MANAGEMENT OF SPECIFIC CONDITIONS

Part I

DEVELOPMENT OF SURGICAL INTENSIVE CARE

CHAPTER 1

HISTORY OF INTENSIVE CARE

Henrik H. Bendixen, M.D.

John M. Kinney, M.D.

Between 1950 and 1970 there was extraordinarily rapid growth of an approach to therapy that has been called by many names, including "intensive care" and "critical care." Prior to 1950, few general hospitals had an intensive care unit; by 1970, these units had sprouted to the extent that literally every acute hospital had at least one. All bigger hospitals now are likely to have several units, each aimed at a different patient population, such as those with coronary disease, burns, or trauma. The organization of care in an acute hospital would be inconceivable without intensive care units, for the reason that they have realized a life-saving potential. Hard data are scarce, but there is little doubt that a large number of patients survive today because of intensive care units, patients who a generation ago would have died.[52]

What prompted the efforts to provide intensive care? What made the spectacular growth possible? The answers to these questions are complex, and in order to provide answers, the intellectual and technological roots of intensive care must be examined as well as the conditions of public interest and availability of funds that were needed to support a form of therapy which was inherently expensive, although often highly cost-effective.[7] In searching for the roots of intensive care, the primary interest is not in the first spectacular demonstration in animals, nor in the first daring application in humans. What is significant is the beginning of sustained clinical application.

Intensive care covers a large range of activities and defies any attempt to define it with precision. However, characteristics of intensive care, and of intensive care units, can be listed. Intensive care is a form of treatment of patients with serious, often life-threatening, trauma or illness, demanding special resources of manpower and technology. The practical way of delivering such care has been by centralizing patients and resources in areas where expertise can be developed and maintained, where the necessary manpower

3

categories can be deployed, and where the required technology can be assembled and kept working.

A common threat to the life of a patient in an intensive care unit is failure of the respiratory system in the broadest sense. Although other support systems are available or under development, ranging from the artificial kidney to circulatory assist devices, it is certainly the case that effective treatment or prevention of failure of ventilation or oxygenation, and the maintenance of a free airway, have been at the core of activities in most intensive care units. This historical sketch traces the roots of centralization of airway management, oxygen therapy, and artificial ventilation.

CENTRALIZATION OF PATIENTS AND RESOURCES IN SPECIAL UNITS

The centralization of those patients who cannot be handled elsewhere may be traced back to the origin of hospitals. The first "public" hospitals provided a place to care for those patients who could not be cared for in their homes because of a lack of resources. These early hospitals from the period 1750 to 1850 were characterized by their 12 to 20 bed wards for the poor, making supervision and care practically and economically feasible. It was much later that the well-to-do moved from their homes into hospitals for treatment, and then to single or double rooms in private pavilions.[18] This happened around the turn of the century, as the hospitals grew in resources, especially with respect to diagnostic and surgical facilities.

As any house officer knows, it is difficult or impossible to provide intensive care for seriously ill patients in private rooms. Therefore, to the other reasons for having intensive care units must be added the fact that resource-demanding care of illness and trauma, involving vital organs and systems, requires a concentration of patients to be handled economically. The single or double room is viewed as the hallmark of upper class care, which should be universally available. At the same time, the hospital planner must provide intensive care areas for that fraction of the patient population that is seriously ill, and reserve the single and double rooms for those less ill. It helps that often the ward can be rearranged and equipped for intensive care fairly readily.

Centralization of patients with special illnesses or conditions goes back so far as to be lost in antiquity. The first purpose undoubtedly was to separate individuals with infectious diseases and mental afflictions for the protection and comfort of the rest of the community. Much later came centralization of patient categories because of therapeutic possibilities—examples are the gas poisoning units of World War I[4,33] and the shock units of later wars.[61] Also, in the face of civilian disaster, special units were promptly opened so that patients and resources could be centralized. A well reported example is the unit that opened at the Massachusetts General Hospital when the

Coconut Grove disaster struck in 1942.[22] Major outbreaks of poliomyelitis elicited a similar response, and large treatment units were created almost instantaneously; a spectacular example was the epidemic in Copenhagen in 1952.[37,40] In recent decades we have seen special units open to receive special patient categories. Burn units have proved their usefulness,[1,47] as have coronary care units.[14]

A special unit that may be viewed as a precursor of the surgical intensive care unit is the recovery room.[55] Even Florence Nightingale recommended holding the patient in a "corner" to allow recovery before returning him to his ward.[35] Whether this was for the sake of the patient operated on or for the sake of other patients is not clear. Such units for care of surgical patients during the period of immediate recovery from anesthesia and surgery began to appear sporadically between the world wars, but it was not until about 1950 that their numbers grew. They are now found in every hospital where surgery is performed. The rapid growth, starting after World War II, most likely resulted because there were older and sicker patients requiring more complex procedures, and also because surgeons had become accustomed to the benefits of recovery rooms in the military during the war and pushed the civilian hospital to update itself in this respect. Reports of a high incidence of postanesthetic mortality also stimulated the demand for recovery rooms.[54]

Another reason that recovery care became a necessity at this time was the change in anesthetic technique. For almost a century, most general anesthesia could be characterized as the single agent–deep anesthesia type, often using ether or cyclopropane. This technique was well tolerated by patients in good to fair condition, but led to hypotension or circulatory collapse when the patient was elderly, in poor condition, or lacking sympathetic system protection.[17] By 1950, new techniques employing muscle relaxant and narcotic drugs in combination with "light" inhalation anesthesia were rapidly gaining in acceptance. Although muscle relaxant drugs do not have an inherent toxicity,[6] respiratory function certainly must be watched with vigilance in the recovery period. The risk is even greater when muscle relaxant and narcotic drugs are used together. The anesthesiology literature of the 1950s contained many papers on "mysterious" prolonged apneas. As the understanding of physiology, postoperative evaluation, and recovery care improved, these reports disappeared.[8] Modern anesthetic techniques that involve significant physiologic trespass upon the respiratory system would not be possible if the modern recovery room could not be relied upon to monitor and support respiration.

The recovery room has gradually changed its role. From a relatively quiet room in which patients slept off their ether, safely on their side and with the head positioned to free the airway, and with a kidney basin in readiness on every bed, it has evolved into a unit bustling with activity, which ranges from checking blood gases and setting respirators to management of circulating volume and fluid balance. Not surprisingly, many surgeons made the discovery that the recovery room was better prepared to give "intensive" care than was any other area of the hospital. Soon the sickest patient would stay overnight in the recovery room, then several days. For many hospitals, the recovery room was the first intensive care unit.

A SKETCH OF THE HISTORY OF AIRWAY MANAGEMENT

The history of airway problems and resuscitation must begin with a reference to the prophet Elijah, who restored to life the son of the Shunammite woman by "putting his mouth upon his mouth."[26] Next we observe the dramatic discoveries and demonstrations. As an example, Vesalius reported in 1543 on passing into the "rough artery" (as the trachea was then called) a reed through which he could blow intermittently. Hooke, in 1667, demonstrated that he could keep a dog alive by using bellows to blow into the opened trachea.[30,33,60,63]

It may be of equal or greater interest to determine what led to the first therapeutic efforts in man, and when such efforts became successful and widespread. Active airway management in man may be traced to the period 1760 to 1780, when great advances in the knowledge of respiration occurred with the discovery of oxygen and carbon dioxide and their physiologic roles, the principal contributions being made by Black, Priestley, Scheele, and Lavoisier.[3,30,33] It was also a time of concern with resuscitation. In 1767, a Dutch society for the saving of drowning victims was founded, evidently in response to a public concern, and it rapidly led to similar activities in other countries, among them the Humane Society (1774) in London. Here, John Hunter (1776) recommended bellows for insufflation of air for resuscitation.[30,38] A review on resuscitation dating from 1796 showed remarkable insight and practical skills, including mouth-to-mouth and mouth-to-nose resuscitation, the introduction of a curved tube into the windpipe, and even tracheotomy. Other measures that we must find ludicrous were also recommended, including the rubbing of the body with oil, the use of emetics, and the insufflation of tobacco smoke into the rectum.[34]

At about the same time, another therapeutic imperative was present in the form of diphtheria, which occurred widely and resulted in many deaths. All accounts suggest that physicians realized that lives could be saved if only the airway could be kept open. Francis Home described diphtheria in 1765, calling it croup and suggesting tracheotomy.[36] Apparently, one reason for the lukewarm acceptance of the procedure was its high mortality rate, and not many were done until Bretonneau in 1826 reported the success with his technique of tracheotomy in this disease.[10] For another century, diphtheria continued to supply a therapeutic imperative to further improve tracheotomy techniques and to explore endotracheal intubation as an alternative. Endotracheal intubation through the mouth was introduced by

Macewen[42] (1879), who had an oral endotracheal tube made and reported on its successful use in patients needing surgery on the airway. O'Dwyer[50] (1885) introduced an apparatus for inserting metal tubes into the glottic opening of patients with diphtheria, leaving these in place for many days.

The transition to the modern era of endotracheal intubation came gradually, prompted by two therapeutic imperatives: the plastic surgical reconstruction in the wake of World War I,[30,43] and the advances of thoracic surgery over several decades. For such surgery, the endotracheal technique became recognized as superior.[28,29,39]

A SKETCH OF THE HISTORY OF OXYGEN THERAPY

Oxygen was a latecomer among physiologic discoveries, becoming known during the years 1770 to 1790. The use of oxygen in the Pneumatic Institute of Beddoes and Davy appears to have been prompted more by the urge to experiment and to know rather than by the urge to treat.[46] For the next century, oxygen was occasionally mentioned as beneficial in the treatment of one condition or another, but did not have much of an impact on patients or the profession. We do not have many detailed descriptions of how oxygen was made or administered, but it appears that the chemist would heat potassium chlorate in the presence of manganese dioxide, collecting and storing the gas in airtight bags; for home use, hydrogen peroxide could be heated.[5] One may wonder if the inspired concentration of oxygen was increased more than marginally with such methods. Mostly for technical reasons, oxygen therapy did not become easily applicable until high-compression techniques made it possible to provide tanks of compressed oxygen on a commercial basis, which happened after World War I. Also, there does not seem to have been a strong urge to treat during this period, except for sporadic instances. One therapeutic effort was initiated by Haldane[33] and by Barcroft,[4] who used oxygen in treating the pulmonary edema secondary to war gas poisoning.

During the next several decades, the use of oxygen was recommended for the treatment of conditions ranging from leg ulcer to pneumonia and myocardial infarction.[3,60] However, it remained a very sporadic application. We know of no hospital that had piped oxygen available prior to 1950, and of very few prior to 1960. The imperative to treat with oxygen undoubtedly came so late because recognition of hypoxia was not placed on a quantitative basis until the electrode for measuring partial pressure of oxygen in arterial blood had been perfected and put on the market. This occurred during the period 1960 to 1965.[19,41] It is difficult to document, but it is likely that the blood gas measurements have been far more effective than is usually perceived in making possible the rapid growth of intensive care in recent decades, since it had not been possible to document the presence or absence of respiratory failure until the blood gas measurements became available.

A SKETCH OF THE HISTORY OF
ARTIFICIAL VENTILATION

Here, again, we may distinguish between the urge to know, which led to brilliant demonstrations of what is possible, and the therapeutic imperative, which led to the treatment of patients. Some of the early demonstrations have been mentioned previously. It was not until this century, however, that the clinical development started. Throughout the nineteenth century, the emphasis was on resuscitation—from resuscitation of the newborn led by the French obstetricians to a variety of other applications.

By the end of the century, the physiologic and mechanical principles of artificial ventilation had been established, and the stage was set for progress. The first major therapeutic imperative apparently was provided by tuberculosis. Sauerbruch,[57] in his memoirs, mentions the thousands of patients waiting to be operated on, if only the problem of the open thorax could be managed. Undoubtedly, surgeons at the turn of the century were projecting a large number of pulmonary, esophageal, and even cardiac operations,[24] but it still seems that tuberculosis loomed largest as a therapeutic imperative, especially in Europe. Sauerbruch[56] and Brauer[16] understood the importance of transpulmonary, pleural, and airway pressures. Sauerbruch's first invention was the negative pressure box surrounding the open thorax. It was cumbersome, but it worked and stayed in use for decades. Brauer's approach was a box that surrounded the patient's head, creating a positive airway pressure. This also worked, and a variety of modifications and variations appeared, both in Europe and in the United States. With time, simplicity won in the form of a positive airway pressure applied by mask or by endotracheal tube combined with intermittent positive pressure ventilation. Two pioneers of note were George Edward Fell of Buffalo[28] and Franz Kuhn of Kassel,[39] whose understanding of physiology and methods of simplicity were the closest to present-day techniques. Excellent and entertaining accounts of artificial ventilation in thoracic surgery are provided by Northrup,[49] Matas,[44] Green,[31] Robinson and Leland,[53] and Green and Janeway.[32] The piston-pump respirator designed by Matas (1902)[44] seemed sound and of a simple enough design to be practical, but piston-pumps did not gain favor for another 50 years. Another approach was taken by Meltzer and Auer (1909),[45] who used high flow insufflation into the trachea to produce continuous respiration, but without respiratory movements. This approach, although physiologically acceptable for short procedures, never found much application in man, except in a modified form.

It is interesting that now, seventy years later, so-called CPAP (continuous positive airway pressure) is used so effectively in the treatment of the infant respiratory distress syndrome. The method consists of having the patient breathe spontaneously against a positive airway pressure. Similarly, the now so popular IMV (intermittent mandatory ventilation) consists of having the patient breathe spontaneously against a positive end-expiratory pressure (PEEP) while the machine provides only one or a few breaths per minute. The use of a positive pressure mask in the treatment of pulmonary edema is also related.[3] These methods are modern variations on a theme composed at the turn of the century. We have to go from Sauerbruch and Brauer (1904) to Crafoord's[23] modification (1938) of Frenckner's[29] spiropulsator before we find an intermittent positive pressure respirator that works for anesthesia and surgery. A large-scale use of the respirator in the care of surgical patients did not begin until the period 1950 to 1960. It may be that one reason for the long delay was less effective communication than we have today, or that many different factors had to be brought together and made to work before sustained clinical activity became possible. It may also be, as Comroe[20,21] has suggested, that powerful individuals held back science for many decades.

In addition to thoracic surgery, first for tuberculosis and then for other intrathoracic problems, the only other major therapeutic imperative for supported ventilation was poliomyelitis. It is ironic that the knowledge and techniques for effective long-term ventilation were finally ready when the polio vaccine was also ready. The recognition of respiratory failure as a cause of death in poliomyelitis came slowly and was not clearly spelled out until about 50 years ago,[51] at the same time when experiments with tanks began. First came Thunberg's tank,[59] which fully enclosed the patient. In short order followed Drinker and Shaw's[25] tank, in which the head of the patient protruded through a snug neck collar. This device was simple, rugged, and reliable enough to maintain ventilation for days, weeks, and months. Although nursing care was difficult, positioning was a chore, and what we now know as chest physiotherapy was nearly impossible, it was the therapeutic mainstay for 25 years. The next important advance occurred when Bower[15] reported improved survival when the tank respirator was combined and coordinated with intermittent positive pressure via a tracheostomy. The tank continued its supremacy, however, until the Copenhagen epidemic,[37,40] when the volume of patients was so large that ventilation had to be supplied by intermittent positive pressure breathing, via endotube or tracheostomy, provided manually by medical students working in shifts. Soon it was clear that survival statistics were more favorable with the newer methods, and the tank was retired.

In short, the therapeutic imperative to provide artificial ventilation (for more than resuscitation) was provided in large measure by two diseases: the first was tuberculosis, seconded in time by other pulmonary and cardiac conditions; the other was poliomyelitis. Although it may seem that the use of respirators in treating chronic obstructive pulmonary disease should also be mentioned, it is quite likely that the respirator has been of relatively small importance in this situation. Undoubtedly, some patients have been helped by the respirator in conditions such as status asthmaticus and intercurrent infections, and after operations. However, in the face of advanced disease, the respirator at best plays a delaying action. Despite Emerson's[27] early suggestion (1909), the use of positive airway pressure in treating pulmonary edema came decades later.[3]

CHANGES IN ATTITUDE TOWARD THERAPY

It is difficult to define the attitude toward intensive care therapy with any degree of precision. Whereas only a few decades ago there was less of a tendency to try heroic efforts in the face of fatal illness or trauma, several factors have cooperated to bring about a change in attitude, which now favors active intervention under most circumstances. One factor is the ability to resuscitate. Only in the last two decades have the tools of resuscitation been perfected, making available everything from airway management, ventilation support, oxygenation, cardiac defibrillation, and pacing and drug support to the circulatory assist devices being tried on patients in shock after a myocardial infarction. Another factor is the increasing survival of patients receiving long-term respirator support. We are able to prevent death in a substantial number of patients who would have died only a generation ago. This advance has brought with it a host of problems, from ethics to cost, but these are outside the scope of this chapter.

At the same time, as the profession has become more aggressive in therapy, the public opinion, in fact, has been supporting such aggressiveness. As Lewis Thomas[58] says (1977), in a society adoring technology and wishing good health to be a human right, dying is regarded as the ultimate failure. The aim of the intensive care unit is to prevent death when death is not inevitable, and to restore the patient to his former state of health. Needless to say, nothing could better reflect the aim of public opinion.

Another factor, often overlooked, in the rapid growth of intensive care is the role played by research support, much of it from the National Institutes of Health[12,13] and also from many other public and private foundations and organizations. The pioneers of intensive care often worked in teaching hospitals and were able to support the early units by making available manpower and equipment from research laboratories. With time, some units were supported in full from research funds. Whatever form the research support took, the investment has paid off handsomely by providing a treasure of pathophysiologic information that could not have been obtained in any other way. The publication of good clinical research helped establish the foundation of knowledge that made the growth of intensive care possible.

THE LAST TWENTY YEARS

What are the main events of the last 20 years? Perhaps we are too close to give a valid answer, but we may try, knowing that contradiction may follow in time. Essentially, we have progressed sequentially, taking one hurdle at a time.

Twenty years ago it was a generally held opinion that pneumonia must follow when a patient had a tracheostomy and was given artificial ventilation. The patients with neuromuscular disease did a special service, because they made it possible to disprove the inevitability of pneumonia as a consequence of treatment. In patients, often young and with normal lungs, who received tracheostomy and artificial ventilation following thymectomy for myasthenia gravis, the mortality rate has been zero in our experience, and the morbidity has been very low. Results nearly as good have been obtained in patients with polyradiculitis and similar conditions. What was required to achieve this first win? It took the elaboration of sound basic nursing routines, positioning, chest physiotherapy, suctioning, tracheostomy or tube care, and effective humidification. Also, proper patterns of ventilation, which would minimize ventilation-perfusion problems, were elaborated. Today,[9,48] with effective preventive care, no patient should die from airway obstruction or respiratory failure.

Placing oxygen toxicity in a proper perspective was another hurdle. This was a surprisingly emotional issue, but one that generates little heat today. We have not solved the riddle of the mechanism of oxygen toxicity, but we know enough to avoid it in the vast majority of cases. We also have better respirators and measuring devices, so the accidental exposure is eliminated.[48,52]

We have come far toward understanding some of the mechanisms behind the terms "shock lung," "wet lung," "heavy lung," and so on. The emphasis is on using positive end-expiratory pressure to maintain a nearly normal lung volume, to support the heart, and to counteract the commonly occurring interstitial pulmonary edema by accelerating fluid removal. Fluid overload often plays a role, and weighing the patient remains the soundest method of checking fluid balance,[62] taking into consideration the catabolic loss of tissue mass that occurs in the ill patient.[48]

Another hurdle that has not been scaled but is being vigorously attacked is that of nutrition. Just a decade ago it was often true that patients were starved in intensive care units. Despite gaps in basic knowledge, we have come far in providing nutrition, even to the patient who does not possess a functioning gastrointestinal tract.

By 1970, it became clear that few patients in intensive care units died from respiratory or circulatory failure. In this decade, most deaths are associated with sepsis, often involving gram-negative organisms. At a time when successful management of respiratory, circulatory and renal failure, singly or in combination, is well within reach, sepsis is a major roadblock to a further increase in patient survival. Perhaps the interplay between nutrition, infection, and antibiotic use may be the key question for the next decade.

The modern history of intensive care spans little more than two decades. Its roots go far back, but thoracic surgeons and polio physicians must receive the credit for setting the stage for the modern era. We may wonder why it should have taken so long for the modern era to begin, when most of the prerequisites were present at the turn of this century. Perhaps half a century was required to bring all individual components together. Or it may be that one important discovery was that the gradual deterioration of the patient following major surgery, ending in respiratory and circulatory failure, could be interrupted or prevented by respiratory system support. Björk

saw that a patient could live following radical lung removal, provided he
could be tided over the immediate postoperative period by intensive care
with mechanical ventilation.[11] Cardiac surgeons uniformly had similar experiences. The patient following major surgery and the patient who sustains
major trauma probably constitute by far the largest groups of patients who
have benefited from intensive care. A dramatic report on the use of mechanical ventilation in treating the crushed chest came from Avery.[2] Today,
the prognosis is much improved for the patient after major trauma, in large
part because of intensive care.

REFERENCES

1. Artz, C. P., and Yarbrough, D. R., III.: Major body burn. J.A.M.A., 223:1355, 1973.
2. Avery, E. E., Mørch, T. E., and Benson, D. W.: Critically crushed chests. J. Thorac.
   Surg., 32:291, 1956.
3. Barach, A. L.: Inhalation therapy—historical background. Anesthesiology, 23:407, 1962.
4. Barcroft, J., Hunt, G. H., and Dufton, D.: The treatment of chronic cases of gas poisoning
   by continuous O_2 administration in chambers. Q. J. Med., 13:179, 1920.
5. Bartholow, R.: A Practical Treatise on Materia Medica and Therapeutics. 6th Ed. New
   York, D. Appleton and Company, 1888.
6. Beecher, H. K., and Todd, D. P.: A Study of the Deaths Associated with Anesthesia and
   Surgery. Springfield, Illinois, Charles C Thomas, 1954.
7. Bendixen, H. H.: The cost of intensive care. In Bunker, J. P., Mosteller, F., and Barnes,
   B.: Costs, Risks and Benefits of Surgery. New York, Oxford University Press, 1977.
8. Bendixen, H. H., and Laver, M. B.: Hypoxia in anesthesia—a review. Clin. Pharmacol.
   Ther. 6:510, 1965.
9. Bendixen, H. H., Egbert, L. D., Hedley-Whyte, J., Laver, M. B., and Pontoppidan, H.:
   Respiratory Care. St. Louis, C. V. Mosby Company, 1965.
10. Billington, C. E., and O'Dwyer, J.: Diphtheria, Its Nature and Treatment, and Intubation in
    Croup. New York, William Wood, 1889.
11. Björk, V. O., and Engstrom, C. G.: The treatment of ventilatory insufficiency after pulmo-
    nary resection with tracheostomy and prolonged artificial ventilation. J. Thorac. Surg.,
    30:356, 1955.
12. Black, E. A., and Deming, P. A.: The Study of Injured Patients. A Trauma Conference
    Report. Bethesda, Maryland, Department of Health, Education and Welfare Publ. No.
    (NIH) 74-603.
13. Black, E. A., and Deming, P. A.: Anesthesiology: Its Expanding Role in Medicine. A
    Research Conference Report. Bethesda, Maryland, Department of Health, Education
    and Welfare, Publ. No. (NIH) 76-918.
14. Bloom, B. S., and Peterson, O. L.: End results, cost and productivity of coronary care unit.
    N. Engl. J. Med., 288:72, 1973.
15. Bower, A. G., Bennett, V. R., Dillon, J. B., and Axelrod, B.: Investigation on the care and
    treatment of poliomyelitis patients. I and II. Ann. Western Med. Surg., 4:561, 686,
    1950.
16. Brauer, L.: Die Ausschaltung der Pneumothoraxfolgen mit milfe des ueberdruck ver-
    fahrens. Mitt. Grenzgeb. Med. Chir., 8:483, 1904.
17. Brewster, W. R., Jr., Isaacs, J. P., and Andersen, T. W.: Depressant effect of ether on
    myocardium of the dog and its modification by reflex release of epinephrine and
    norepinephrine. Am. J. Physiol., 175:399, 1953.
18. Crichton, M.: Five Patients—The Hospital Explained. New York, Alfred A. Knopf, Inc.,
    1970.
19. Clark, L. C., Jr., Wolf, R., Granger, D., and Taylor, Z.: Continuous recording of blood
    oxygen tensions by polarography. J. Appl. Physiol., 6:189, 1953.
20. Comroe, J. H., Jr.: Retrospectoscope. Inflation—1904 model. Am. Rev. Resp. Dis.,
    112:713, 1975.

21. Comroe, J. H., Jr.: Retrospectoscope. How to succeed in failing without really trying. Am. Rev. Resp. Dis., *114*:629, 1976.
22. Cope, O.: Management of the Coconut Grove burns at the Massachusetts General Hospital. Ann. Surg., *117*:801, 1943.
23. Crafoord, C.: On the technique of pneumonectomy in man. Acta Chir. Scand., Suppl. 54, 1938.
24. Cutler, E. C.: The origins of thoracic surgery. N. Engl. J. Med., *208*:1233, 1933.
25. Drinker, P., and Shaw, L. A.: An apparatus for the prolonged administration of artificial respiration. J. Clin. Invest., 7:229, 1929.
26. Elijah, prophet: 2 Kings 4, 34: Restored the son of Shunammite woman to life, "putting his mouth upon his mouth."
27. Emerson, H.: Artificial respiration in the treatment of edema of the lungs. Arch. Intern. Med., *3*:368, 1909.
28. Fell, G. E.: Artificial respiration. Forced respiration, with comments on the cabinet methods of Sauerbruck, Unger and others; also a new method in thoracic surgery. Surg. Gynecol. Obstet., *10*:572, 1910.
29. Frenckner, P.: Bronchial and tracheal catheterization. Acta Otolaryngol., Suppl. 20, 1934.
30. Gillespie, N. A.: Endotracheal Anesthesia. 2nd Ed. University of Wisconsin Press, 1950.
31. Green, N. W.: A positive pressure method of artificial respiration, with a practical device for its application in thoracic surgery, together with a report on transpleural operations on fourteen dogs. Surg. Gynecol. Obstet., *2*:512, 1906.
32. Green, N. W., and Janeway, H. H.: Artificial respiration and intrathoracic oesophageal surgery. Ann. Surg., *52*:58, 1910.
33. Haldane, J. S.: Respiration. New Haven, Yale University Press, 1922.
34. Herholdt, J. D., and Rafn, G. G.: Life Saving Measures. Copenhagen, H. Tikiøb, 1796. (Translation: Aarhus, Stiftsbogtrykteriet, 1960.)
35. Hilberman, M.: The evolution of intensive care units. Crit. Care Med., *3*:159, 1975.
36. Home, F.: An Enquiry into the Nature, Cause and Cure of the Croup. Edinburgh, Kincaid and Bell, 1765.
37. Ibsen, B.: The anesthetist's viewpoint. Polio, 1952. Proc. R. Soc. Med., *47*:72, 1954.
38. Keith, A.: Three Hunterian Lectures on the mechanism underlying the various methods of artificial respiration. Lancet, *1*:745; 825; 895, 1909.
39. Kuhn F.: Perurale Tubagen mit und ohne Druck. I and II. Dtsch. Z. Chir., *76*:148; 467, 1905.
40. Lassen, H. C. A.: A preliminary report on 1952 polio epidemic. Lancet, *1*:37, 1953.
41. Laver, M. B., and Seifen, A.: Measurement of blood oxygen tension in anesthesia. Anesthesiology, *26*:73, 1965.
42. Macewen, W.: Introduction of tracheal tubes by the mouth instead of performing tracheotomy or laryngotomy. Br. Med. J., *1*:122, 1880.
43. Magill, I. W.: Appliances and preparations. Forceps for intratracheal anaesthesia. Br. Med. J., *2*:670, 1920.
44. Matas, R.: Artificial respiration by direct intralaryngeal intubation with a modified O'Dwyer tube and a new graduated air-pump, in its applications to medical and surgical practice. Am. Med., *3*:97, 1902.
45. Meltzer, S. J., and Auer, J.: Continuous respiration without respiratory movements. J. Exp. Med., *11*:622, 1909.
46. Miller, A. H.: The pneumatic institution of Thomas Beddoes at Clifton, 1798. Am. Med. History, *3*:253, 1931.
47. Moncrief, J. A.: Burns. N. Engl. J. Med., *288*:444, 1973.
48. Moore, F. D., Lyons, J. H., Jr., Pierce, E. C., Jr., Morgan, A. P., Jr., Drinker, P. A., McArthur, J. D., and Dammin, G. J.: Post-traumatic Pulmonary Insufficiency. Philadelphia, W. B. Saunders Company, 1969.
49. Northrup, W. P.: Apparatus for artificial forcible respiration. Medical and Surgical Report of the Presbyterian Hospital in the City of New York, *1*:127, 1896.
50. O'Dwyer, J.: Intubation of the larynx. N.Y. Med. J., *42*:145, 1885.
51. Petren, K., and Sjövall, E.: Eine Studie über die tödliche akute Form der Poliomyelitis. Acta Med. Scand., *64*:260, 1926.
52. Pontoppidan, H., Geffin, B., and Lowenstein, E.: Acute Respiratory Failure in the Adult. Boston, Little, Brown and Company, 1973.
53. Robinson, S., and Leland, G. A.: Surgery of the lungs under positive and negative pressure. Surg. Gynecol. Obstet., *8*:255, 1909.

54. Ruth, H. S., Haugen, F. P., and Grove, A. P.: Anesthesia Study Commission. J.A.M.A., *35*:881, 1947.
55. Sadove, M. S., and Cross, J. H.: The Recovery Room. Philadelphia, W. B. Saunders Company, 1956.
56. Sauerbruch, F.: Zur Pathologie des offenen Pneumothorax und die Grundlagen meines verfahrens zur seiner Aussehaltung. Mitt. Greuzgeb. Med. Chir., *8*:399, 1904.
57. Sauerbruch, F.: Master Surgeon. New York, Cromwell, 1953.
58. Thomas, L.: On the Science and Technology of Medicine. Daedalus, Proceedings of the American Arts and Sciences, *106*:35, 1977.
59. Thunberg, T.: Der Barorespirator, ein neuer Apparat für künstliche Atmung. Skand. Arch. Physiol., *48*:80, 1926.
60. Tovell, R. M., and Remlinger, J. E., Jr.: History and present status of oxygen therapy and resuscitation. J.A.M.A., *117*:1939, 1941.
61. U.S. Army Medical Services: Surgery in World War II. Washington, D.C., Office of the Surgeon General, Department of the Army, 1955.
62. Wangenstein, O. H.: Care of the patient before and after operation. N. Engl. J. Med., *236*:121, 1947.
63. Waters, R., Rovenstine, E. A., and Guedel, A. E.: Endotracheal anesthesia and its historical development. Anesth. Analg., *12*:196, 1933.

CHAPTER 2

HOW TO START AN INTENSIVE CARE UNIT

Henrik H. Bendixen, M.D.

The planning process that was used to develop the early intensive care units just one or two decades ago is no longer adequate. A far more comprehensive and professional process than that employed in the past is required. A brief look at the thinking that has gone into past planning is still useful, however, because it is the good ideas of the past that must be combined with new ideas and be presented in a modern context by those who today are planning new units or modernizing old units.

The first of the modern intensive care units were started during the decade following the polio epidemics of the 1950s. The pioneering physicians and surgeons who started these units recognized that the time had come to treat vital system failure in many patient categories on a large scale. Typically, the pioneers spent a varying length of time badgering their colleagues, their chiefs, and their hospital administrators, trying to explain what they had in mind. In the end, they often were granted the use of some already existing space that did not need expensive remodeling. An outmoded 10- to 20-bed ward served the initial purpose well. Usually, some equipment was already on hand, and a few respirators and monitors could be added. It remained only to persuade the director of nursing to provide the planned unit with adventurous nurses, preferably at a nurse/patient ratio of 1:1.5.

From all written and verbal accounts it would appear that the early ICU physicians were in remarkable agreement about the main features of an intensive care unit, namely, centralization of patients with certain common denominator conditions in a special area that possessed special resources in both manpower and equipment. With respect to manpower, most of the early units were directed on a more or less full-time basis by physicians with special interest in respiratory and circulatory pathophysiology. The availability of a full-time director capable of setting the standards of care was seen as clearly desirable. Similarly, most of the early units had as an essential feature the 24-hour coverage by house staff assigned to the intensive care unit with no other responsibility. From the outset, such close coverage gave ample return in the form of excellent training for the house staff involved. At both the staff and the house staff levels, it was recognized that multi-disciplinary collaboration was desirable and perhaps necessary.

The importance of meticulous nursing care for patient survival was obvious to the early ICU directors, and with time it was apparent to everyone. Twenty years ago it was a firmly held thesis that anyone who had a tracheostomy and was connected to a respirator would inevitably contract pneumonia. We now know that patients can be taken care of for weeks or months without getting pneumonia, provided basic preventive nursing care and chest physical therapy are first-class. The two early battles concerning nurse coverage raged over the ratio of nurse to patient and over specialization. From the outset, it was apparent that the intensity of nursing care would have to be considerably greater in the intensive care unit than in the general wards. Quite early it was recognized that the intensity of care would vary, depending on the patient population, from the fairly slow pace of caring for a myasthenic patient in a steady state to the very fast pace of caring for a patient with severe burns, multiple trauma, or a multiple-drain septic condition. But even the pace that is relatively slow for an intensive care unit would be faster than that in the general wards. Soon it became recognized that the required ratio of nurse to patient might vary from 1:0.66 to 1:2, with most surgical intensive care units averaging 1:1.5. Before the era of intensive care, most of the patient's special needs were met by the so-called special nurse. The intensive care unit helped boost the drive toward nurse specialization, which today has proceeded much further than most people realize. Today's nurse specialist in intensive or critical care is superbly trained, receives excellent continuing education, and is very well organized. The special nurse of the past is known today as a private duty nurse.

The intensive care unit set a new pattern of life for physicians. Instead of making rounds and prescribing for the next 12 to 24 (or more) hours, the physician now stayed with the patient and titrated treatment against assessment on a moment to moment basis. For such titration, monitoring and measurements had to be developed. To be useful, results of measurements had to be available promptly. Arterial blood gas measurements had to be calculated quickly enough for the turn-around time (from arterial stick to result in hand) not to exceed 10 minutes. Such requirements were not consistent with the pace of the central laboratory, which was and is geared to receiving the bulk of samples in the morning and delivering the bulk of results in the afternoon. Almost uniformly, the determination of blood gas and certain other measurements became decentralized to a back room of the ICU (or "acute" laboratory nearby), where it must remain as long as there is no better way to provide the results within 10 minutes.

The concept of the intensive care unit has been so successful that it is difficult today to find a general hospital that does not have one or more such units. The era of the special nurse attempting special treatment in a single room is past. No longer is it acceptable practice to provide mechanical respiratory support to patients outside an intensive care unit or recovery room. Today, as a matter of course, the critically ill patients are cared for in intensive care units, as are many patients who are at risk of becoming critically ill. However, the incorporation of such a unit into the hospital's pattern of life has not been painless. First, a conflict exists between the social goal of providing every citizen in a democracy with care in a single or double hospital room and the impossibility of caring for any patient with a significant illness in such a facility. The single or double room, that hallmark of equal access to high-level care, allows diagnostic work-up or the uneventful recovery from routine surgery in healthy patients, but not much more. Second, the hospital administrator likes the hotel-like uniformity of similar double or single rooms, which permits a flexible admission policy and in turn yields the highest occupancy rate. This concept is fine, provided all patients are in a good risk category and admitted for trivial procedures or treatment. Third, a gap is often apparent between the care provided by the high-powered ICU and that available in single rooms (or on the general ward, where it still exists). In most hospitals, the lack of intermediate care units is becoming painfully apparent. Such units could be constructed (or converted) at much lesser expense than the high-powered ICU, and they could help in giving the hospital flexibility of a different kind. Some of the old 12- to 20-bed wards should be considered candidates for low-cost conversion to intermediate care units.

Much has been learned about intensive care units in the past 20 years, and a body of knowledge is available to any group charged with planning an intensive care unit. In a way, then, the task today is easier than it was 20 years ago, when there was little or no past experience. Yet, so much more is demanded today that the planning must be professionally detailed and time-consuming. Exhaustive documentation may well be needed to obtain permission from outside agencies to construct a unit or to ensure future reimbursement. Twenty years ago, units were started by enthusiastic and persuasive individuals. Today, unit planning is a demanding cooperative enterprise involving doctors, nurses and administrators, and often outside professional consultants.

THE PLANNING PROCESS

The first step in the planning process is to realize that real planning will be required; that the planning process must be professional and competent; and that the planning process must include representatives from every group that will work in the intensive care unit in addition to architects, engineers, safety experts, efficiency experts, and reimbursement experts. Clearly, any one intensive care unit must be considered in the context of the hospital's overall need for intensive care unit beds. Much of what planners must deal with is described in other chapters. Here we shall consider the framework only, and proceed methodically to answer precise questions.

Who Is the Patient?

What is characteristic of the patients who will be cared for in the unit? What will be the philosophy with respect to admission? Each hospital will answer the first question somewhat differently. In some locations, highway trauma predominates, in other areas urban warfare. But in most hospitals, the surgical intensive care unit is dominated by the postoperative patient. In almost every case it should be possible to estimate the yearly number of postoperative and trauma patients who require intensive care, taking into account that the need is usually underestimated. The total environment must be considered. Will the unit have to be available to patients from other services, and, in reverse, are there other units that can serve as buffers or backups for the one you are planning? Are there special units already for burns, open heart surgery, pediatric surgery, and so on, or must the unit span a number of special functions?

With respect to philosophy of admission, the planners must decide whether the unit should admit only patients who are critically ill, or whether the unit should admit also those patients who are at risk of becoming critically ill. In most hospitals, preventive intensive care is becoming more frequent, but still the typical intensive care unit patient is all too often in the "catastrophe" category. On the whole, the incidence of "catastrophes" is likely to decrease as preventive intensive care is used more. Also, the role of the ICU is not only to perform lifesaving heroics. More often, its role is the calm and competent conversion of a dramatic disease course into an uneventful course. This role of the ICU is far from fully exploited, and it should be stressed that economies may be achieved, in part because a short stay is cheaper than a long stay, and in part because the uncomplicated course is less demanding in nursing care, tests, blood and blood products, and everything else that makes intensive care expensive. Such an approach is also important for personnel reasons. Both nurses and doctors have difficulty coping, physically and mentally, when they are surrounded only by desperately ill patients with a high rate of mortality. It is good for an ICU to have the right mixture of patients, with a preponderance of preventive admissions, that can give the personnel the sense of professional achievement. We do not hesitate to recommend that a deliberate effort be made to follow an admission policy that results in at least 75 per cent of patients surviving. In any case, these matters of patient selection deserve the most careful consideration. Similarly, the truly hopelessly ill should not be admitted, but careful considerations should be given to definitions. If in fact there is no hope, everyone will know what to do and what not to do. Too much has been said by healthy philosophers about "death and dignity" and "prolonging life unnecessarily." Patients who survive an ordeal in intensive care may be critical of details, but generally are grateful for the effort. A small committee may advise in matters of when to resuscitate and when to keep trying on the margin of the impossible.

How Large a Unit?

This is the same as asking how many patients there are, at any given time, in the patient categories briefly mentioned previously. Various quotations are available, suggesting that anywhere from 3 to 15 per cent of surgical beds should be in intensive care units. Clearly, this depends on the patient population of the individual hospital, on the admissions policy, and on whether intermediate care units are also available. Most units that we see are too crowded, both with respect to the space around each patient and with respect to total unit size. A unit can be too large, and the general consensus is that no one team can handle more than 12 to 16 patients of the type usually found in the surgical unit. If more patients need intensive care, there should be more than one unit, perhaps with subspecialization, but with enough flexibility for mutual support.

Related to the question of how large a unit is needed is that which asks how long the patient will stay. The average surgical ICU will have a mean length of stay in the range of 7 to 12 days, which is long enough to make it mandatory that the patient's psychological welfare be taken into consideration in every aspect of the planning process.

Who Will Take Care of the Patients?

Under this heading we discuss the manning of the unit. The following questions must be answered: Will the unit provide merely increased coverage by nurses, or will it provide intensive care by full-time physician experts and nurse specialists, with chest physiotherapists, respiratory therapists, and multidisciplinary consultants participating? Will the unit have house staff coverage dedicated 24 hours a day? Will teaching take place, involving not just house staff, but all manpower categories? Will research take place, or at least basic data collection? Most units are deficient in space for conferences and teaching, and grossly deficient in space for equipment, both around the patient's bed and in storage or parking areas. Last, but not least, very few units are able to offer any waiting area for the families of ICU patients, not to mention a quiet room where family and ICU physicians can talk in privacy.

What Will Be Done for the Patient?

The general answer is vital systems support. The planners must try to be more specific and also take into consideration the technological potential of the next decade. It is hazardous to assume that miniaturization of existing equipment will keep pace with development of new equipment. Respiratory system support is basic and, together with transfusion and infusion therapy, taken for granted. We must prepare for an increase in renal dialysis and for counterpulsation support of the circulation. The extracorporeal oxygenator may be good technology, but has failed to find good indications for its use. What will be done for the patient, from isolation to multiple vital systems support, determines manpower and space needs, lay-outs, and traffic patterns. In the same context, the planners must define monitoring and support equipment needs at the bedside, at control stations, and in the ICU laboratory. The ICU must protect the patient against accidents, not only those that are immediately fatal, such as a respirator disconnection, but also those that may result "only" in transient complications. Safety engineering must be included in the planning process and must span the entire spectrum from oxygen line failure alarms and closed circuit television to the development of quality control and proper written standard procedures, and the means of seeing to it that these are followed. It is well also to anticipate computer-assisted decision-making procedures.

What Comes Next?

As the answers to the above questions begin to come in, the planners proceed to the next phase, which consists of (1) defining organizational framework and management patterns; (2) determining personnel requirements, the needs for training personnel before opening the unit, and the need for continuing education; (3) preparing equipment lists, planning at the same time the checking, servicing, and safety engineering requirements; (4) anticipating isolation needs and traffic patterns; and (5) preparing the architectural drawings, which should not take final form until all the above have been completed.

Human Relations

Much has been said about ICU psychoses among personnel as well as among patients. Even though an increasing degree of professionalism is improving the overall picture, good planning calls for special measures to ensure patient and personnel sanity. The basic measure is education of all personnel so that they come to realize the importance of professional behavior in the presence of patients. The most common complaints by ICU patients concern, first, the pain of intratracheal suctioning (too many ICU personnel are oblivious of just how exquisitely painful that is), and second, idle nonprofessional chitchat or arguments. By a peculiar twist of logic, doctors and nurses alike seem to conclude that if a patient is prevented from talking by an endotracheal tube or tracheostomy cannula, then the patient is barred from all comunication, including hearing.

Another special measure must be directed toward establishing and keeping good relations among the personnel. Always the most tender is the relationship between the highly experienced and competent nurse specialist and the knowledgeable but inexperienced house officer on rotation. This relationship requires anticipation and constant tactful attention.

INSTITUTIONAL RELATIONS

Good planning requires considering also how the new ICU will fit into the pattern of life of the hospital and the community. Under this heading come such elementary matters as establishing smooth working relations with administration, nursing office, laboratories, blood bank, engineering and electronics laboratories, respiratory and physical therapists, and so on. The proper use of the unit by physicians and surgeons is essential, and the unit must communicate its anticipated role in any way from newsletters to grand rounds to corridor conversations. Such communications are essential if the unit is to be used optimally. It must also be anticipated whether the ICU can play a role in serving the community. In some areas there is little tendency to refer; in other areas, a competent ICU can serve as a referral ICU for a wide area. An ICU is a major resource, and it is unfortunate if it is not used as such.

CHAPTER 3

THE DESIGN OF AN INTENSIVE CARE UNIT

JOHN M. KINNEY, M.D.
CARL W. WALTER, M.D.

Toffler in *Future Shock* wrote that hardly a meeting or conference in science or industry takes place without some ritualistic oratory about the challenge of change. Nowhere are design changes for medical care more important than in the intensive care unit, where construction is always in danger of becoming outdated as new procedures and equipment become established parts of intensive care.

The design of an intensive care unit for surgical patients is usually not considered to be a matter of concern for the busy practicing surgeon. In fact, many surgeons fail to take an active interest in the day-to-day quality and availability of intensive care for survival. Every surgeon has a growing responsibility for the quality and availability of intensive care in his institution. Surgical operations are becoming more complex and are being applied to the very young, the very old and poor-risk patients with preoperative complications. Postoperative intensive care may be a major determinant in their survival.

The well-designed ICU allows a level of acceptance and efficiency that can never be attained, regardless of the hard work and dedication of the staff, when they are forced to function in a poorly designed unit. However, various kinds of local roadblocks may prevent the initiation or upgrading of surgical intensive care. Therefore, each surgeon owes to his patients an effort to be informed to the degree that he can speak to the hospital administration in defense of the principles of intensive care which may be sacrificed in the absence of an informed and persuasive professional staff.

A modern intensive care unit should segregate and concentrate all of the assets available for managing the critically ill patient in that institution. Too little attention is paid to the fact that a poorly designed and carelessly run

ICU can segregate and concentrate the liabilities of the institution, such as congestion, noise, medication errors, electrical hazards, infection exposure and psychological trauma. Perhaps the most important step in minimizing these liabilities is by careful planning and proper physical design of the unit.

The surgical intensive care unit must be planned with the help of architects and engineers as well as manufacturers of various kinds of equipment. These individuals may have the best of intentions and great expertise, yet often find themselves working on an ICU design without real insight into the clinical reasons behind what they are doing. A prevalent feeling among them is that as long as they plan within conventional building codes and prescribed guidelines, their plans are therefore correct. The field is too young and professional opinions too varied to expect an architect to produce the best design for an ICU with the same assurance that one would expect him to design more conventional areas of a hospital. The interested professional staff have a special obligation to study the matter themselves and to guide the architect toward the type of ICU they desire. The architect has as great a need for medical guidance as the medical staff has for architectural and engineering guidance! Nowhere in hospital planning will detailed study by physicians yield greater dividends than with an ICU, where patient care, staff relationships and operative expenses are intimately involved.

SIZE OF THE UNIT

The design of an intensive care unit must begin by a careful institutional review of how large the clinical need is for intensive care. Clarity of objectives and accuracy of information regarding potential demand for ICU care will greatly assist both staff and consultants in deciding between conflicting alternatives as to size, location and staffing. This means not only the types of patient but the volume of patient days per year. It is generally felt that an acute hospital for medicine and surgery should have approximately 4 to 5 per cent of its total beds committed to the provision of intensive care. Their use will vary a great deal from service to service. Some will have minimal demands, whereas postoperative open-heart patients in most cases will require specialized care for several days and 20 per cent of them may require more prolonged intensive care.

The 15-year period from 1945 to 1960 saw the introduction and acceptance of the post-anesthesia recovery room. The 15-year period from 1960 to 1975 was a corresponding transition period for the introduction and acceptance of intensive care units, particularly with regard to the care of surgical patients.[7] There is now sufficient experience with intensive care units throughout the United States to make certain observations regarding their role in the hospital. An ICU tends to have larger and more unpredictable fluctuations in patient census than any other area in the hospital. This emphasizes the importance of proper selection of the number of beds for a proposed ICU.

A unit which is filled year round with patients needing intensive care would imply a significant number of additional patients who are denied intensive care because of the lack of accommodations. However, an ICU with enough beds to always meet occasional peak demands has an unnecessarily high operating cost per bed resulting from the periods with lower than average occupancy. Therefore each institution must determine the number of ICU beds that is an appropriate compromise between maximum bed occupancy and maximum hospital service. The process requires educating the professional staff to expect a few periods during the year when peak demands cannot be fully met and educating the hospital administration to expect an occasional occupancy which is lower than considered optimum.

LOCATION OF THE UNIT

The location of the surgical intensive care unit depends upon the locations of related services, plus other local factors, and is to some degree a matter of philosophy. If a given hospital has a large emergency service with many trauma cases, its planners may wish to locate the surgical ICU near the emergency department or near the operating rooms, in order to expedite the handling of severely injured patients. A more common desire is to have the post-anesthesia recovery room and the surgical ICU adjacent to each other, so that there can be sharing of equipment and staff and common supporting services, such as the acute clinical laboratory and radiology.[8] Another option is to locate the surgical ICU next to other specialty ICU's for economy of sharing equipment, staff and supporting services.

The logical extension of this concept is to group all of the special care units into a large integrated critical care center, with maximum sharing of staff and equipment, and presumably the maximum opportunity for specialty consultation between services.[13] The center concept requires a relatively large area which may be available only in a new building. Some experts feel that geographic grouping of specialty units is of greatest benefit when the patients require similar management (for example, the medical chest patient and the patient with postoperative pulmonary failure who both require mechanical ventilation). The neonatal intensive care unit appears to be sufficiently different from adult intensive care to lessen the benefits of their being in the same area.

A surgical intensive care unit usually has between 6 and 12 beds. The small hospital will recognize that a separate intensive care unit of fewer than four beds is usually not practical to operate. Therefore the intensive care facilities may be combined with the post-anesthesia recovery area to gain the advantages of sharing staff and equipment. The upper limit appears to be 12 to 15 beds for a single intensive care unit. It is difficult to administer a larger number of beds from a single nursing station. Therefore, if more ICU beds are needed for a large hospital, it is better to divide the total beds around two nursing stations which may be planned in an integrated way.

Combined ICU and Recovery Room.   The relationship of a surgical ICU to the recovery room is partly a matter of the size of the institution. Hospitals of less than 75 beds usually keep intensive care patients in the recovery room facilities, utilizing the same nurses and equipment. The ICU's in the hospitals of 75 to 150 beds are often located in space adjacent to the recovery room, with certain nursing staff and equipment in common. Hospitals of intermediate size (150 to 400 beds) usually find their needs for intensive care broad enough to warrant building a surgical ICU independent of the recovery room. Larger hospitals usually decide that their requirements for intensive care are sufficiently diversified to justify the construction of multiple ICU's, each oriented to a particular type of patient. The advantages of sharing nurses and equipment when multiple units adjoin each other must be weighed against the greater convenience and frequency of visits by the medical staff to a specialized ICU located closer to the area of their customary activity.

Since not all hospitals require, or can afford, a separate surgical ICU, it is important to consider carefully the advantages and disadvantages of a combined ICU-recovery room. The equipment (beds, utilities, monitoring devices and resuscitative aids) is identical for the most part. Patient disorders may differ, but there are certain similarities in the nursing care which is required. The advantages of this combination for the smaller hospital are threefold: (1) economy of space, equipment and personnel; (2) increased flexibility of operation—beds which are not needed for one phase may be utilized for the other; and (3) availability of post-anesthesia care on a 24-hour basis, which is not practical for the post-anesthesia recovery room of most smaller hospitals. There is the added convenience for the anesthesiologists and surgeons of having a location near the operating rooms.

Unfortunately, the disadvantages of this combination are often not as carefully considered. It is obvious that there may be some interference with recovery room functions by intensive care requirements and vice versa. Patients who might infect others cannot be treated in an intensive care unit-recovery room combination since the recovery room is technically part of the operating room. This rule denies admittance to seriously ill patients who have infection although they may require intensive care even more than other patients who are admitted. Curtains are available for privacy in a recovery room, but they are often not drawn. Such a facility may be satisfactory when the patient spends a few hours recovering from anesthesia; his awareness of those around him and his need for privacy are minimal. Some ICU patients are sick enough to be oblivious to their surroundings, but others are fully conscious. Their fears are heightened by their own illness and by seeing acutely ill patients around them. The lack of privacy and the extra apprehension which may be aroused in a patient residing in an open recovery room for many days can be a significant deterrent to recovery.

ARRANGEMENT OF THE UNIT

The unit which is built with two to four beds per enclosure often finds that with the very sick or infected patient, the entire area is utilized for one patient alone, thereby wasting the use of the adjacent beds. Single rooms offer the maximum chance for handling each patient without regard to their sex, clinical problem or the presence of infection. However, it is more difficult for one nurse to pay close attention to two or three patients as she must move from room to room. A reasonable compromise would appear to be rigid wall partitions between beds with the space opening to the corridor made up of folding doors which can function to close that area into a room or to open it for the treatment of crisis problems. Double paned windows in these folding doors and windows in the side partitions which have venetian blinds between the two panes of glass allow a flexibility from maximum surveillance to maximum privacy depending upon the condition of the patient and the degree of surveillance required from the nursing station. The patients who need continuous surveillance as they first come into the unit may require intensive care for many days afterward, when the need for privacy throughout part of each day becomes an increasingly important part of their convalescence.

The area devoted to each bed in a large open room is usually less than 100 square feet per bed. This area is clearly inadequate when bulky equipment needs to be stationed at the patient's bedside. Rigid wall cubicles usually require 120 to 150 square feet per bed, while separate rooms traditionally utilize 150 to 200 square feet per bed. The total area of an ICU generally approximates two and one-half to three times the area required for bed space alone. Thus a 10-bed unit with 1400 square feet alloted to bed space might require a total of 3000 or 4000 square feet for the complete unit. This would allow space for supporting area which might include a utility area, an area for clean linen storage, an area for storage of major equipment such as ventilators, fluoroscopy units and other portable equipment to be taken to the bedside but not routinely in use, a small conference area for doctors and nurses, a small laboratory area, a lounge area for the staff and a visitors' waiting area.

THE ICU NURSING STATION

The nerve center of a busy ICU is, of course, the nursing station. This should have a central location, approximately equidistant from each bed. Reconstruction of a narrow rectangular area may make this difficult. The nursing station of an ICU is of necessity the focal point of a high-activity area. Having the distance between the nursing station and patient as short as possible contributes to nursing efficiency and to the patient's sense of security. But the size of the corridor around a central station must be a compromise between excessive distance to the patient and adequate space to accommodate traffic of equipment, housekeeping, sterile supplies and so on, as well as the movement of medical personnel.

The nursing station must be kept patient-oriented and not allowed to become a lounge for coffee, a social center for off-duty chatter, or a telephone desk for non-professional calls. There must be adequate horizontal writing surface for doctors and nurses near the patient records, but out of the main stream of nursing activities. The head nurse will benefit from her own office adjacent to the nursing station, yet readily available for private conversations. A nearby lounge area with rest rooms will provide moments of relaxation during a hectic working day without leaving the area of the unit.

A seldom discussed problem in hospital care is the matter of medication errors which have been estimated to equal 10 to 20 per cent of all medications administered. Two major causes of medication errors are hurry and interruption. Since the nursing station is, of necessity, a high-activity area, interruptions are common. An increased chance of error is coupled with the greater seriousness of an error in some critically ill patients. In order to minimize the chances for error, the medicine preparation area should be located where a nurse may be partially protected from the frequent interruptions at the nursing station. It should not have a telephone, and it should be deliberately positioned so that visual surveillance of patients cannot be performed while preparing medications.

A conference area is an important addition to an ICU and should be positioned adjacent to the nursing station. This is important to display x-rays and hold small conferences without obstructing the station. Such a conference room will contribute greatly to the teaching and training potential of the unit.

Remote television monitoring of each bed at the nursing station has become more practical with television cameras which function at extremely low light levels. Such remote monitoring can assist the nursing service when understaffed and when patients are located in relatively isolated areas of the unit. However, a surgical ICU requires a great deal more bedside nursing than a unit for coronary care, and thus will gain less benefit from remote TV monitoring than a unit with less professional time spent at the bedside.

THE PATIENT AREA

Appropriate design of each bed area will depend to some degree on the type of patient to be cared for. The general surgical patient will often require two suction outlets and occasionally three (the trauma patient with a chest tube and abdominal sump tube who requires tracheal suctioning). There are seldom too many wall electrical outlets near the bed: two duplex receptacles should be available on each side of the bed. Some of the electrical outlets and lights should be connected to an emergency power system that is appropriately labeled.

The lighting of the ICU patient area requires extensive thought. The patient, the nurse and the physician each require a different level of illumination. Lighting levels required in the bed area range from a fraction of a footcandle for night lighting up to 100 footcandles or more for emergency examination and treatment. Several steps of lighting levels between these extremes are needed for patient use and for routine nursing care. Central lighting should be arranged for appropriate intensity and color tones. Ceiling lighting above each bed should be designed to minimize the glare in a patient's eyes but still provide bright lighting promptly in an emergency. A dimmer can add flexibility and comfort to a standard lighting arrangement.

Before actual construction is begun on an ICU, it is extremely helpful to have a life-size mock-up constructed of a standard bed area and the nursing station. Physicians and nurses will take more interest in such a model than in a blueprint, and thus it will elicit the kind of suggestions and criticisms that should be considered while changes are relatively inexpensive.

ARCHITECTURAL PROGRAM

An architect can develop a "program" for use in planning a new ICU. The details to be considered in such a program require background information from both the architectural and the medical side before the best decisions can be reached.[9] When either the architect or the medical staff take a "leave the matter to me" attitude, the end product will be less than optimum. In addition, the education for medical personnel of certain of the physiologic principles involved in ventilation, lighting, electrical safety and so forth, may carry over into safer and more informed operation of the new unit.

An example of an "architectural program" for an ICU is presented here. This program was prepared by Mr. Fred D. Hickler, of Medical Facilities Planning Associates, Inc., of Boston. Such a program can be developed by a planning committee or by questioning and modifying the one presented here.

Ten Patient Bedrooms at 162 Square Feet each = 1620 Square Feet

1. The clear unobstructed space in the patient bedroom should measure 11 by 12 feet minimum (132 square feet) with the 11 foot dimension being the patient headwall. The balance of 30 square feet should be alloted to the following: (a) clothing closet; (b) lavatory with elbow blades and germicide dispenser; (c) storage and work counter.

2. The headwall should contain the following as a minimum: (a) four oxygen outlets; (b) four vacuum outlets; (c) one medical air outlet; (d) eight 110 volt outlets (four on each side of the bed); (e) two grounding jacks for equipment (one on each side of the bed).

3. Optional on the headwall are the following: (a) central physiological monitoring jacks; (b) TV monitoring outlets; (c) exam light; (d) 220 volt outlet for portable x-ray equipment.

4. The corridor wall should be designed to provide visual supervision

by the professional staff. The door should be located so that the patient's head is visible from the corridor. (In actual practice, bedroom doors are usually restrained in the open position. Such restraint does not comply with fire and safety codes unless it is by a magnetic type hold open device with an automatic smoke-actuated door closer.) A properly designed and maintained ultraviolet light barrier around the opening to the corridor is an effective deterrent to environmental sepsis.

5. Many authorities recommend that the corridor walls be largely glass. (Several proprietary systems providing fully retractable glass walls are available in designs that comply with most codes.) If these are used, curtain tracks are required to provide for the possibility of visual privacy. When deciding how much glass to use the following factors should be considered:

(a) Patients ought to be able to see professional activity fairly frequently so that they do not feel abandoned but should not be subjected to a "fishbowl" environment.

(b) In actual practice the members of the nursing staff are generally at the patient's bedside. Some authorities are beginning to believe that the constant and simultaneous view of many patients in great distress has a disturbing effect on the staff and that large areas of glass do not necessarily improve the level of patient care.

(c) Functional design of the core of supporting services around which the patient rooms are grouped has to be seriously compromised just to maintain uninterrupted sight lines.

6. The exterior wall should have a view to the outside. The windows should have a thermal "U" factor of not more than 0.52 to prevent condensation. They should be manually vented in case of air conditioning failure, and the top section (at least) should be vented to exhaust smoke in case of fire.

7. The two remaining partitions should be arranged to provide visual and acoustical privacy between patients without occluding visual supervision by the staff. One of these walls should contain a clock located so that it can be seen by the patient.

Central Station of 480 Square Feet

1. This unit should consist of the following areas: (a) nurses' area of 180 square feet; (b) doctors' area of 180 square feet; (c) administrative area of 120 square feet.

2. Low counters and screens should divide the central station into discrete areas but not so as to interfere with easy communication. The nurses' and doctors' areas should have quick access to patient bedrooms. Ideally the administrative area should overlook the entrance to the unit. Patient charts should be easily available to all staff members.

3. Central monitoring, if provided, should be arranged so that it is visually accessible to staff.

Conference Room of 160 Square Feet

Dietary Area of 80 Square Feet

1. Unless the central food service of the hospital indicates otherwise, the dietary area of the ICU should be a small refreshment area with a sink,

hot plate, refrigerator, ice-maker, and a minimum amount of base, counter and wall cabinets.

2. Many proprietary package units are available between 4 and 8 feet long.

Drug Preparation Area of 80 Square Feet

1. This should be a discrete area centrally located but not a part of the nurses' station. Prescription errors are reduced significantly when they are prepared in a secluded area.

2. This area requires a small sink, an undercounter explosion-proof refrigerator, a lockable narcotics cabinet, a work counter and storage contained in wall and base cabinets, arranged to suit the hospital pharmacy system.

3. Many proprietary units are available between 5 and 7 feet long.

4. If sterile solutions are to be stored in this area, it will require additional space and separate shelving. Allow as much as 6 to 7 linear feet of storage, approximately 18 inches deep and 8 feet high. Some well designed proprietary systems are available for this function.

5. Sterile solutions may be alternatively stored in the utility area.

Utility Area of 120 Square Feet

1. This is basically a clean storage area but should contain a work counter and a sink for setting up equipment and supplies. The balance of the area should consist of adjustable shelving. Typical items to be stored are: (a) tracheotomy sets; (b) venesection sets; (c) urinary catheterization trays; (d) dressing kits; (e) sterile solutions (if not stored in drug preparation area).

Linen Cart Storage of 80 Square Feet

Soiled Holding Area of 120 Square Feet

1. This area should be zoned for the following functions: (a) holding of wastes and disposables—usually bagged; (b) holding of items to be returned to central supply for reprocessing; (c) used linen—usually bagged.

2. A work counter and sink should be provided for sorting, disposal of liquid wastes, and rinsing.

3. This area may also be used for the disposal of bedpan wastes, in which case a bedpan washer/sanitizer may be provided. It should be noted that the use of toilets with devices for rinsing bedpans should not be encouraged because of the resulting aerosol effect.

Equipment Storage Area of 140 Square Feet

1. This should preferably be a single room and not distributed throughout the unit in alcoves, but in either case, it represents a significant amount of space usually not accounted for. Without intending to limit the equipment normally found in an ICU, the following list is typical: (a) mobile bedside electrocardiograph oscilloscope monitors; (b) direct writing electrocardiographs; (c) cardiac defibrillators; (d) transvenous pacemaker; (e) emergency carts; (f) mechanical ventilators; (g) oxygen therapy equipment; (h) respirometers; (i) oxygen analyzers; (j) scale for supine patients.

Two Toilets for Staff at 60 Square Feet

1. It is assumed that patients in an ICU will generally be too ill to use the toilet so that only staff toilets are provided here.

2. The provision of toilets for patients is optional.

3. Visitors' toilets are included below under Visitors' Reception Area.

Janitor's Closet of 80 Square Feet

1. This closet should contain a mop receptor, storage for cleaning supplies, and a wet vacuum cleaner. Ideally, it should be located near the entrance to the unit.

Visitors' Reception Area of 280 Square Feet

1. This function should be located outside of but adjacent to the patient care area. It should be easily accessible to staff members and should contain the following: (a) a family waiting room of 120 square feet; (b) two small acoustically private cubicles of 60 square feet each for discussions between staff and family members, or for family members to confer together or to express grief without disturbing others; (c) a unisex toilet of 40 square feet designed to meet the physically handicapped code; (d) two acoustically private telephones; (e) a coffee maker.

Optional Areas

1. Staff lockers.

2. Staff lounge.

3. Blood gas lab.

4. On call rooms.

The total net area without the options just listed is 3300 square feet, to which 2000 square feet should be added for open space, utility shafts and so on.

ELECTRICAL SAFETY

Most health care personnel are familiar with the desired performance of an electrical appliance but have little appreciation of the hazards of electricity. This is particularly true when these hazards are compounded in a complex of appliances hastily assembled to support a critically ill patient.[10] Knowledgeable behavior is crucial for the safe use of electricity in the ICU, but this statement presumes that the institution concurrently provides an appropriate electric distribution and grounding system and electrical appliances that are tested to demonstrate electric safety.

The details of an electric distribution system that can be used safely in patient care areas of increasing complexity are described in Chapter 2 of *Safe Use of Electricity in Patient Care Facilities* (National Fire Protection Association Publication 76-BT, 1973). Performance specifications for appropriate electrical appliances can be found in Chapter 3 of the same handbook. The use of electricity for the care of the critically ill requires a continuous supply of power. *Essential Electric Systems for Health Care Facilities* (NFPA 76-A) describes basic systems.

Technical and administrative information for the organization and operation of a program of inspection and preventive maintenance for electric appliances and electric distribution systems in health care facilities is available.[5,6]

This discussion is concerned with the use of electric appliances ranging in complexity from the bedside lamp or electric bed to monitoring systems and external cardiac pacers. It focuses responsibility on all personnel in the intensive care unit.

Electrical Properties of the Human Body.   A simplified model of the electrical properties of the human body is an insulating bag of skin filled with a core of markedly lower electric resistance traversed by neurovascular bundles of even less electric resistance.

Dry skin has an electric resistance high enough to protect vital functions (40,000 ohms) except where mucous membranes are exposed. Wet skin loses this insulating property and transmits enough electric current to be hazardous at voltages conventionally used in the ICU. The effects of electric current vary with the current path. This is determined by the anatomic location of the contacts with the electric power, the maximum current being in the path of lowest resistance, i.e., the shortest neurovascular pattern. When vital organs lie in the path of the current, aberrant function or lethal malfunction results.[2,3] Categorizing specific effects provides insight into the pathophysiology of electric shock, but it must be remembered that combinations of the various noxious effects are common. The effects of electric current in the body can be listed:

1. *Contraction of Muscles.* The tetanic contraction of muscles may make it impossible to "let go" the source of electric power. The continuous contraction of respiratory muscles stops respiration.

2. *Respiratory Failure.* The nervous system involved in the mechanics of breathing may be damaged, or the central nervous system may be destroyed by the passage of an electric current through the brain.

3. *Circulatory Failure.* Current applied to the conduction system of the heart causes ventricular fibrillation.

4. *Hemorrhage.* Heating of the neurovascular bundle due to the concentration of electric current in the poorly resisting blood and lymph results in destruction of tissue and hemorrhage. Peripheral ischemia follows vascular thrombosis.

5. *Burns.* Burns of the skin or mucous membranes may occur where the current is concentrated by a point contact or low resistance of tissue. Burns of the mouth in children who suck electric connectors, burns of the skin in contact with the indifferent electrode of the endothermy, or burns about a needle electrode inserted through the skin are illustrative.

Obscure effects result from the application of electric currents of marginal power to patients who are susceptible to electric current because of medication, metabolic derangement, obtundation, or instrumentation of the heart, gastrointestinal tract or respiratory tract. Violation of the protective insulation of the dry skin predominates in increasing the hazard of electric shock. Skin wet with perspiration, incontinence or discharge provides a large low-resistance contact that is often overlooked.

Sources of Electrical Hazard.   Except for phenomena that intrude into the ICU, such as a lightning strike, electric power surges, or low voltage, electrical accidents are not spontaneous occurrences. Carelessness, expedience, ignorance and negligence set the stage. Because safety depends upon the user of each electric appliance in the vicinity of the patient, education of everyone is of critical importance. Everyone must learn to ensure electric safety.

As they approach an ICU patient, most people appreciate that they are about to share a microbiologic environment with him. In a more subtle way each individual joins the electric environment of every patient. Because everyone is a conductor of electricity, he becomes the electric connector between current-carrying surfaces that are touched simultaneously. Such surfaces can be classified as to hazard.

Obviously a bare electric power wire presents the greatest hazard. These are encountered where insulation is damaged, a plug or connector is broken, the enclosure of an appliance is open or heating elements are exposed.

Low-voltage terminals and electrodes present lesser hazards depending upon the source of electric power, the circuit of the appliance, and what other appliances are used at the time. Battery powered appliances present minimal hazard if ungrounded.

Metal surfaces in the vicinity of the ICU patient must be suspected because it is impractical to identify their relative electric potentials other than by periodic checks. Metal surfaces of portable appliances such as lamps and electric beds are more hazardous than metal surfaces fixed to the structure that have "hard-wired" electric connections.

Metal surfaces of portable appliances are usually grounded by a grounding wire (green) in the power cord.[12] Depending upon the effectiveness and integrity of the insulation of the electric circuits of the appliance, an electric potential may be impressed on the metal enclosure. An intact grounding circuit carries harmlessly to ground both fault current and the leakage current that inevitably penetrates insulation. A defective grounding circuit permits an electric potential to accumulate on the metal case.

A different hazard—a return path for electric power—is inherent in permanently installed metal surfaces. In a modern ICU such surfaces are electrically interconnected, are at ground potential, and are connected to the neutral (white) wire of the conventional AC distribution system at the service entrance ground. Hence contact between the live (black) wire and a grounded surface results in sparking and arcing. A person contacting both the live wire and grounded metal will experience an electric shock. Permanently installed metal surfaces include plumbing and heating fixtures, metal cabinets, electric fixtures, and structural metal, such as door and window frames. These surfaces are usually inadvertently interconnected during construction or installation and approximate ground potential unless there is a positive connection with the grounding bus of the electric distribution system.

A member of the staff who approaches a patient joins the electrical environment in his vicinity. The patient can be unwittingly involved in a hazardous circuit by simultaneously touching the patient and a metal object.

A valuable safety habit upon approaching a patient is to inspect the assemblage of appliances grouped about him for obvious faults. Malfunctioning appliances should be disconnected. Housekeeping appliances should be removed. Dangling power cords or patient cables should be secured. Kinks in wires, loose plugs, faulty receptacles, worn or frayed cords should be noted. Appraise the dryness of the patient—perspiration, spillage, a wet dressing or bed warns of increased vulnerability to shock because of the loss of the insulating value of the dry skin. When an instrument is adjusted or electrodes are checked, do not touch anything else at the same time. When the patient is handled, do not touch electrical appliances with the other hand. The bedside lamp and the electric bed are the most hazardous. These commonplace appliances are exposed to wear and damage. Faulty performance is tolerated, and hazard is not anticipated.

HIGH RISK PATIENTS.   Patients with indwelling catheters or electrodes in the heart or great vessels are highly vulnerable to electric shock. AC current levels that are undetectable when applied to the dry intact skin may induce ventricular fibrillation when applied to the endocardium. The hazardous area is specific: the exposed wire or terminals of catheters or electrodes. Special precautions include:

1. Wear rubber gloves when handling bare metal contacts or stylets.

2. Cover exposed metal terminals with insulating sleeves.

3. Intracardiac electrodes and catheters should only be connected to instruments or transducers with high impedance or isolated electronic circuitry.

4. Nonconductive stopcocks should be used on catheters.

5. Do not touch exposed pacemaker leads or stylets with one hand while adjusting instruments or contacting electric appliances with the other.

6. All electric appliances in the vicinity should be grounded by a three-wire cord. Double insulated appliances are the exception.

HIGH RISK OF MULTIPLE APPLIANCES.   Each assemblage of electric appliances poses unique electric incompatibilities. Any appliance may be a current source and another metal surface may be the ground, with the patient caught in a current path between the two. Appliances with two-wire cords such as the bedside lamp, TV set or electric fan may operate properly yet have dangerous levels of leakage current. A poorly maintained electric bed may introduce a ground potential that differs from that of the other properly grounded electric appliances. Its metal parts are convenient handholds for patients and personnel alike. The patient may touch the metal surfaces directly or indirectly through wet bedding. An attendant may become the pathway for electric current by simultaneously touching the patient and a metal surface that is at a disparate potential.

It is well to remember that the patient who is being monitored is usually grounded because he is connected to ground through the indifferent (right leg) lead of the ECG or a column of conductive saline in a catheter attached to a grounded pressure transducer. Patients suspended in traction may be grounded by the apparatus.

Certain precautions can be enforced in the ICU to protect patients who are surrounded by a complex of electrical appliances:

1. Ground all electric appliances through three-wire cords and three-prong plugs connected directly to grounding receptacles. Never use a cheater or adapter to match the three-prong plug with a two-slot receptacle.

2. Inspect electrical appliances periodically for leakage current.

3. Connect all the electric appliances in a patient vicinity to adjacent receptacles.

4. Do not use an extension cord.

5. Disconnect appliances which malfunction or display interference or faulty recording.

Vigorous programs of education and maintenance should be continually integrated to insure the safe use of electricity in the ICU. Safety does not happen; it must be pursued by everyone who enters the vicinity of each patient.

MEDICAL CLIMATOLOGY

There is an increasingly pertinent and growing literature on medical climatology, a subject that concerns the design, construction and operation of facilities to provide a benign climate for the patient with critical illness or injury. Air conditioning and ventilation complement biologic processes for the exchange of heat and water and remove most of the hazardous particles or offensive products of human activity from the environment. Advances in construction of buildings have included higher elevators, decreased window space and artificial lighting with all of these things contributing to a separation of man from his natural environment. None of these architectural features have more physiologic significance than modern ventilation and air conditioning. The ease of manipulating temperature, humidity and air flow in modern hospitals has outdistanced our knowledge of physiologic requirements and how they are altered in a critically ill patient. Too often the ventilation and air conditioning are regulated for the comfort of the professional staff rather than the physiologic needs of the patient. It is obvious that patients benefit when not obliged to combat a wasteful, hostile climate. Occupational advantages also accrue to harried, emotionally stressed personnel. A climate that aids the patient is not always achieved by the design of modern hospitals, and circumstances can readily be found where the medical climate complicates rather than assists convalescence.

Temperature. A thermoneutral zone of ambient temperature exists from approximately 27 to 31° C.; body heat production is increased below this range and active sweating begins above this range. Within the relatively small range of thermoneutrality, body temperature is regulated by small changes in vasomotor tone and the resulting small increases or decreases in heat loss by radiation. Below an ambient temperature of 28° C., vasoconstriction rapidly becomes maximal. Then shivering obtains as the major, and perhaps only, thermoregulatory response to the negative thermal load. In the intensive care unit, it is important to remember that the critically ill patient may have abnormalities of heat production with or without changes in body temperature and a decreased capacity for heat transport to the body surface where it can be lost to the environment.

An analysis of patients in a partially air-conditioned hospital where the ambient climate is normally hot and humid has revealed an improvement of vital signs in those patients hospitalized in air-conditioned wards as opposed to the group assigned to the non-air-conditioned part of the hospital.[1] The air-conditioned group was quieter and had more rapid physical improvement. The greatest difference was in the perspiration rates, a factor of importance to cardiac patients in particular. Patients with thyrotoxicosis or other hypermetabolic conditions tolerate hot humid conditions very poorly. When the metabolic rate is increased the heat production is increased, and the patient may be unable to eliminate heat from the body surface as rapidly as it is produced and transported to the skin. The patient develops hyperthermia with tachycardia and increased demand for blood flow to the skin. The increased body temperature leads to increased cell metabolism which in turn produces more heat. This vicious cycle may threaten life if the cardiopulmonary or circulatory systems begin to fail. A cool, dry environment favors the loss of heat by radiation and evaporation from the skin, and may save the life of the patient.

Environmental factors exert a profound effect on the response to injury in the rat and other small mammals. Qualitatively similar changes can be expected to occur in larger mammals such as man, although exploration of this area is still in its early stages. A reduction in post-injury nitrogen loss and a more normal plasma protein metabolism have recently been shown in both the rat and man[4] following fracture of a long bone if convalescence was in an environment of 28 to 30° C. rather than 20 to 21° C. The mechanism of this improvement is not clear, although an ambient temperature below the thermoneutral zone in the patient area may cause an increased nitrogen loss as the result of a greater food intake, or of some unidentified neuroendocrine stimulus such as increased catecholamine output.

One suggestion has been that the thermoneutral zone (27 to 31° C.) for seminude man should be the guide for the ambient temperature of the intensive care unit. Perhaps in the hospital, graduations of patient care from the recovery room and the ICU to intermediate care and then to an area of limited care during late convalescence should be accompanied by changes in ambient temperature, from 25° C. for an area of intermediate care to conventional indoor temperature for late convalescence. Thus the transition in graduated medical care could have a parallel stepwise return toward the mild environmental stress associated with conditions of ordinary indoor living.

Ventilation.   The range of air flow which is planned for different parts of a hospital depends upon the purpose in mind.[11] Apparently six air changes per hour are required for minimum odor control. Recirculation of air makes it economically feasible to increase the rate of ventilation to a bacteriologically effective level. This involves 30 to 60 air changes per hour.

A misconception has persisted for 60 years that decries airborne contagion while simultaneously demanding ventilation of critical areas of hospitals by fresh air to avoid spread of infection. Airborne contagion has been documented for all forms of microorganisms. Sterile air is just as effective in dispersing contagion as contaminated air. Properly managed, sterile air can dilute contagion particles to the point where infection no longer occurs ("threshold sanitary ventilation"). This concept recognizes the disinfection of air within a space as by germicidal aerosols or ultraviolet radiation as equivalent of replacement with sterile air. Threshold sanitary ventilation requires 60 air changes per hour or its equivalent in simultaneous disinfection. The hygienic effect is measured by determining the disappearance of bacteria aerosolized into the air as droplet nuclei. Because volume is a factor in dilution, the cubic footage of a space in relation to its occupancy is significant.

Design and Cost Considerations. Hospital designs are developed by architects who may have preeminent esthetic qualifications which may not correlate with competence in ventilation and air conditioning. Drawings for the system are sometimes lacking in detail and in sufficient attention to potential sources of contamination. There are few urban areas where air pollution is not a problem. Most hospital designs result in pollution of the air in the vicinity of the structure. The location of the air intake for the ICU is critical to avoid external recirculation of noxious fumes, odors and microorganisms.

The cost of an air conditioning system depends upon the ventilation rate specified as well as upon the performance required in terms of control of temperature, humidity, odor and airborne microorganisms. The equipment to move, purify and condition large volumes of air is expensive. Depending upon climate, the cost of energy to heat, cool and control humidity can exceed that of moving the air. Ridding the air of pollution adds to the operating expense. Hence it is advantageous to recirculate conditioned air to minimize the cost of energy exchange and purification.

Modern techniques of disinfection permit 85 per cent of the air to be recirculated safely, making high rates of ventilation economically practical. Where ambient air pollution is great, recirculation is highly advantageous. The penalty inflicted for recirculation is meticulous maintenance of a system that disinfects the air. High efficiency filters, or filters and ultraviolet radiation, or filters and scrubbers must be maintained at peak efficiency. Because an air conditioning system is costly (one-fourth of the structure) and faulty operation so wasteful, skilled maintenance is a justified but seldom accepted expense.

The ventilation rate and other specified factors are not detectable without testing equipment, and specifications can be imperceptibly trimmed to lower the budget. The bidding procedure may allow substitution of inferior equipment. Preacceptance performance testing of installed systems is seldom required in the frenzied climate preceding the opening day. After the unit is in operation, it is important to remember that poor maintenance ultimately permits even the best system to destroy itself. Hospital maintenance often consists of crisis repairs, rather than adhering to preventive maintenance schedules. None of these mistakes should be allowed by the ICU planning committee.

Studies that relate deviation in climate to physiologic stress are not compelling because their significance is hidden and often not appreciated by physicians, administrators, architects and engineers. The patients' symptoms are alleviated by a temporary expedient or obtunded by medication or ultimately by disease. Symptoms are rarely related directly to faulty engineering or architectural concept.

How can the physician marshal the complex forces essential to the provision of a benign climate for his patient? First, he must understand the concept. Second, he must insist on satisfactory answers to questions seeking reasons for deviations from ideal temperature, relative humidity and air flow. Third, he must appreciate the economic implications of his requirements. Moving air is expensive, and adjusting the relative humidity is expensive, in terms of energy consumed as well as initial cost of equipment and installation. Maintenance is expensive both in terms of qualified manpower and supplies such as filters and detergent germicides.

SUMMARY

The therapeutic assets of an ICU may be offset by possible liabilities inherent in the design such as congestion, noise, medication errors, infection exposure, electrical hazards, improper ventilation and psychological trauma. The surgeon, along with other professional colleagues, should take an active part in preparing the architectural designs of the ICU that will care for his surgical patients. This chapter presents the need for certain basic space requirements; emphasizing the fact that the available space for patients must be accompanied by one to two times that amount of space for an adequate nursing station, supporting areas and a free flow of traffic. The nursing station is often constructed in a way which makes efficiency and discipline difficult to maintain. The single most common defect is inadequate storage for equipment and supplies, seldom adequate after two to three years of operation of a unit. A modern ICU should be constructed to allow each individual patient the balance between surveillance and privacy which is optimum for his condition at that time. The physiologic basis for new attention to ventilation and air conditioning is presented. Electrical safety is outlined with emphasis on the fact that everyone who approaches the bed of an ICU patient enters his electrical environment, as well as his microbiologic environment. In brief, the physical design of an intensive care unit will enhance or retard the ability of even the most dedicated staff to render modern, safe intensive care.

REFERENCES

1. Burch, G. E., and DePasquale, N.: Influence of air conditioning on hospitalized patients. JAMA, 1959.
2. Burke, J. F., Quinby, W. C., Jr., Bandoc, C., McLaughlin, E., and Trelstad, R. L.: Patterns of high tension electrical injury in children and adolescents and their management. Amer. J. Surg., *133*:490, 1977.
3. Butler, E. D., and Gant, T. D.: Electrical injuries, with special reference to the upper extremities. Amer. J. Surg., *134*:95, 1977.
4. Cuthbertson, D. P., and Tilstone, W. J.: Metabolism during the post-injury period. *In* Sobotka, H., and Stewart, C. P., eds.: Advances in Clinical Chemistry, vol. 12. New York, Academic Press, 1969.
5. Electricity in Patient Care Facilities. Publication 76-BT. Boston, National Fire Protection Association, May 1973.
6. Kilpatrick, D. G., and Kilpatrick, L. B.: Electrical safety standards in the health care delivery system. CRC Critical Reviews in Bioengineering, October 1972, pp. 289–332a.
7. Kinney, J. M.: The intensive care unit. Am. Coll. Surg. Bull., *51*:201, 1966.
8. Kinney, J. M.: Design of the intensive care unit. *In* Berk, J. L., Sampliner, J. E., Artz, J. S., and Vinocur, B., eds.: Handbook of Critical Care. Boston, Little, Brown and Company, 1976, p. 3.
9. Tagge, G. F., Salness, G., Thams, J., Whipple, G. H., and Shoemaker, W. C.: Experience with a multidisciplinary critical care center in a community hospital. Crit. Care Med., *2*:231, 1975.
10. Walter, C. W.: Fire in an oxygen-powered respirator. JAMA, *197*:44, 1966.
11. Walter, C. W.: Ventilation and air conditioning as bacteriologic engineering. Anesthesiology, *31*:186, 1969.
12. Walter, C. W.: Electrical hazards in hospitals, and that green wire. Lab Data, vol. 3, no. 1, 1972, published by Underwriters' Laboratories, Inc., Chicago. (Reprinted from Fire Journal, vol. 65, no. 6, November 1971.)
13. Weil, M. H., and Shubin, H.: Centralized hospital care for the critically ill. *In* Safar, P., ed.: Clinical Anesthesia. Philadelphia, F. A. Davis Co., 1974.

CHAPTER 4

ADMINISTRATION AND OPERATING PROCEDURES

JOHN M. KINNEY, M.D.

HENRIK H. BENDIXEN, M.D.

Introductory material in this volume has emphasized that the term "intensive care unit" refers to a growing variety of special care units which vary in location, design, equipment and operation, depending upon the types of patients to be cared for and the size and character of the hospital and staff where the unit is to function. Early special care units made major contributions to the lowering of mortality for patients undergoing neurosurgical and open-heart operations. However the development of units for the intensive care of general surgical patients was uncommon until one to two decades later. Part of this delay was related to the wide variety of clinical problems which could be encountered in a general surgical unit.

In some respects, the general ICU represents the opposite requirement from a coronary monitoring unit. The latter involves "intensive surveillance" to a much larger degree than "intensive care" at the bedside. It has the advantage of dealing with the disorders of a single organ system, the cardiovascular system, around which to plan a staff, monitoring equipment and physical design. The well defined electrical signal of the heart makes the ECG of unusual monitoring value.

In contrast, the general surgical patient may require intensive care for a wide variety of problems, the majority of which require intensive bedside care as well as continuous surveillance. The life of the patient in a coronary monitoring unit is usually at risk from ventricular fibrillation or failure of the left ventricle. The life of the surgical patient may be at risk due to peripheral or central circulatory failure, ventilatory failure, renal failure, overwhelming infection or upper gastrointestinal hemorrhage. The wide variety of lethal patterns among surgical patients means that the surgical ICU staff must be trained in a wide variety of procedures, and the related support of vital organs requires a correspondingly large amount of specialized equipment.

41

The most important general principle underlying an ICU is that the unit be designed and operated in a way which is "patient oriented." This statement appears trite and unnecessary. However, examination of the design, administration and daily operation of intensive care units often reveals that decisions regarding these subjects have been made for the convenience of the staff or considerations of the general hospital budget, which are essentially unrelated to the quality of intensive patient care. Nowhere is this more evident than in examining the various ways in which fear and pain may be unnecessarily aggravated by lack of sufficient privacy for each patient, a high monotonous noise level, thoughtless behavior and noisy communication between staff members—all usually justified in the name of quick and efficient operation of the unit.

COMMITTEE FOR ICU POLICY AND PROCEDURES

It is important to have a policy committee responsible for each ICU, with representatives from every major group that is involved in the daily operation of the unit. This committee should be charged with establishing policy and standard procedures and making this policy available in written form for the general understanding of the hospital staff. Above all, the policy committee is responsible for the overall quality of care in the unit. In addition, the policy committee should assume responsibility for providing a data handling system which is effective and convenient.

If specialized forms or computerized data handling are to be employed, the committee should accept responsibility for the education necessary to make the system work effectively. This will require periodic survey of the ICU records and decisions regarding which portion will be part of the permanent record and which part is appropriate to discard at the time of the patient's discharge from the ICU. The administrative arrangement for the unit should be such that there is free and open communication between the committee and the people responsible for the day-to-day operation of the unit.

It is helpful to have the supervisor of the sterile supply service, the chief of the pharmacy, the head of the clinical laboratories and the heads of the respiratory therapy service and the chest physical therapy service meet with the policy committee and discuss the particular problems presented by the extra service load that intensive care patients place on their particular hospital service.

The problem of how to manage the critically ill vs the hopelessly ill patient needs thoughtful review. A sensitive but rational approach is needed, particularly when and how to give orders not to resuscitate a patient. A group of three articles dealing with this area should stimulate every ICU committee to accept an approach as stated in these references or develop an alternate approach considered acceptable by that institution after appropriate legal consultation.[1-3]

RESPONSIBILITY FOR AN INDIVIDUAL PATIENT IN THE ICU

The development of intensive care units for general surgical patients has proceeded more slowly than the development of other units because of the uncertainty within the surgical community as to the proper way to handle responsibility for the surgical patient being transferred to such a unit. Much of the early reluctance and uncertainty in this development is understandable. Surgical residency training over the past 50 years has been based upon the cornerstone of personal responsibility that each surgeon felt for his patient. The surgeon might call a consultant when he desired help in an area outside his own expertise, but the consultant became involved with the patient only upon his request and not otherwise.

After World War II, a certain amount of conflict remained regarding the proper division of responsibility in the operating room between the surgeon and the anesthesiologist. In time, the agreement of the surgeon to share ultimate responsibility with the anesthesiologist in the operating room was followed by a similar sharing of responsibility in the post-anesthesia recovery room. The concept of giving up further responsibility for his patient by transferring that patient to an intensive care unit represented for some surgeons a disturbing further abdication of responsibility.

Perhaps there is no single correct way for the sharing of responsibility in such a unit. The sharing of responsibility in the ICU should be based on the size of the hospital, on the patient population, on the available staff and on the economic support available to specially trained physicians or surgeons interested in spending major portions of time in intensive care work.

Responsibility for the management of an individual patient in the surgical ICU can be thought of as either of two extremes or some position midway between them. One approach might be termed the "open shop" arrangement, where the surgical ICU is essentially little more than a group nursing unit. The hospital designates a certain ward as the surgical intensive care unit and agrees to provide extra nursing coverage with extra equipment for monitoring and treating acutely ill patients. Any surgeon is free to admit his patient to this unit within the limits of the bed capacity. The surgeon or the house officer representing him leaves orders each day in the order book and deals with the nurses in exactly the same relationship as he would if his patient were hospitalized elsewhere in the hospital.

The opposite extreme might be called the "closed shop," where the surgical intensive care unit has a staff of doctors and nurses who spend their entire time working in this unit and accept total responsibility for any patient transferred into the unit. This type of arrangement can sometimes lead to the referring surgeon's being left in the role of a visitor or friend rather than continuing to have professional responsibility for the patient's care.

Proponents of the permanent full-time staff with full patient responsibility point out that with this arrangement, advanced procedures are introduced more quickly, skill is developed more rapidly and a higher quality of care can be provided for complicated clinical situations. Certain difficulties must also be recognized, particularly the loss of continuity between the referring surgeon and his patient which sometimes deprives the staff of important background information and the patient of the psychological support of someone with whom he has built rapport. In addition, the adherence to a rigid closed shop may result in certain patients not being transferred at all when their clinical condition needs intensive care.

It seems obvious that there are certain advantages and disadvantages to both the open and closed shop approaches. Therefore some institutions have sought an intermediate arrangement. One such intermediate arrangement has been termed "consultants in residence." This arrangement requires that a small group of attending physicians and surgeons with appropriate training and interest be willing to accept assignment in the intensive care unit. This would include responsibility for daily rounds of all ICU patients and discussion of their progress with the ICU staff. Such attending physicians should not only represent certain skills which are important in intensive care, but should be responsible for good working relationships with the various other services or individual physicians who might provide important services or consultation. These "consultants in residence" would not necessarily assume legal responsibility for any of the ICU patients. But they would be available in the event of any emergency care which might be required before the referring surgeons could be reached. They would naturally assume a central role in the education of the professional staff working in the unit.

Another approach is to have a director of the ICU who is in charge of the day-to-day operation of the unit. The question then arises as to what medical specialty should be represented by the person who might be placed in charge of a surgical ICU. Surgeons often feel that another surgeon should be in charge of the unit, while other disciplines have frequently taken the point of view that life support systems are sufficiently complicated that anesthesiology would more logically be the field of training for the administrator of a surgical ICU. With the experience of the past decade, it seems clear that no single discipline automatically provides the breadth of expertise which may be needed for surgical intensive care. Therefore, the director should be that individual who is a tactful professional having the combination of personal training and interest, together with the greatest ability to mobilize and integrate all of the necessary strengths of a hospital in behalf of any patient in the ICU.

The best way of sharing responsibility in the surgical ICU does not lie in a single, dogmatic approach. The best way is that arrangement which allows the professional staff of a given hospital to provide the highest level of intensive care of which that institution is capable.

PROCEDURES AND PRACTICES

The surgical intensive care unit represents a unique challenge because of the wide variety of patients requiring care and the various types of organ failure requiring management and possibly resulting in death. Thus the number of procedures for monitoring and treating patients is broader than usual, and they often carry associated risks when improperly carried out. It is necessary for effectiveness of care and efficiency of educating new staff that procedures be carefully standardized with uniform equipment. A loose-leaf notebook of procedures should be developed when a surgical intensive care unit is opened. This notebook should be under constant review so that updated procedures can be added and unused procedures removed.

Nowhere is standardization of approach to the critically ill patient more important than during the time of acute resuscitation. The entire staff should be aware of where all vital equipment is located, and all equipment should be left only where it belongs. It is important that each shift be equally familiar with clinical procedures, and detailed communication is needed from one shift to the next regarding the status of each patient and the function of the equipment which is in use with that patient. All too often an apparently sudden change in hemodynamic or blood gas values will turn out to have been associated with the beginning of another shift, when the new nurse used equipment in a different way or perhaps discovered malfunctioning equipment.

The surgical intensive care unit provides a special challenge to the conventional way in which patient information is kept in the hospital record. Life-threatening problems require more types of information and more frequent information in order to make proper clinical decisions. Careful thought should be given to the frequency of obtaining data so that the frequency is appropriate to the rate of change of the variable when clinical deterioration occurs. The bedside electrocardiograph is an example of continuous or "seeing-eye" monitoring; its importance in the unit has to do only with the appearance of significant abnormalities. There should be a way of permanently indicating the appearance and type of such abnormalities with representative ECG strips, but the majority of the 24 hours will require no permanent record. Similar considerations apply to continuous strip chart recordings of other physiologic variables unless summarized by a trend chart or other means. For patients on mechanical ventilation it is important that certain information such as the setting of the ventilator, peak inspiratory pressure and average tidal volume be included at the time that arterial blood gases are drawn. Only in this way can appropriate modifications be made and the results analyzed after obtaining blood gases which are unsatisfactory.

Relation to Consultant Services   The consultant services in a surgical ICU include the needs of the entire unit as well as the needs of individual patients. One of the most obvious areas for the entire unit requiring special attention has to do with infection and hospital epidemiology. A hospital bacteriologist or perhaps a nurse epidemiologist should have a standardized procedure worked out for periodic evaluation of bacterial growth in certain special areas of the intensive care unit as well as providing month-to-month data on the bacterial strains in the hospital population and their antibiotic sensitivities. The hospital bacteriologist can often make valuable contributions to ICU rounds on the basis of his overview of infection problems throughout the hospital.

Another area where there is general need for help is in the field of acute therapeutic nutrition. Many patients in the intensive care unit are receiving good or even outstanding care of ventilatory or circulatory problems but at the same time are being allowed to develop extensive deficits in both calories and nitrogen. In the ideal circumstance there should be a nutrition service available with professional staff interested in the problems of acute therapeutic nutrition. The team should be capable of instituting total parenteral nutrition and providing adequate follow-up. It usually includes one or more interested doctors, a nurse with special training, and the services of the hospital pharmacist. In this way solutions for total parenteral nutrition can be made up in an aseptic manner with various additives inserted under sterile conditions. A central venous catheter requires not only skill in insertion but extreme care in aseptic technique. The nurse can be trained to provide frequent aseptic care of the catheter in order to minimize the problem of catheter sepsis.

Patients with renal failure may be managed in various ways; however, therapeutic programs usually require a staff with special training in the use of unique equipment. The management of renal problems in the ICU is nearly always done most efficiently by having one consultant or one group who is willing to spend time working out procedures for the special renal problems presented by the ICU patient. When hemodialysis is required there must be general agreement about which patients can be moved to a special area and which may have to be hemodialyzed in the ICU because of other life support systems which make movement of the patient difficult and hazardous.

Relation to Supporting Services   The intensive care unit represents a special type of demand on the supporting services of the hospital, particularly the clinical laboratory and the radiology department. In each case the requested services are usually only a small proportion of the services provided in those departments. However, the volume of services per ICU patient is relatively high.

The director of the clinical laboratory and the director of the department of radiology naturally seek to centralize their activities in one area as much as possible for the efficiency of their staff and economic use of equipment. The clinical laboratory commonly processes a large number of samples in one batch with the results being distributed to the patient areas around the hospital eight hours or more later. Doing blood measurements on an emergency basis in the intensive care unit means interrupting the efficient batch processing of regular hospital samples in the laboratory.

Therefore the responsible people in the hospital administration must meet with the director of the clinical laboratory and the staff of the intensive care unit to work out what represents the best compromise for efficient laboratory services to the intensive care patient. In some institutions this involves establishing a section of the main hospital laboratory for emergency procedures 24 hours a day where the turn-around time is 10 minutes or less.

Other institutions have found it more satisfactory to establish satellite laboratories in the various special care areas of the hospital. Such satellite laboratories cannot be numerous; however, such a laboratory can function well to perform the particular measurements most frequently requested on an emergency basis. If the satellite laboratory concept is utilized, it is important that the main laboratory accept responsibility for some form of quality control and equipment maintenance on a regular basis.

The relationship of the radiology department to the ICU is one of special importance because of the rapidly expanding diagnostic technology which has recently become available. The patient in the ICU may benefit the most from some of these diagnostic procedures, yet be the most difficult to move because of the sophisticated life support systems which are in use. Therefore, special procedures are needed for moving the occasional critically ill patient to the radiology department when absolutely necessary, and avoiding unnecessary delays or periods of inadequate professional attention.

The intensive care unit which takes patients on mechanical ventilation places large demands on the respiratory therapy or inhalational therapy service. It is common practice to have a member of the service assigned to the ICU or at least spending part of his time each day in the ICU in order to change inhalational therapy equipment as frequently as is needed to minimize infections and also to guarantee the functioning of ventilators, spirometers and humidifiers. The matter of chest physical therapy is of sufficient importance that the physical therapy service should also have a representative in the ICU part of each day or actually assigned to the unit.

The role of the psychiatrist in the ICU includes counseling and therapy for both patients and staff. The physicians caring for ICU patients must be constantly alert to psychological responses which would benefit from the care of a psychiatrist. Scheduled rounds with an interested psychiatrist will tend to turn up psychological problems previously unrecognized or ignored as trivial. The presence of a psychiatrist in the ICU on a scheduled basis insures a chance to observe the emotional climate and personal interactions between patient and staff and between members of the staff. The unit staff may all benefit from having a skilled psychiatrist lead a discussion around certain emotionally charged problem areas in the unit.

Services such as occupational therapy, social service and the clergy can play an important role which is often overlooked in the need for immediate life-saving measures. The fear of death can be a larger problem on the ICU than it would be elsewhere in the hospital and particularly with the patient who has difficulty communicating because of a tracheostomy.

TEACHING AND TRAINING IN THE ICU

The ICU should represent a constant opportunity for education and training, perhaps greater than in any other place in the hospital. This is true for a number of reasons, three of which will be mentioned here.

The ICU may be thought of as the "hospital's hospital." Here all of the assets of an institution for managing the critically ill patient should be available in one place. Many of these assets involve new procedures and new equipment, so that a continuing education program is required for the ICU staff and staff replacements assigned to the unit. A growing collection of audiovisual teaching aids are available, which can assist staff members who seek to make the best use of short periods of time while waiting to start or resume work on the unit. The ICU not only concentrates all of the assets of the institution, it has a mindless way of concentrating the liabilities as well. The problems which are part of an institution's daily operation—whether related to personnel, supplies, supporting services or many other areas—may normally exist at an annoying but tolerable level. The intensive care unit often concentrates these problems until they become intolerable. Electrical hazards, medication errors, infection and psychological reactions are all hospital problems which might become of concern in the intensive care unit. Part of the responsibility for reducing these hazards depends upon effective teaching programs for the ICU staff, which need repetition at relatively frequent intervals.

The ICU often has the patients in whom organ failure of a given type carries the highest mortality, since the patients have so many complicating circumstances. Thus there is the added stimulus to teach and learn as much as possible about the pathophysiology of each type of organ failure which one sees in an ICU, in the hope of decreasing the mortality associated with such patients.

Medical schools are beginning to recognize the ICU as a particularly exciting area for undergraduate medical teaching. Since it is often not practical to take large groups of students to visit an ICU patient, increasing numbers of institutions are utilizing color video tapes of such patients away from the bedside. A patient with multiple organ failure offers a special challenge to the student. Much of the explosive growth in medical knowledge over the past 50 years has resulted from intensive study of one or another isolated organ or tissue. The student may not be stimulated to struggle with the complex problems of multiple organ failure in the same individual unless he is actually assigned the study of such a case. Only then will he begin to appreciate the number of times when the best way to treat one type of organ failure may be by providing further damage to the already inadequate function of another organ. The educational process in medicine is ultimately concerned with how to help the student transform factual information into clinical judgment. The ICU has a unique and important role to play in such education.

THE SPECIAL IMPORTANCE OF COMMUNICATION

The intensive care unit represents a special challenge to communication in three different ways: between the patient and the ICU staff, the ICU nurses and other ICU staff, and the ICU staff and the referring physicians.

When a patient is critically ill, it is all too common for the professional staff to expend great effort in the technical details of proper management and forget some of the amenities of communication which are normally in use in other areas of the hospital. This is sometimes justified by saying that the patient is "too sick" to be aware of his surroundings. It seems reasonable that a patient can have his condition aggravated by a failure of the staff to recognize the degree of apprehension which is present. This degree of fear may cause the patient to misinterpret innocent comments of the staff which a few thoughtful words could go far to correct. Naturally the communication problem is more critical when the patient is on a ventilator and fear of malfunctioning of the ventilator and sudden death is added to the communication problems caused by the tracheostomy. Thus, the "talking" tracheostomy would appear to be a useful device for certain patients where a small secondary line provides a stream of humidified air or oxygen which is directed upward through the vocal cords for phonation at the same time that the balloon is inflated properly for mechanical ventilation.

The skilled ICU nurse spends more time and often develops a closer relationship with the ICU patient than anyone else on the staff. It is important that the rest of the professional staff be aware of the fact the nurse may have important suggestions to make regarding management at the time that the patient's case is under discussion by doctors responsible for writing orders. In a teaching hospital where house staff is given considerable responsibility in the intensive care unit, the relationship with the older ICU nurse is of particular interest. The maturity of the young doctor who is assigned to the ICU is often tested by his ability to learn from the skilled ICU nurse rather than feel a threat to his professional status.

The ICU staff may be organized as a "closed shop" as described above. Under these circumstances it is obvious that the physicians elsewhere in the hospital will not be familiar with the activities of this unit and may feel ill at ease in seeking to become more informed. Therefore, the ICU staff has a particular responsibility to seek ways of communicating with other physicians on the staff, partly to encourage the transfer of acutely ill patients as promptly as possible when the ICU could benefit them and partly in order to provide an educational resource for the hospital staff in general. The effort at extra communication should come from the ICU staff and this can be not only from formal teaching conferences and case discussions but also by special attention on the part of the ICU staff to encourage the participation of other members of the hospital staff in regular ICU activities whenever possible.

REFERENCES

1. Bok, S.: Personal directions for care at the end of life. New Eng. J. Med., *295*:367, 1976.
2. Clinical Care Committee of the Massachusetts General Hospital: Optimum care for hopelessly ill patients. New Eng. J. Med., *295*:362, 1976.
3. Rabkin, M. T., Gillerman, G., and Rice, N. R.: Orders not to resuscitate. New Eng. J. Med., *295*:364, 1976.

CHAPTER 5

STAFFING PATTERNS AND EQUIPMENT

AKE GRENVIK, M.D.

PETER SAFAR, M.D.

PHYSICIAN RESPONSIBILITY AND COVERAGE

Responsibilities for medical care in an intensive care unit (ICU) depend on local circumstances. The Society of Critical Care Medicine (SCCM) and the Joint Commission on Accreditation of Hospitals (JCAH) recommend that every ICU should have a *medical director*. He should be chosen on the basis of experience, competence, interest, and availability rather than specialty affiliation. Ideally, for a surgical ICU, the director should have completed residency training in surgery, anesthesiology, or both, and have acquired advanced skills and knowledge in life-support techniques and patient monitoring through additional training in critical care medicine (CCM).[7,8,11,12] However, presently there are surgical ICUs directed also by internists with additional CCM training. This may have the advantage of supplementing the attending surgeon's knowledge in the field of internal medicine, since many of the complications that occur with the surgical patients are indeed of an internal medical nature, such as myocardial infarction, renal failure, or pulmonary infection. If and when certification of "special competence in critical care medicine" becomes available, it is recommended that the ICU medical director be able to display such competence.

In an AMA Category I hospital general or surgical ICU, the director should be geographic full-time in the unit and thus devote the majority of his time to the unit. In a Category II or III hospital, the ICU director may be part-time employed for the unit. A Category IV hospital is not required to have an ICU.[1] The ICU director should be responsible for patient care matters to the staff and for administrative matters to the chief administrator of the hospital. One or more ICU codirectors, whose primary specialties may be different from that of the director, may share full-time supervision as well as responsibility for teaching and patient care.

The medical director or his designate should approve all admissions and discharges, be responsible for monitoring, resuscitation and life support, and ensure that patient care involving multiple services is coordinated. He should have the right to request consultation from other physicians or services and determine which patients will require isolation. He is responsible for education and administration in the unit. The latter includes proposing the annual budget, supervising record-keeping, and evaluating care.

In specialized intradepartmental ICUs, such as surgical units, it may be possible for every patient admitted to be transferred to the service of the ICU medical director and his house staff, with the admitting surgeon becoming the consultant. This would free the surgeon to conduct his operative activity without interruption by his need to remain with one critically ill patient, whom he would continue to visit at least once daily, thereby ascertaining continuous care of that patient's surgical problems.

In advanced medical intensive care units—both multidisciplinary and specialty ICUs, e.g., the surgical ICU—the complexity of modern critical care makes it unlikely that one person is competent in of all its aspects. Therefore, continuous surveillance and management of patients should be provided by a team of CCM physicians of various disciplines experienced in CCM, together with specially trained nurses and allied health personnel. The team should always include the patient's personal surgeon, the director of the ICU, and other specialists as indicated.

A team coordinator with ultimate authority and responsibility for the patient's general care is essential. The patient's personal surgeon could retain responsibility for his patient's general care and coordination of the team, provided he is available at all times for guidance of the team. If not, he should delegate this role at least temporarily to the ICU director and his staff or to a colleague or a senior resident who is available and familiar with critical care. The coordinator could be that team member who is most experienced in managing the patient's predominant problem. Ideally, all orders should be channeled through a member of the unit's full-time staff or a physician trainee assigned full-time to the unit. Other options would include: general orders by the attending surgeon, who acts as team coordinator; respiratory orders by the full-time ICU physicians; and emergency orders by any physician who is present at the time of the crisis. General and specific care orders in an intensive nursing care unit of a Category III hospital should be written by the patient's primary attending physician, and nonmedical staff carry out emergency measures according to standing orders.

Because of the traditional "possession" of his patient by the attending physician or surgeon in the health care system of this country, patient care authority has evolved in our general ICUs and in many others elsewhere according to the following compromise: orders are written jointly by the attending physician or surgeon or his house officer and the ICU director with his block-assigned ICU physician trainees. The ICU physicians are automatically involved in the care of all patients as team members and are responsible for all respiratory care, life-support monitoring, cardiopulmonary resuscitation, administration, and teaching. Automatic team membership involves more than being a consultant, since the latter must wait until called upon (which may be too late) and may not be permitted to assume responsibility for any phase of the management. Attending staff and mature house staff of various disciplines have collaborated well in this system, but immature and inexperienced house staff sometimes fail to cooperate in a satisfactory manner.

To provide optimum care of the patient and ensure efficient operation of the unit, it is advisable to have a list of consultants, for instance, in cardiology, gastroenterology, infectious diseases, nephrology, neurology, pulmonary diseases, neurosurgery, orthopedic surgery, metabolic diseases, radiology, and psychiatry. Such specialists should manifest an interest in applying their specific skills to patients with life-threatening illness and injuries and work cooperatively with members of the unit's staff.

Physicians who provide 24-hour coverage in ICUs should already be competent in CCM or at least be in training in this field of medicine. They should have at least two years of approved postgraduate training. Care of the critically ill by inexperienced house staff or by physicians who do not personally or through experienced designates remain with the patient should be strongly discouraged.

In Category I hospitals, 24-hour coverage within the general ICU should be provided by CCM physicians (trainees or staff men) who are responsible to the director of the ICU and assigned full time to the unit without additional responsibilities in other areas of the hospital.

In Category II hospitals, ICU-assigned house officers should also be responsible to the unit's medical director, but around-the-clock physician coverage may be provided by regular house officers responsible to the attending physician or surgeon.

In Category III hospitals, physicians admitting patients to the ICU retain responsibility for general care of these patients. They should delegate responsibility for ongoing life-support and emergency services to nonphysician personnel who act according to standing orders. They should also delegate responsibility for special problems that are beyond their competence to consultants, including the ICU medical director.

It is important that final responsibility for ICU patient care reside with the physician who provides continuous patient observation and care, who is aware of the patient's overall problems, and who has acquired greatest experience in CCM.

CCM PHYSICIAN EDUCATION

Manpower Needs.   Job opportunities for physicians with special expertise in CCM are ample in traditional departments, but there are few for autonomous interdisciplinary ICU directors in spite of JCAH and SCCM recommendations. However, there are about 1400 acute care general hospitals with over 200 beds in the United States. With an average need of at least one CCM director and one codirector for each hospital's general ICU (counting on 24-hour in-house coverage help by additional physicians), about 2800 CCM experienced, trained, and committed physicians are needed in this country now. However, there are probably not many more available than the 500 members of the SCCM. Furthermore, there are only 26 reported CCM fellowship training programs that approach the SCCM education guidelines. These programs trained about 70 CCM physicians in 1975–1976 and therefore need to be expanded.

At the University of Pittsburgh, we have developed educational objectives separately for medical students, traditional residents, and CCM physician trainees in terms of knowledge, skills, experience, ability, and attitude.

Medical Students. Most medical schools have inadequate educational programs in resuscitation, emergency care, and intensive care. Only one-third of the medical schools in the United States and Canada offer a formal emergency medical care course. Most are conducted by the Department of Surgery, focused on trauma, and limited to emergency room experience. Between 1963 and 1975, at the University of Pittsburgh, a combined emergency and critical care medicine program evolved for medical students, which is coordinated by a multidisciplinary faculty committee. First-year students receive a 20-hour emergency care course; second-year students are taught cardiopulmonary resuscitation (A, B, C, and D) and instructed in the management of different emergencies, e.g., trauma, shock, and acute respiratory failure; third-year students have an obligatory three-week clerkship in Anesthesiology/CCM for acquisition of basic life-support skills in the treatment of circulatory, respiratory, and central nervous system failure; and fourth-year students may take a six-week elective ICU rotation.

Traditional Disciplines. Although some critical illnesses are covered well by conventional specialties and their house staff (e.g., cardiology/cardiac care unit; nephrology/dialysis unit; cardiac surgery; neurosurgery), experience has shown that most traditional residencies, including anesthesiology, medicine, pulmonary diseases, cardiology, pediatrics, general surgery, surgical subspecialties, and obstetrics/gynecology, do not adequately prepare graduates for modern care of the critically ill and injured patients with multiple organ failure. An American Medical Association conference in 1974 recommended that all residents of traditional clinical disciplines should have available to them CCM training by full-time assignment to ICUs with training programs. This should be obligatory for anesthesiology and emergency physician residencies. However, making it mandatory for all clinical specialty residents would presently be unrealistic, because of the limitations of suitable ICU facilities and the number of patients available.

CCM Physician Specialist Fellowship Program. Such a program was started at the University of Pittsbugh in 1963 with the objective of training physicians who would staff and lead ICUs in community and teaching hospitals. The CCM physician is a traditional specialist with additional interest and training in cardiopulmonary resuscitation, life support, and CCM organization and education, who has special expertise in supportive care, i.e., in the maintenance of vital organ system homeostasis when autoregulation fails. He is both a specialist and a generalist, the latter because of his interest in patients with multiple organ failure, even though he is involved in their management only in the life-threatening phase. This interdisciplinary approach of critical care medicine is in agreement with present public pressure for more comprehensive rather than specialized and disease-oriented practice.

The CCM physician needs a *base specialty* because CCM is not a recognized specialty in itself, because he needs in-depth scientific background in a traditional discipline to function as a team member, and because full-time clinical practice in critical care may be too demanding to be tolerated for the entire professional lifetime.

The University of Pittsburgh CCM Fellowship Program is flexible to meet the needs of physicians with different specialty backgrounds. Fellows are accepted after a minimum of three years of training in anesthesiology, internal medicine, pediatrics, or surgery. The CCM Fellows' basic experience is in the general ICU. In addition, they selectively rotate through cardiology, nephrology, neonatalogy, EMS (emergency medical service, including mobile ICU), and CCM-oriented research. One-year Fellows are encouraged to participate part-time in clinical research, and two-year Fellows in full-time laboratory, clinical, or health care delivery research. So far, the American Boards of Anesthesiology, Internal Medicine, and Pediatrics have accepted our first Fellowship year as the elective year within the three- to four-year residency programs in anesthesiology, medicine, and pediatrics. However, only six months of CCM training counts for Board eligibility in surgery.

Even with intensification of EMS and CCM training within medical schools and conventional residencies, traditional specialists are unlikely to sustain their EMS and CCM experience, since they are not involved in large enough numbers of appropriate cases. In addition, rapid progress in knowledge and technology may be beyond their ability or willingness to assimilate. Further, they may not be able to provide 24-hour life support for titrated care, especially if this prevents them from practicing their base specialties with the traditional rounding and order-prescribing type of care. They may also lack ability and training to look after education, budgets, organization, administration, quality control of life-support, and the CCM/EMS links with the community, which would not necessarily prevent them from providing care. Finally, they may be unable to innovate and perform research in CCM.

At a 1974 American Medical Association Workshop, an evaluation and approval system of CCM Fellowships and "Certification of Special Competence in CCM" was recommended as a cooperative venture of the American Boards of Anesthesiology, Medicine, Pediatrics, and Surgery and SCCM. It was recommended that candidates for "Special Competence in CCM

Examinations'' should be physicians who have passed one of the above four specialty board examinations and who, in addition, have completed an approved CCM training. Certification in CCM could be granted by an interdisciplinary body, for instance, the American Board of Medical Specialties. Special competence in CCM would then be considered a subspecialty of each individual's base specialty.

NURSING SERVICE

Responsibility and Coverage. Nursing services provided to intensive care patients should be under the direction of a professionally qualified head nurse who is competent in both clinical nursing and administration. The individual selected must have the ability to organize, coordinate, and evaluate the ICU nursing service on a full-time basis, including: the design and formulation of nursing policies, procedures, functions, and standards of care; the establishment of criteria for staffing and policies regarding staffing; the provision of nursing coverage and teaching personnel; the supervision of nursing care within the unit; and the development of a complete teaching program.

A sufficient number of properly trained registered nurses who have demonstrated abilities in problem-solving and have developed specialized skills in critical care nursing must be on duty at all times to provide high-quality nursing care. The basic intensive care unit nursing requirement is one registered nurse for every two patients. However, special consideration should be given to patients whose life-support system is not yet stabilized, such as those who are comatose, those who require mechanical ventilation or assisted circulation (e.g., intra-aortic balloon pumping) or hemodialysis, unstable arrhythmia patients, and others. These conditions generally require one registered nurse per patient, which may not always be possible. To provide adequate intensive care in such situations, allied health personnel (e.g., licensed practical nurses, nursing assistants, respiratory therapists, and technicians) may give bedside care within their fields of training.

The unit's staffing patterns should be developed and implemented with the purpose and goals of patient care as defined within the intensive care unit. Periodic evaluations should be conducted by utilizing such mechanisms as nursing audits to determine nursing care effectiveness.

Each registered nurse should be able to demonstrate the ability to plan, implement, and evaluate the quality of nursing care and to supervise other nursing personnel who may provide such nursing care not requiring the skill and judgment of a registered nurse.

Education. ICU nurses' training should include an orientation course, in-service training, and a critical care nursing course.[5]

In addition to general hospital orientation, intensive care nurses should have a two-month ICU orientation course including both theory and clinical application.

In-service training in an ICU should include a clinical specialist whose primary responsibility is staff development; the head nurse who makes rounds daily or at least every other day with the unit's director or codirector; and weekly patient-oriented conferences for all ICU nurses.

AMA Category I and II hospitals should arrange critical care nursing courses at least twice a year. These courses should also be available to clinical specialists and ICU nurses from Category III and IV hospitals in the area so that these nurses may become knowledgeable about new diagnostic, monitoring, and therapeutic techniques.

The American Association of Critical Care Nurses (AACN) has designed a core curriculum for training in Critical Care Nursing (CCN).[2] Completion of such training and successful examination in CCN leads to certification as Critical Care Registered Nurses (CCRN). The first such examination took place in January 1976.

Based on the level of training, the following categories of ICU nurses have been proposed:

Critical Care Nurse I is the bedside ICU nurse who has completed her orientation course and passed a written CCN I examination.

Critical Care Nurse II has had at least one year's experience and has taken the advanced critical care course and passed the pertinent examination. The CCN II nurse may be a team leader or the nurse in charge of a shift.

Critical Care Nurse III is a CCRN who has passed the AACN examination for specialty certification in critical care nursing. She is usually on the ICU head nurse level.

A CCN III nurse with an M.S. degree may become a *clinical specialist in CCN* to be the bedside teacher, for instance, who trains ICU registered nurses during their orientation course and teaches new techniques to all ICU registered nurses.

Policies. Policies for ICU nursing care should be contained in a manual that includes nursing philosophy and objectives, functions and guidelines defining criteria for staffing assignments, admissions, discharges and transfers, definitive therapy, equipment, emergencies, nursing procedures, and general standards of care. Policies for medical management are particularly important in those ICUs where physicians are not present around the clock, e.g., in Category III hospitals.

Registered nurses in an ICU must be trained in performing the following procedures, as described in the ICU Nursing Manual: cardiopulmonary resuscitation, including defibrillation and administration of antiarrhythmia drugs, and emergency tracheal intubation; electrocardiogram interpretation; arterial and venous puncture; intravenous catheter insertion; intravenous therapy; peritoneal dialysis; isolation techniques; and different types of respiratory care.

Nursing standards of care should be established for patients with acute myocardial infarction, acute respiratory failure, acute renal failure, brain injury, spinal cord injury, multiple injuries, shock, gastrointestinal bleeding, total parenteral nutrition, and postanesthesia/surgery recovery, including surgical, cardiovascular and neurosurgical patients.

Detailed standing orders for treatment of emergencies are needed. These should include cardiac arrest, emergency intubation, life-threatening arrhythmias, pulmonary edema, acute respiratory failure, adjustment of ventilators, arterial blood sampling and blood gas analysis, emergency medication, and the like. There should also be standing orders for nonemergency situations regarding patient monitoring, laboratory blood work, daily weighing, chest x-ray examination, intravenous fluid administration, and routine sampling of tracheal bronchial secretions for culture and sensitivity tests.

ALLIED HEALTH PROFESSIONALS

Respiratory Therapists.   The majority of critically ill patients have respiratory problems, no matter what the primary disease is. Therefore, these patients are often treated with mechanical ventilation during the most critical phase of their disease. The management of mechanical ventilation and other sophisticated respiratory care, as ordered by the physicians and surgeons, is the responsibility of respiratory therapists.[4] These are very important ICU team members who have become physician assistants in respiratory care. They receive an associate degree after two years of college education, with a high-school diploma as a prerequisite. After passing the National Board of Respiratory Therapy Examination, they become registered in the American Registry of Respiratory Therapists.

Other Ancillary Staff.   No doubt, respiratory therapists are the most important allied health professionals in intensive care. However, there is a large number of other personnel, including physical therapists, biomedical electronics technicians, laboratory technicians, social workers, bacteriologists, physiologists, and computer technicians. They all serve important functions related to patient care, either directly (physical therapists and social workers) or indirectly via the environment (bacteriologists) and equipment (biomedical electronics technicians and computer technicians). An electrical safety officer should also be appointed to provide preventive maintenance of all electrical equipment and systems in the unit. Further, a clerk-typist should assist the head nurse during daytime shifts to facilitate efficient patient and administrative record-keeping, purchase orders, phone calls, and physician page calls. Finally, if the hospital utilizes unit managers, there should be an ICU manager who is responsible for control and ordering of supplies and equipment, as well as coordination of other administrative functions, including budgets.

EQUIPMENT

Minimum equipment requirements for a Category III ICU include the following installations per cubicle/bed: two oxygen outlets, one compressed air outlet, three vacuum outlets, eight electrical outlets, one sink, bedside and central monitoring and recording devices, and air conditioning. Category I and II ICUs should meet these minimum requirements and should also be equipped with a computer connection.

In Category I and II hospitals, x-ray facilities should be sufficiently comprehensive to provide nearly all of the patient's x-ray requirements. Since patients in need of constant monitoring and life-support equipment can seldom be transported out of the unit to a routine x-ray facility, improved patient care and lower mortality should be achieved by locating x-ray facilities within the unit. In Category III hospitals, the minimum requirement is a portable x-ray machine for the ICU.

ICU beds must be adjustable for various positions, and the patient must be accessible from the vertex. Further, these beds should be translucent to permit use of image-intensifiers to simplify positioning of various intravascular catheters and other devices in desired positions. ICU beds should also be equipped for continuous or at least intermittent measurement of the patient's weight.

There is no evidence at this time that use of computers in ICU monitoring decreases morbidity, mortality, or cost, mainly because there are no useful cost-effectiveness studies. Physiologic titration of care is enhanced by on-line computerized monitoring, but the great impact may not come until computerized techniques "close the loop" from sensors to therapy, so-called servo-controlled life support.

Modern critical care techniques necessitate a more vigorous electrical safety program than in regular patient units. This program, supervised by the electrical safety office, should include necessary electrical equipment maintenance, a program for regular checking of equipment, heavy-duty three-prong plugs on all equipment, regular checking of defibrillator output, analysis of unexplained recorder or monitoring interference, prohibition of electrical beds in the ICU, special rules for external pacemakers, and regular documentation of safety testing.

Electrocution hazards should be minimized by following national standards. These call for equipotential grounding plus isolation transformers for each bed, and current leakage no greater than 10 microamperes from any equipment.[6]

APPENDIX

Crash Cart: Equipment and Drug Requirements

The following recommendations were made by the American Heart Association/National Research Council in May 1973, and are applicable to the hospital crash cart.

Respiratory Management.   For airway management and artificial ventilation, all life-support units should be equipped with the following: (1) oxygen supply (two E cylinders) with reducing valves capable of delivering 15 liters/minute and with mask and reservoir bag; (2) Steiner spray cannula; (3) mask for mouth-to-mask ventilation; (4) oropharyngeal airways; (5) S-tube (optional); (6) laryngoscope with blades (curved and straight, adult and infant) and extra batteries and bulbs; (7) assorted adult-size (cuffed) and child-size (uncuffed) endotracheal tubes with stylet and 15/22 mm adaptors; (8) syringe with clamp or plastic two-way or three-way stopcock or valve for endotracheal tube cuffs; (9) acceptable bag-valve-mask unit (adult, child, and infant), with provisions for 100 per cent oxygen ventilation; (10) bite blocks; (11) adhesive tape (1 inch and 0.5 inch); (12) suction (preferably portable), with catheters sizes 6 to 16 and Yankauer-type suction tips; (13) nasogastric tube; (14) esophageal obturator airway (optional); (15) cricothyrotomy set.

Circulatory Management. To provide adequate management of the circulatory system, all advanced life-support units should be equipped with the following: (1) portable defibrillator-monitor with ECG electrode-defibrillator paddles or portable DC defibrillator and portable ECG monitor; (2) portable ECG machine, direct writing, with connection to monitor; (3) venous infusion sets (micro and regular); (4) indwelling venous catheters (regular and special units); catheter outside needle (sizes 14 to 22), catheter inside needle (sizes 14 to 22), CVP catheters; (5) intravenous solutions (5 per cent dextrose in water, lactated Ringers); (6) cut-down set; (7) sterile gloves; (8) urinary catheters; (9) assorted syringes and needles, stopcocks, venous extension tubes; (10) intracardiac needles; (11) tourniquets, adhesive, disposable razor and similar items; (12) thoracotomy tray.

Essential Drugs. All life support units must have these drugs available: sodium bicarbonate (prefilled syringes, 50 ml ampules, or 500 ml 5 per cent bottles); epinephrine (prefilled syringes); atropine sulfate (prefilled syringes); lidocaine (Xylocaine prefilled syringe); morphine sulfate; calcium chloride or calcium gluconate.

Useful Drugs. These drugs are recommended for hospital and nonhospital life-support units: aminophylline; dexamethasone (Decadron); dextrose 50 per cent; digoxin (Lanoxin); diphenhydramine HCl (Benadryl); dopamine (Intropine); ethacrynic acid (Edecrin); furosemide (Lasix); isoproterenol (Isuprel); lanatoside C (Cedilanid); meperidine HCl (Demerol); metaraminol (Aramine); methylprednisolone (Solu-Medrol); naloxone HCl (Narcan); norepinephrine (Levophed); phenylephrine HCl (Neo-synephrine); potassium chloride; propranolol HCl (Inderal); procainamide HCl (Pronestyl); quinidine; sodium nitroprusside (Nipride); succinylcholine Cl; tubocurarine.

REFERENCES

1. American Medical Association, Commission of Emergency Medical Services: Categorization of hospital emergency capabilities, Chicago, 1971.
2. American Association of Critical Care Nurses: Core curriculum for critical-care nursing. 1975. P.O. Box DN, Irvine, California 92664.
3. Comprehensive Health Planning Association of Western Pennsylvania, Inc.: Guidelines for

the planning and development of adult intensive care in Western Pennsylvania. Pittsburgh, 1974.

4. Grenvik, A.: Role of allied health professionals in critical care medicine. Crit. Care Med., *2*:6, 1974.

5. Kahn, J. N.: Trends in the educational process for the critical care nurse. Crit. Care Med., *3*:123, 1975.

6. National Electrical Code. National Fire Protection Association, Boston, 1971.

7. Safar, P., and Grenvik, A.: Critical care medicine, organizing and staffing intensive care units. Chest, *59*:535, 1971.

8. Safar, P., Benson, D. M., Esposito, G., Grenvik, A., and Sands, P. A.: Emergency and critical care medicine, local implementation of national recommendations. *In* Safar, P. (Ed.): Public Health Aspects of Critical Care Medicine and Anesthesiology. F. A. Davis Company, Philadelphia, 1974.

9. Shoemaker, W. C.: Interdisciplinary medicine: accommodation or integration? Crit. Care Med., *3*:1, 1975.

10. Society of Critical Care Medicine: Guidelines for organization of critical care units. J.A.M.A., *222*:1532, 1972.

11. Society of Critical Care Medicine: Guidelines for training of physicians in critical care medicine. Crit. Care Med. *1*:39, 1973.

12. Safar, P., and Grenvik, A.: Organization and physician education in critical care medicine. Anesthesiology, *47*:82–95, 1977.

INTENSIVE CARE MONITORING

SAMUEL R. POWERS, M.D.

The aim of monitoring is to maintain mechanical surveillance of a seriously ill patient so that the physician may have early warning of a change in the patient's condition. Ideally, the surveillance should be accomplished without the patient or the medical personnel surrounding him being aware of the physical presence of mechanical equipment. Monitoring should provide frequent, highly reliable data concerning specific physiologic abnormalities. It cannot supplant or compete with careful human surveillance carried out by nursing personnel or, to a lesser extent, by a physician. The prime goal of monitoring equipment is to bring nursing and physician personnel to the bedside of the seriously ill patient when their services are most urgently required. Under no circumstances should monitoring interfere with or supplant the human contact of medical personnel with their patients. Only rarely will a monitoring device provide accurate diagnosis of the cause of the trouble or suggest appropriate therapy. If intensive care monitoring equipment is to perform this function of rapid, reliable surveillance, there are certain conditions that must be considered.

The variable to be monitored should be appropriate for the anticipated physiologic derangements of the particular patient. Continuous monitoring with an electrocardiogram is appropriate for a patient in the coronary care unit but will merely get in the way of personnel caring for a young patient with multiple trauma. Surveillance of the timed urine volume is more appropriate in the latter case. Monitoring equipment should be flexible and should include a wide variety of parameters that can be measured. Specific monitoring requirements for each patient should be ordered with the same understanding of the underlying disease process as in the selection of appropriate laboratory and x-ray examinations in a careful diagnostic work-up.

Monitoring equipment in an intensive care ward should make the job of the medical personnel easier, not more difficult. Equipment that demands constant readjustment, mechanical manipulation, or complicated interpretation is a hindrance to good medical care, not an asset. Generally speaking, monitoring equipment gets in the way. It should not be used unless the information provided is essential for the proper care of the patient and cannot be obtained in any other way.

The selected monitoring equipment must be reliable. If the equipment signals a disaster when none is present, then it will be ignored when a real disaster occurs. True reliability is a form of respect that must be earned. When the monitoring equipment has correctly predicted a catastrophe at a time when the professionals were unaware of impending trouble, then the monitoring equipment will have earned its place as a member of the intensive care team.

Monitoring equipment should pose little, if any, increased risk to the patient. The ideal of noninvasive sensors coupled to remote devices for data acquisition and processing is unfortunately an unrealized dream of the future. Present equipment will pose some finite risk each time it is applied. The physician must repeatedly inquire as to whether the risk of a possible complication is greater than the risk of detecting it. The risk of acute renal failure in the usual postoperative patient is significantly less than the risk of infection that may be introduced by a urethral catheter necessary for its detection. Routine catheterization is not good monitoring. If, on the other hand, the risk of a specific complication is significant, then monitoring should proceed with every precaution to minimize the risk of a diagnostic invasion. Monitoring of unnecessary physiologic variables or of those that have a low probability of providing useful clinical information should be avoided. The number of physiologic and biochemical variables that can be monitored has increased in recent years to the point where an undiscriminating physician might easily be overwhelmed with a mountain of useless data. Good monitoring practice demands that the needs of each patient be carefully considered so that risks to the patient will be minimized and the medical personnel will be alerted only when urgent action is required.

The prime requirement for selecting appropriate monitoring equipment is to define the time course of the anticipated complication. Cardiac arrhythmias may cause death in a matter of minutes, and therefore the monitoring equipment for cardiac arrhythmias should have a turn-around time from detection to alerting signal of no more than several seconds. If the anticipated complication is the acute respiratory distress syndrome, then the monitoring requirements for this complication need not involve on-line, real time analysis and report, but should consist of off-line, intermittent spot analysis of blood gases. When the anticipated complication is acute renal failure, appropriate monitoring for the early detection of this condition requires only the hourly determination of urine volume. Complex and expensive devices for moment-to-moment determination of urine output are available, but since the evolution of acute renal failure requires many hours, this expensive equipment not only is unwarranted but may interfere with good care, since it provides a large quantity of irrelevant numbers. Thus, the specifications for monitoring equipment for different types of patients in our intensive care unit will vary from clinical observation by the nursing personnel to sophisticated on-line computer analysis.

A convenient method for classifying the many varieties of monitoring systems is in terms of the anticipated abnormalities that may occur. Typical examples include the circulatory system; the respiratory system, including both ventilation and gas exchange; the central nervous system; renal function; and systemic sepsis. Monitoring the patient who has sustained multiple trauma is unique because all of these systems may easily be involved.

MONITORING THE CIRCULATORY SYSTEM

Failure of the heart, the driving force of the circulatory system, can occur suddenly owing to a cardiac arrhythmia or more slowly owing to myocardial failure. The former complication is detected by changes in the electrical activity of the heart as monitored by the electrocardiogram, whereas myocardial failure is detected from changes in the filling pressure of the left side of the heart and the ability of the left ventricle to maintain an adequate cardiac output for the metabolic needs of vital organs. Sudden, severe cardiac arrhythmias are generally treatable conditions; therefore, the requirement of instantaneous detection, reliable alarm, and prompt corrective action is demanded. These conditions may be met if the electrocardiogram provides a display in the nurses' station where continuing surveillance is possible. It should be emphasized that clinical situations that may result in death in a matter of moments following detection of the abnormality require that the ward personnel be properly trained and equipped to correct the abnormality as soon as it is detected. Monitoring devices for detecting cardiac arrhythmias must include an alarm system, since the visual display cannot be under observation at all times. Most alarm devices depend upon measuring the R-R interval and responding to a sudden change in this value. The precise abnormality cannot be diagnosed by most monitoring equipment, so it is necessary that the intensive care unit nursing personnel be skilled in the interpretation of the electrocardiographic tracing.

Most of the catastrophes that take place in the surgical intensive care unit, including bleeding, infection, pulmonary embolus, respiratory insufficiency, renal insufficiency and hepatic failure, do not produce a change in the electrocardiogram. Monitoring systems that depend primarily on analysis of the electrocardiogram have limited use in the surgical intensive care unit and serve only to sound an alarm after all opportunity for corrective action has already passed.

Failure of the circulatory system that may result in the death of a patient within a matter of hours is generally associated with a change in intravascular pressure of either the arterial or venous side of the circulation. Pressure-sensing devices are, therefore, the mainstay of monitoring equipment in the surgical ICU. The interpretation of pressure measurements depends on an understanding of the physiologic principles involved in the Starling-Sarnoff ventricular function curve. There must be a sufficient blood volume to ensure an adequate filling pressure for the left ventricle, and the left ventricular myocardium must be capable of ejecting an adequate volume of blood at a reasonable mean arterial pressure. In more technical terms, there is a relationship between the filling pressure of the left ventricle and the ability of the left ventricle to perform work. The essential inputs for this evaluation include measurement of filling pressure, cardiac output, and mean aortic pressure. Filling pressure of the heart can be estimated from a central venous pressure measurement or determined more directly from the pulmonary capillary wedge pressure. Both forms of measurement should be available in the surgical intensive care unit. The central venous pressure line is generally inserted percutaneously and consists of a long, flexible catheter that is passed through the lumen of a large-bore needle. Under most circumstances, the catheter will pass into the superior vena cava or right atrium, and if this position is confirmed by a chest roentgenogram, then a reliable measurement of the filling pressure of the right side of the heart can be obtained. Although this catheter measures only the filling pressure of the right side of the heart, it will usually reflect the filling pressure of the left ventricle. Important exceptions to this generalization include patients with increased pulmonary vascular resistance due to chronic obstructive lung disease, congestive heart failure, sepsis, and the acute respiratory distress syndrome. The central venous pressure catheter has uses and limitations in the surgical intensive care unit. It is usually quite accurate for the initial resuscitation and primary management of the surgical patient but often becomes less reliable if respiratory complications or generalized sepsis develop in the subsequent days or weeks.

The pulmonary artery catheter (balloon-tipped flow-directed catheter) provides a more direct estimation of filling pressure of the left ventricle. This catheter is best inserted by surgical cutdown over an antecubital vein. The catheter is advanced approximately 30 cm, and then a small balloon is inflated. The inflated balloon is swept forward by the bloodstream as if it were an embolus carrying the catheter through the right ventricle and into the pulmonary artery. No fluoroscope is necessary. Observation of a pressure tracing obtained from the tip of the catheter will provide the final assurance that the catheter is in the pulmonary artery. When the catheter is advanced as far as it will pass and the balloon is reinflated, this catheter becomes a device for sensing left atrial pressure. Even this measurement may be in error, as, for example, when the terminal branches of the pulmonary artery are occluded either by multiple small fibrin aggregates or by a major pulmonary embolus. In most circumstances, however, this measurement is vastly to be preferred over the measurements of central venous pressure. Adequate filling of the left ventricle will generally take place when the pulmonary wedge pressure is between 0 and 5 mm Hg.

The measurement of cardiac output was once a laboratory curiosity performed only in the most sophisticated research facilities. The recent development of the thermal dilution technique for estimation of cardiac output has now put this measurement within reach of any surgical intensive care unit. The detecting device is located on the tip of the same pulmonary artery catheter that is used for an estimation of left atrial pressure. A small quantity of cold saline is injected into the proximal lumen of a double-lumen Swan-Ganz catheter, and a dilution curve is recorded from a thermistor placed at the catheter tip. A cardiac output computer supplied by the manufacturer performs all the necessary calculations and provides an immediate digital display of the output of the heart. Since this technique does not require the removal of any blood and demands only the injection of a small quantity of saline, it can be repeated at frequent intervals and may be carried out in duplicate or triplicate in order to minimize the chances of a spurious result. The normal value is at least 3.3 liters/min.

The final measurement necessary for evaluation of circulatory function is the mean arterial blood pressure. This is obtained from a cannula that is inserted into a peripheral artery and is thus connected to a strain-gauge transducer for continuous recording of arterial pressure. Most monitoring devices contain a small switch that permits electrical integration of the pressure wave form with the display of a single number representing the mean arterial pressure. The normal value is about 80 mm Hg. The same pressure transducers, amplifiers and recorders as are used for measurement of filling pressure of the heart can also be used for measurement of mean arterial pressure. All the elements necessary to describe circulatory function adequately are now available.

Patient monitoring utilizing pulmonary artery and peripheral arterial catheters is invasive and should be used only when clearly indicated. There are three classes of patients in whom the risk of such invasive techniques may be warranted. The first and largest group is composed of those patients who are not responding to standard therapy in the manner that was expected. The second group comprises those patients who initially responded well to resuscitative measures but were then unable to maintain their vital signs without extraordinary supportive measures. Finally, the third group includes those patients in whom an outright catastrophe has occurred. Each of these classes will require the judgment of experienced physicians and surgeons, but the rule of thumb is that when a patient is not responding to a particular treatment in an expected manner, then additional procedures must be instituted. Patients who have suffered multiple trauma or a misadventure in the operating room resulting in extensive blood loss are prime candidates for these techniques, since the anticipated incidence of organ failure warrants extraordinary measures to assist in its prevention.

Estimates of left ventricular function by noninvasive techniques is a continuing dream of the intensive care physician. Although a reliable technique for such evaluation has not yet been developed, certain indirect methods are under current investigation and may hold promise for the future. Many such techniques depend upon an estimate of the internal mechanical events associated with ventricular contractions and the production of an adequate peripheral pulse. Monitoring devices that are necessary to carry out such measurements include an electrocardiogram, a phonocardiogram, and an external pressure-sensing device to record the form of the carotid pulse. The duration of systole is measured from the onset of the QRS complex on the electrocardiogram to the second heart sound detected by the phonocardiogram. This is referred to as left ventricular systolic time (LVST). The duration of left ventricular ejection is obtained from the elapsed time for the up-stroke of the externally recorded carotid pulsewave. This value is referred to as ventricular ejection time (LVET). The difference between these two numbers (LVST−LVET) represents the lag period between the onset of electrical activity of the heart and the onset of mechanical activity and is referred to as the pre-ejection period (PET). The PET/LVET ratio is quite constant for normal hearts, with a value of approximately 0.35. This number increases in the presence of left ventricular failure. Unfortunately, this value is also dependent upon the degree of peripheral vascular resistance, and therefore the method cannot as yet be accepted for monitoring in the surgical intensive care unit.

Monitoring the peripheral tissues provides an assessment of the adequacy of the peripheral circulation. An ideal monitor of the peripheral circulation would provide continuous estimation of the tissue oxygen partial pressure. Unfortunately, such devices are currently limited to a few highly specialized research laboratories and there is no reliable equipment available for this direct measurement. A highly satisfactory substitute can be obtained using the indirect measurements of temperature and muscle pH. Inadequate blood flow to the periphery can easily be detected by a widening of the temperature gradient between the body core (rectal temperature) and the interdigital space of the hand or foot. Inexpensive thermistors are available that can be placed in a noninvasive manner and provide almost foolproof information about this important function.

Inadequate tissue perfusion results in the accumulation of the products of anaerobic glycolysis, including lactic acid. There is a fall in muscle pH. A tiny pH electrode can be applied to the surface of a muscle bundle by means of a small incision. Correlative studies have indicated a close relation between muscle pH and the level of tissue oxygenation. This technique has not been widely applied, in large part because of its invasive nature and the extreme fragility of the sensing device. Its greatest use will be in situations in which a single extremity may have diminished blood flow owing to skeletal or soft tissue injury and the adequacy of peripheral circulation requires continued surveillance.

MONITORING THE VENTILATORY SYSTEM

Failure of the ventilatory system to provide an adequate supply of oxygen to the blood and to ensure removal of carbon dioxide is one of the commonest causes of serious physiologic derangement in the surgical intensive care unit. These abnormalities may also be divided into those that may produce death of the patient within a matter of minutes and those that may result in death in a matter of hours or days. Immediate death due to ventilatory failure almost invariably results from inability of the lungs to exchange

an adequate quantity of inspired gas. The usual reason is mechanical interference to the movement of air as a consequence of obstruction of the upper
or lower airways. Sudden failure of ventilation may result from aspiration of
blood or vomitus, formation of mucus plugs, or sudden misplacement of an
endotracheal tube or esophageal balloon. Unfortunately, there is currently
no adequate method for the detection of such acute ventilatory emergencies.
Constant surveillance of the patient by trained personnel is the only satisfactory method. If the patient has an endotracheal tube and is being maintained
on a mechanical ventilator, then a satisfactory monitoring device consists of
a spirometer attached to the expiratory side of the system. There is a great
need for a simple noninvasive device to estimate the patient's tidal volume.
This is one of the few situations in clinical medicine in which prompt recognition and immediate corrective action will result in the saving of a life.

A more common variant of ventilatory insufficiency is depression rather
than complete cessation of ventilation. Inadequate ventilation may result
from excessive pain medication, the presence of a head injury, the occurrence of multiple fractured ribs, or even a painful upper abdominal incision
with inadequate pain medication.

Many cases of apparent sudden death in the intensive care unit are in
reality due to a relatively prolonged period of inadequate ventilation. The
hallmark of ventilatory insufficiency is an elevation of the arterial P_{CO_2}. All
patients whose clinical condition suggests the possibility of inadequate ventilation require frequent determinations of blood gases and immediate treatment of the arterial P_{CO_2} in excess of 45 mm Hg. The arterial P_{O_2} may be
misleading because many patients in the intensive care unit are receiving
supplemental oxygen by mask or nasal catheter. These measures may raise
the arterial oxygen to relatively normal levels at a time when carbon dioxide
elimination is seriously impaired. Proper treatment requires the use of a
mechanical ventilator.

Respiratory failure, as indicated by an arterial P_{O_2} of less than 75 mm
Hg, may occur at a time when total ventilation is adequate but the inspired
gas does not come into contact with blood perfusing the lungs. The lungs of a
seriously ill patient, particularly those who have been subjected to multiple
trauma or prolonged sepsis, show great variation from region to region.
Some areas may have normal or supernormal ventilation but receive very
little of the pulmonary blood flow. Other areas may receive large quantities
of pulmonary blood flow but be poorly ventilated or not ventilated at all.
These patients demonstrate arterial hypoxemia that is associated with a
normal arterial P_{CO_2}, since total ventilation is within normal limits. The low
arterial P_{O_2} results from mixed venous blood passing through the lung without coming into contact with ventilated alveoli. This mechanism is referred
to as an intrapulmonary shunt. The shunt may be calculated from a knowledge of concentration of oxygen in the inspired gas, the arterial P_{O_2}, and the
mixed venous P_{O_2}. The blood gases are obtained from the same arterial and
pulmonary artery catheters that are used for pressure monitoring. The actual
magnitude of the shunt is easily estimated by means of a nomogram such as
that described by Bartlett (Fig. 1).

A significant intrapulmonary shunt (greater than 15 per cent) is an indication for mechanical ventilatory support, frequently with the addition of positive end-expiratory pressure (PEEP). Although the measurement of shunt fraction requires a pulmonary artery catheter, the occurrence of a decreased arterial Po_2 in association with a normal arterial Pco_2 suggests the presence of an intrapulmonary shunt. A good rule is that when the arterial Po_2 cannot be maintained above 75 mm Hg with a face mask utilizing 50 per cent oxygen, then a pulmonary artery catheter should be passed and the magnitude of the shunt determined. If the shunt is above 15 per cent, mechanical ventilatory support is indicated. Prompt detection of increased intrapulmonary shunting followed by correction with mechanical ventilation is highly successful in preventing the acute respiratory distress syndrome. Application of these techniques represents one of the significant advances in surgical care in recent years.

Patients with an endotracheal tube in place who are being supported with a mechanical ventilator may be monitored for alterations of the mechanical properties of the lung. Abnormalities of the lung parenchyma, as distinguished from disorders in the control of ventilation, are associated with an increased stiffness more correctly referred to as a decreased compliance of the lung. In simple terms, the compliance of the lung is determined by the increase in lung volume that results from an increase in inflation pressure. The units of compliance are liters/cm H_2O. Most volume-cycled ventilators contain a pressure gauge as well as a method for determining the tidal volume. Dynamic compliance is obtained by dividing the tidal volume by the observed inflation pressure. Normal compliance is 0.1 liter/cm. If the patient is maintained with a constant tidal volume, then an increasing inflation

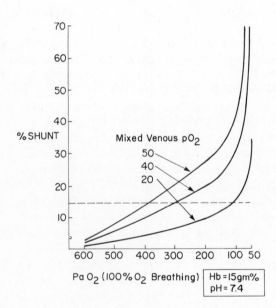

Figure 1. Relation of Pao_2 to shunt fraction at different levels of mixed venous Po_2. Note that a 15 per cent shunt may result in a Pao_2 of any number from 100 mm Hg to 400 mm Hg.

pressure observed on the gauge of the ventilator indicates an increased stiffness of the patient's lungs, whereas a decrease in inflation pressure is generally associated with an improvement.

There are numerous other measurements that can be performed to further assess the ventilatory function of seriously ill patients. These include measurement of dead space, airway resistance, and diffusing capacity. These methods are not readily performed, and therefore cannot be considered as a part of monitoring in the intensive care unit.

MONITORING THE RENAL SYSTEM

Of all the organ systems that may be kept under surveillance in the surgical intensive care unit, the kidneys are the easiest and the most informative to study. Observations on renal function provide a window into the function of the visceral organs. When the kidney is functioning normally, it produces and delivers to the outside of the body its metabolic end-product—the urine. Monitoring the quantity and chemical composition of urine provides information on the function of the kidney and also provides an estimate of the adequacy of perfusion of the other visceral organs. The kidney is the guardian of the internal environment so that analysis of the urine provides information not only on the function of the kidney but also on the functional state of the interior of the body. Normal renal function demands that a proper quantity of fluid of proper composition be presented to the kidney at the proper pressure so that filtration may occur. When an adequate quantity of filtrate is produced, this fluid is operated upon so that its composition becomes significantly different from that of plasma. A key principle for monitoring renal function derives from this consideration that the composition of urine will be different from that of plasma. If this is not true, then the kidney has failed. Monitoring renal function depends on hourly measurements of both the volume and composition of the urine. The simple measurement of hourly urine volume alone may be inadequate or misleading.

A normally functioning kidney produces urine with a composition significantly different from that of plasma. These differences can be quantitatively stated in terms of urine plasma ratios. Common substances that are readily measured in most clinical laboratories include sodium, creatinine, and osmolarity. When the urine plasma osmolar ratio is equal to 1, the urine plasma sodium ratio is less than 2, and the urine plasma creatinine ratio is less than 10, then renal failure has taken place irrespective of the urine volume. On the other hand, a low urine volume below 30 ml/hour that is associated with a urine plasma osmolar ratio of greater than 1.5, a urine plasma sodium ratio greater than 50, and a urine plasma creatinine ratio greater than 100 describes a kidney that is normal but is operating on an internal environment that is depleted. It is not practical to obtain chemical determinations on each hourly urine specimen. Chemical analysis of the urine is indicated, however, when the urine volume is inappropriate for the patient's clinical state. A patient who has received sufficient intravenous fluids to correct a presumed volume loss but remains oliguric deserves these measurements. Of equal importance is a patient who appears to be volume-depleted yet produces a urine volume of over 100 ml/hour. This patient may be suffering from the high output form of renal failure.

Of all the physiologic functions that can be monitored in the intensive care unit, the observations of the quantity and composition of urine have produced the most striking improvement in patient care in recent years. Early detection and rapid correction of abnormalities in renal function have rendered acute renal failure a vanishing disease.

NOTES ON CURRENT MONITORING EQUIPMENT

Modern monitoring systems consist of a series of detectors that produce signals generally electrical in nature which are then processed, analyzed, and displayed. The portion of the system of most interest to the user is a display device, since it is this output that is used for monitoring. Display devices vary from a simple alarm bell which is triggered when a pre-set condition is met to multi-channel, high speed print-outs of computed values obtained from mathematical manipulation of several input channels. In general, the more clearly a physiologic process is understood, the simpler will be the display device. It is desirable to have a display device that makes a permanent record so that a time course of the monitored variable is available. A low value has an entirely different meaning if it is progressively deteriorating or if it is rapidly improving. A strip chart recorder provides the cheapest and most reliable method for such sequential observations. A large oscilloscope is of value only if the pathologic process being monitored may result in changes within a matter of seconds or a few moments. For all other purposes, the large and usually expensive oscilloscope is of limited value. The ideal monitoring hardware for the usual surgical intensive care unit is a four-channel system involving one electrocardiogram, two pressure channels, and a fourth channel for recording of dilution curves, temperature, or other single measurements. The simpler the system, the more likely it is to be correctly used and correctly interpreted. Any system that cannot be effectively operated and interpreted by the nursing personnel in the intensive care unit will be a source of frustration rather than an aid in the management of the patient.

REFERENCE

1. Powers, S. R., Jr., and Gisser D.: Monitoring the traumatized patient. *In* Brown, Jack H. U. (Ed.): Advances in Biomedical Engineering. Vol. 4. New York, Academic Press, 1974, pp. 151–207.

CHAPTER 7

DATA HANDLING SYSTEMS

John E. Brimm, M.D.
Richard M. Peters, M.D.

DATA HANDLING IN THE INTENSIVE CARE UNIT

The intensive care unit (ICU) is a medical microcosm with its own special problems, procedures, and patients. Data handling in the ICU must cope with those special requirements. The term "data handling," in the sense employed in this chapter, includes not only recording information into patient's charts, but also organizing and interpreting that information for their care. Similarities clearly exist between data handling in the ICU and in other medical environments. Weed's observations[26] on traditional data handling methods, particularly for keeping medical records, pertain in the ICU setting. He states two fundamental criteria that the record system ought to meet: it must be structured with well defined rules, and it must be useful for analysis of patient care. The purpose of this chapter is to discuss how ICU data handling methods, given their special requirements, can be both structured and useful, and to illustrate how computers may enhance or supplant traditional methods.

DATA CLASSIFICATIONS

An understanding of the possible data types and recording organizations is necessary for designing a data handling system. ICU data can be classified in a variety of ways. They may have qualitative or quantitative information. Blood pressures and chemistry laboratory values are quantitative; state of consciousness and type of respiration are qualitative. Regularly collected data include measurements of blood pressure, heart rate, and urine output. Drug administration records, chemistry laboratory determinations, cardiac output measurements, and x-ray interpretations are irregularly, or intermittently, collected. Data may be primary or derived. Primary data, such as respiratory rate and urine output, are directly measured or observed. Derived data, such as cardiac output and lung compliance, are calculated from primary data.

Data in both patient charts and bedside flow sheets can be structured in two major ways. First they can be arranged to describe the function of a particular organ system. Since cardiovascular, respiratory, central nervous, metabolic, renal, and hepatic functions are essential for sustaining life, information on each should be included in the data organization.

As an alternative, the data can be organized about a series of problems. In the system popularized by Weed,[26] data from a variety of sources are grouped on the basis of underlying disease processes or problems. Each problem may be specific to a particular organ, or it may involve several systems. Septic shock, for example, transcends grouping by organ system because it typically involves cardiovascular, respiratory, and renal function.

For both of these methods of organization, many data can be recorded graphically on the basis of their times of occurrence. This technique, which is used for bedside flow sheets, combines regularly collected data with intermittently collected data, using time as the abscissa and information type as the ordinate. Of course, many different variables can be plotted on the same graph, using a common time axis. One of the major goals of a data handling system must be to make time relationships explicit among data that are only implicitly time-based. A tachycardia associated with the administration of aminophylline, for example, may be missed if the data are not presented to show the temporal relationship.

PROBLEMS IN ICU DATA HANDLING

The problems of data handling in the ICU stem mainly from the complexity of its patients' problems. Caring for them requires the involvement of many people and the accumulation of massive amounts of data.

The development of ICUs has led to a hierarchy of professional and paraprofessional people who make decisions and perform procedures for preserving vital functions. These people are given far more latitude for discretionary action than their counterparts in other hospital areas. Nurses, for example, administer intravenous medications and initiate treament for cardiac and respiratory arrest. The nurse, the physician, the respiratory therapist, and others must all have access to particular information to fulfill their responsibilities. The ICU has become a data-rich environment in order to provide the information necessary for its patients' care.

Unfortunately, the mere accumulation of larger numbers of measurements and observations does not necessarily facilitate decision making. Important information may be obscured by redundant and insignificant data. For example, a blood pressure that varies randomly within narrow limits may have no significance, while a trend downward that exceeds these limits may be predictive of a failing cardiovascular system.

As the frequency and variety of observations on a patient increase, assurance of the quality of each becomes more difficult. If nurses measure a patient's blood pressure once an hour, they can usually determine it reliably. If, however, the frequency is increased to every five minutes and additional, more complex measurements, such as the central venous pressure and the cardiac output, are required, then the overall reliability of measurement and transcription decreases. Uniformly high quality in the collection of larger amounts of data is confounded by competing demands for nursing time, performance of complex measurements, and relatively fixed error rates for transcription. In order to alleviate these problems, the data handling system ought to be designed to identify errors of omission and to minimize errors of commission.

In addition to the problems discussed previously—the fragmentation of care delivery, the proliferation of data, and the difficulty of quality assurance—the data handling system must confront several more specific problems:

1. The collection and recording of patients' data are time-consuming tasks that frequently detract from more valuable nursing services.

2. Important events may be missed by physicians and nurses in interpretation of vital signs.

3. Many of the new and important tests of physiologic function, such as cardiac output, are too complex to be performed manually.

4. Manual data recording requires mental collation and integration to interpret those data; this requirement demands a level of sophistication not necessarily present in all users of the record.

A solution to the problem of providing care in such a complex environment is through the use of protocols, i.e., criteria for a structured system of care. The development of formal protocols for care helps to define and to organize ICU data handling requirements. Komaroff[9] has described the use of protocols for care in primary medicine. In an analogous fashion, ICU protocols can be developed, as has been done by Kirklin[8] for a particular subset of patients. For example, procedures can be established to recognize cardiac tamponade in post–open heart patients,[14] to observe excessive PVCs in postcoronary patients, and to avert volume deficits in posttrauma patients.

DEVELOPMENT OF ICU DATA SHEETS

Historically, the first step in the organization of data in patients' charts was to design individual forms composed of information important to various subspecialties. Multiple individual forms resulted in fragmentation of information; data recording was duplicated when data pertinent to two systems overlapped. Urine output, for example, would be recorded on flow sheets for both renal and cardiovascular function. Because subspecialty records failed to define organ interactions, they have been replaced by the currently used comprehensive records that span 24 hours of data. These are less organ-oriented than the subspecialty forms and require the user to extract information for a particular organ system. They do, however, ease the burden of recording and facilitate evaluation of the total patient state.

Because comprehensive data sheets must account for diverse patient types, flexible design is essential. They must include the sets of data that are common to all patients, such as heart rate and blood pressure, and also provide for data that are specific for certain patient types, such as post-thoracotomy chest tube drainage.

An example of coordinated data sheets has been described by Hilberman.[7] Each pair of sheets contains information for a 24-hour period. The first is composed of vital signs and nurses' notes; the second contains drug administration and fluid balance data. On the first sheet, the vital signs—temperature, heart rate, and systemic arterial, venous, and/or pulmonary arterial pressures—are graphed. Respiratory rate, weight, and incidence of cardiac arrhythmias can be recorded below the graph. Space for discursive nurses' notes is provided, and these notes are often continued to the blank back side of the form.

The bottom portion of the first sheet consists of a check list of state of sensorium, behavior, skin color, type of respiration, and general condition. This part of the form has been less well accepted because of aversion to the check list concept by the clinical staff. The utility of check sheets is greater when the data are used as input to computer systems.

The same 24-hour time base is used for a second page. The administration of up to 11 drugs, the infusion of intravenous fluids, and the output of urine can all be recorded at hourly intervals. Paste-over labels permit easy specification of particular outputs, such as chest or nasogastric drainage. Certain blood chemistry determinations, e.g., electrolytes and arterial blood gases, and respirator settings complete the collected data. Space is provided at the right of the form for 8- and 24-hour summaries of fluid balance, blood loss, and blood replacement.

This method of data recording allows most of the pertinent information to be included on two bedside sheets. The data are highly structured and densely recorded to speed both retrieval and review. Serial observations in a particular parameter can be easily compared to detect important changes. The data have been arranged, wherever possible, to group sets of related parameters; for example, the recording of values for arterial gases near those for respirator settings facilitates assessment of respiratory status. The use of a common time base permits correlation of therapeutic interventions with patients' responses. Each institution should develop its own forms to suit its own particular needs.

The major defects of this recording form are its inflexible time boundaries and its lack of definite problem or organ orientation. It does not provide a simple means of integrating information over more than 24 hours. Slow phenomena that develop over hours or days are easy to overlook because of the inconvenience and fragmentation imposed by the separate pages. Thus, accumulated deficits in chloride intake for patients requiring nasogastric suction, or repetitive fever patterns suggesting developing abscess, may be missed. The inflexibility of the time format is compounded by a lack of a major contextual organization other than time. While events may occur in some time-dependent manner, they may not be related by the user to an underlying process. The data are merely recorded; only minimal provision can be made for arrangement of information into a context. To correct these deficiencies by using manual methods, duplicate data recording would be required. Rearrangements of data and changes of time scales are impractical with manual methods, but are relatively simple if the information has been entered into a computer file.

DATA HANDLING IN MEDICAL DECISION MAKING AND AUDITING

The data handling system must be useful for auditing both ongoing care and ultimate outcomes. Before evaluation can be performed, however, the auditing criteria must be defined for and captured by that system. Patient mortality is the most obvious and common basis, but not the only possible one, for judging care. Frequently, in studies of the effectiveness of ICU care, the initial state of the patients being studied is not taken into account. Different success rates would obviously be expected if one study included patients with complex problems while another did not.

The first requirement for meaningful auditing and decision making, therefore, is clear definition of the status of the patient on admission. Qualitative definitions have been worked out for some disease states, for example, the New York Heart Association method for categorizing the severity of heart disease and various indices proposed for classifying trauma victims.[3] These classifications relate only to a single disease and generally do not provide a complete picture of a patient's status. A type IV trauma or cardiac patient, for example, might have no other complicating disease, or he might have cirrhosis, chronic obstructive airway disease, or some other preexisting complicating process.

Preadmission quantitative evaluation of the functional status of various organ systems would provide a baseline for initiating therapy and for auditing care. A functional status record could be completed for all candidates for elective surgery, and for emergency admissions, the available data should be used to establish a baseline. Periodic updating of this record would provide a means for both evaluating prior and guiding subsequent treatment. Using the information from the admission record, the ICU course, and an evaluation after discharge from the ICU, the late effects of ICU care can be determined. At present, however, the essential components for this record have not been established.

Basic components of the record should undoubtedly include the patient's age, weight, ideal weight, and preadmission injury index. Quantitative and qualitative evaluation of vital organ function should be performed on or before admission, multiple times throughout the ICU course, and after discharge. Measures of the function of each important organ system have to be defined.

The choice of parameters to be included in a patient status record must be made pragmatically. A paramount criterion must be an evaluation of the cost, risk, and benefit to the patient. A measurement of pulmonary capillary wedge pressure might be highly desirable for evaluating cardiovascular function, but it would not be a justifiable risk in some patients. Second, the choice must be based on the ease and completeness of collection of the parameters. Finally, the choice of parameters must be based on clinical judgments of their presumed importance. No guarantees are available that a particular parameter will necessarily be useful in subsequent audit. If cardiac outputs are available on only a small fraction of the patients to be studied, for example, then its use in later audit is statistically limited.

In spite of these pragmatic constraints on the development of patient status records, they have been constructed in limited ways for sets of ICU patients. Friedman, Goldwyn, and Siegel[18,19] have used cluster analysis and multivariate statistical techniques on cardiorespiratory measurements to determine differences among patients in shock. They have developed the concept of multivariate trajectories for graphically depicting retrospective differences in the time course of recovery in normal and abnormal populations. Shubin and coworkers[17] have assessed the prognostic value of various hemodynamic, metabolic, respiratory, and renal variables in patients in various shock states.

Both of these groups, in limited and practical ways, have implemented the conceptual model of data handling in medical audit proposed by Stacy.[21] In this model, a patient has a time-dependent state vector in a status-disease space. If the patient's state can be quantified at a certain time, and if a therapeutic intervention is taken at that time, then the efficacy of the treatment can be evaluated by measuring the patient's state at some later time. Such evaluations would, it is hoped, also identify criteria that presage loss of functional capacity and predict recovery or deterioration. The development and use of functional status records for evaluating prognosis and therapy is still in its infancy. The use of these records is complicated by the presence of co-morbid processes in many ICU patients. Patients with multiple system diseases, for example, frequently require different treatments for a particular problem from those for patients with only that problem. ICU data are so complex that pertinent information sets are scarce. Nevertheless, effective usage of limited medical resources demands that studies to predict treatment cost and patient prognosis be performed. It is hoped that computerized data banks using functional status records will simplify this essential task.

COMPUTERS IN DATA HANDLING

Most of the major computerized ICUs[10,13,24,27] began their work between five and ten years ago. They generally use video terminals for output and keyboards for input. Disk devices are used for short-term mass storage; if computer records are stored permanently, magnetic tape is employed. Most systems do not rely solely on a computer-based medical record; they print an additional paper record for inclusion in patients' charts.

Computers can help to alleviate some of the previously mentioned problems of ICU data handling. Their potential advantages are based on their capacity to store large data bases, to perform complex tasks, and to execute repetitive operations reliably. Specifically, these advantages include the following.

1. The computer can collect continuously monitored signals, such as the ECG and the arterial pressure wave, at regular intervals effectively without regard for competing concurrent activities. This capability is limited only by the accuracy and reliability of the monitoring hardware and patient sensors.

2. The computer can also analyze such signals to recognize abnormal waveforms, e.g., a premature beat in an ECG signal, and to detect ominous trends over time in any data. Except in some ECG monitoring systems, alarms, i.e., the automated recognition and notification of ominous events, remain a largely unfulfilled promise. For applications other than ECG monitoring, satisfactory methods for separating true from false alarms have not been produced, and classification of alarms into priority levels is needed to add discrimination.

3. The computer can perform complex analyses to provide data that would otherwise not be available. The calculation of various parameters of respiratory function, such as compliance and resistance, would be too laborious to be done manually. With a computer, however, these calculations are feasible.

4. The computer can help to decrease error rates in data collection. Errors of omission can be reduced if the computer system detects absent data and prompts users for their entry. Entered data can be checked to see that they are at least reasonable. Finally, since some data, e.g., chemistry laboratory determinations and monitored vital signs, may already be present in other hospital computers or bedside instruments, ICU computers can retrieve them directly without manual transcription.

5. The computer can retrieve and reformat data in a variety of ways. In manual systems, the paper medical record is used both for recording data and for subsequent recall. If different formats are desired, the data must be copied onto a new form. Automated systems uncouple the input and output processes. Once serum electrolyte values have been entered into a computer system, for example, they may be utilized in a variety of ways: they may be retrieved by themselves or in combination with previous electrolyte values, or they may be integrated with other data to provide information about acid-base or fluid balance status. Changes in initial times and time scales for plotting and regrouping by problem type or organ status can be programmed, and so require no effort on the part of ICU personnel. Data densities for computerized bedside displays are, however, far lower than for the previously described comprehensive flow sheets. Multicolor display devices with

higher resolutions may help to alleviate this problem, but they are currently too costly for widespread use.

6. Because the data capture and output functions are separate, computer-generated reports can conform to the level of sophistication and need of the user. Manual systems require all users to garner data from the same record. These data are only roughly structured, and interpretations are not available. Yet the information needed by an experienced physician differs from that needed by a beginning medical student, a nurse, or a paramedic. Computer systems can meet this need by structuring the output into various levels, depending on the user.

7. Computer systems can integrate data from various sources in the patient's record and can combine them with current medical knowledge to interpret them. Programs have been developed for diagnostic interpretation and therapeutic guidance for acid-base status,[2] fluid balance,[20] and antimicrobial agent selection.[15] As medical practice evolves, computer systems have the capacity to provide timely and accurate information about current concepts of diagnosis and therapy. A physician would be alerted that a prescribed treatment is different from current medical practice.

8. Computer systems can, in certain contexts, control therapy, for example, in automating the infusion of blood in post–open heart patients.[13] The use of the computer to provide treatment on the basis of simultaneous measurements, called "closing the loop," has been undertaken in very limited ways. Computer technology is at present not the limiting factor in automating therapy. The problem of providing reliable instruments for measuring patients' responses and mechanical devices for administering therapy precludes widespread use of automated treatment at this time.

9. Computers can be used for review and audit of medical records. ICU records are extremely difficult to audit systematically. Without automation, data at the time of crises may not be recorded because of preoccupation with providing care. Further, even if they have been recorded, they are present in a form that cannot easily be compared with data of other patients. The possibility of learning from experience arises from archiving the patients' records into an intensive care data bank. Monitored parameters, test results, and therapeutic interventions could be correlated with outcome to determine predictors of success or failure.

At this time, no one ICU computer system has obtained all of these potential advantages, and some have barely been broached. Some potentials, such as automated therapy, remain unfulfilled because of the insufficiency of technology, and others, such as reliable automated alarms, because of a lack of specific medical knowledge.

COMPUTERIZED MONITORING OF VITAL SIGNS

The earliest and still most common application of computers in the ICU has been for the repetitive monitoring of vital signs. Because of competing demands on nursing time, computers were thought to be an effective alternative to manual collection of these data. Further, since the computer can measure these signs far more frequently than nurses, the recognition of adverse conditions ought to be more prompt. Early advocates of automated monitoring promulgated the hope for a favorable effect on patient morbidity and mortality. This hoped-for effect has not been demonstrated.[23]

The signals that potentially lend themselves to continuous monitoring are myriad—the ECG, systemic arterial pressure, central venous pressure, pulmonary arterial pressure, left atrial pressure, rectal temperature, urine volume, respiratory rate, respiratory pressure and flow, and others.

Few patients would have more than a small subset of these parameters measured simultaneously. More commonly, a few of them are chosen based on the patient type, the available monitoring hardware, and the orientation of the monitoring group.

With current technology, the need for invasive insertion of the sensor or catheter into the patient limits the number of monitored variables. In only the sickest patients is invasion justified. The high cost of many of the more sophisticated sensors additionally restricts their use. Technical achievements in developing low-cost, noninvasive sensors has been disappointing. Useful inexpensive, low-risk sensors, such as the blood pressure cuff, do exist; however, they require human intervention. Information from this kind of sensor rarely gets entered into the computer because entry is too awkward and time-consuming. Both low-cost, noninvasive sensors and simple, effective manual entry systems are needed to ensure complete collection of patients' data.

The frequency at which various monitored parameters can be sampled is also limited by present technology. To extend the number of patients who can be monitored simultaneously, preprocessing of signals is often done by bedside instruments. The waveforms for blood pressure and ECG, for example, are frequently not sampled directly; rather, bedside hardware, which samples the primary waveforms, generates signals equivalent to the heart rate and systolic/diastolic/mean blood pressures. These transduced signals can be sampled at lower rates, decreasing the processing required within the main computer.

For special types of patients, such as those in coronary care units, the ECG is the most important predictor of crisis. Minicomputer monitoring systems are now commercially available to perform the exclusive task of assessing the ECG. Other special applications could be developed if single parameters so warranted.

Once the data have been sampled, they are stored into a file of limited size so that the most recently acquired data replace the oldest. The time span of vital sign data kept in such files varies from system to system, but it is typically 24 to 48 hours. Most systems permit review of recently monitored data, using plots on video displays or printed outputs, that mimic the traditional ICU graphs.

The sampled physiologic variables may have been contaminated by artifact, spurious data usually of nonphysiologic origin. Artifact can arise in an ECG signal, for example, when the patient is restless or when a lead becomes disconnected, or in the blood pressure when an arterial line becomes kinked or clogged. Both of these cases might be confused with cardiac arrest if the programs processing the data were not able to distinguish artifact from a true signal. Artifact frequently masquerades as patient crisis and causes nurses to disable alarm systems. In order to solve the problem of false alarms, therefore, the first step is to prevent or detect artifact in the sampled signals.

Artifact elimination is an extremely difficult problem. Cox[5] has thoroughly reviewed the difficulties in analyzing the ECG and arterial pressure wave. Two general approaches to minimizing the effect of artifact exist. The first is to eliminate the sources of artifact. Fastidious care of electrodes and transducers is essential; they must be treated as sacrosanct. For arterial lines, slow infusion of heparinized saline can eliminate clot formation[16]; periodic impedance checks can verify ECG electrode contacts.[1] No matter how carefully sensors are treated, however, artifact will arise because manipulation of patients and their sensors cannot be avoided. Once an artifact-contaminated signal has been sampled, computer programs should recognize the data as spurious. Cox[4] has described a method for artifact detection in the ECG, and Glaeser[6] uses a similar method for the arterial pressure. Osborn[11] uses a technique based on interrelationships in the ECG and arterial pressure for detecting artifact in either. Nevertheless, recognition of artifact is sometimes so subtle that highly trained observers have difficulty identifying it. At present, these problems have not been surmounted and some human editing may always be needed.

AUTOMATED ALARMS AND DATA REDUCTION

Even if artifact can be eliminated, intrinsic physiologic and instrumental variations in monitored data create problems in their use. Since the sampling rates for all patients must be sufficiently high to avoid missing significant events in any, data are monitored too frequently for many patients. Manual data collection systems compensate for this problem by having nurses reduce sampling frequency when their patients' vital signs are stable. Methods are needed for discarding data that are not medically important in order to permit efficient data storage, retrieval, and review. Interpretation of primary signals like the ECG and the arterial pressure wave, which have well known morphologies and periodicities, has been possible. For most monitored signals, however, a definition of the medically important features has not been achieved on the basis of either pathophysiologic or statistical models. Specific outcomes, such as mortality, are so infrequent and patients' problems are so complex that clear identification of ominous patterns in monitored data has been difficult. As a result, neither reliable alarm systems nor efficient data reduction algorithms have been developed.

Traditional alarm systems rely on sensing a signal that varies beyond either some preassigned absolute limits or some relative limits within a given time period. Such systems are particularly sensitive to physiologic, instrumental, and artifactual variation resulting in high false alarm rates. If alarm limits are widened to reduce the incidence of false alarms, then discrimination of true medical emergencies is reduced. In an effort to decrease sensitivity to instrumental or physiologic noise, smoothing, or averaging, algorithms have been used.

Taylor[22] has employed time-weighted changes of single monitored variables to provide alarms; recent values of variables are weighted more heavily than past ones. This concept appeals to the heuristic notion that large short-term changes are medically more important than long-term ones. Sacks and coworkers[12] have described a system in which the changes of highly correlated variables are synthesized to produce alarms. Many hemodynamic parameters are highly correlated; for example, changes in the diastolic blood pressure are obviously related to changes in the systolic. When particular parameters change in ways different from what their correlates would predict, then these changes may indicate physiologic instability and, therefore, generate alarms.

COMPUTERIZED DATA INTEGRATION AND INTERPRETATION

Because medical knowledge is constantly increasing, physicians cannot understand the nuances of all specialties. Consultative support is obviously necessary for the general physician seeing patients with diverse problems. Consultation is just as important, however, for a phyisican or nurse confronted by a patient with complex problems in an ICU. The staggering number of diagnostic tests and treatment modalities available in a modern hospital presents a burden of information too great for any individual to encompass. Yet timely decisions based on this information frequently determine patients' survival. If current medical knowledge were integrated into computer systems to aid in decision making, the advantage to the patient in the ICU is obvious. A beginning intern, for example, could consult the computer to aid in the administration of intravenous fluids in a difficult burn patient.

While this potential seems intriguing, it introduces extremely complex logical problems. A first step is to analyze the types of data to be integrated with the knowledge base. To date, the vast majority of ICU computer applications have dealt only with primary, regularly collected data, such as the ECG. The integration and interpretation of medical data are usually even more intricate than those applications because of the complexity of medical decisions and the vagaries of the data.

Since the computer cannot make judgmental decisions, the specification of decision rules, or algorithms, for the processing of incomplete, redundant, inaccurate, and time-sensitive data is required in automated systems. The basis for these rules is often elusive. The prosaic calculation of the creatinine clearance illustrates the difficulties encountered. The creatinine clearance might be used to aid in decisions about the dosage of a drug that is cleared by or toxic to the kidney.

The calculation requires measurement of the plasma and urine creatinine concentrations and the urine flow, i.e., urine volume and hours of collection. These data could be entered by the user at the time he desired the clearance in a fashion similar to that used in acid-base consultation.[2] Since the data for the calculation would probably already be present within the computer record, however, the clearance might be determined automatically. If the proper data are all present and unique in the given time period, then the calculation can be performed easily.

If the data are ambiguous, however, the system must have logical rules for handling the uncertainty. If the time interval contains several plasma creatinine determinations, for example, or if a urine sample has been lost, then the algorithm must be able to deal with these cases. For multiple values, a policy must specify which value to use—perhaps an average or median should be used. If data are missing, the system must know how to proceed—to terminate the process, to assume or calculate a value, or to search for one over a broader time base. Automated decision rules require specification of policies to cover all eventualities.

Computer algorithms can be extremely sensitive to the time of data collection. This sensitivity can seem both rigid and arbitrary. In the example of creatinine clearance, if no plasma creatinine level is present within the hours of collection, then the clearance could not be calculated. The plasma level might have been determined, however, one minute prior to the hours of collection. Analogous problems can arise in ECG and other time-dependent analyses. Computer algorithms must necessarily be rigid; unfortunately, this rigidity can sometimes yield undesirable policies.

If the algorithms used in the system are hierarchical, i.e., if the values or results of a particular step are used in processing at a later step, then inaccuracies introduced at a basic level may be perpetuated or compounded at later stages. In the example of the creatinine clearance calculation, invalid entry of a creatinine level would necessarily yield an incorrect clearance. If the clearance were subsequently used to calculate a drug dosage, then the dosage would similarly be improper. Even in the simple calculation of the creatinine clearance, therefore, complex issues regarding the logical structuring of automated decision rules become apparent.

While these issues are formidable, they are not insurmountable if adequate computing capacity and medical information are available. Warner[25] has described a system in which the medical decision logic is clearly separated from the patients' data and the computer programs. Shortliffe[15] has reported a more complex system for consultation in antimicrobial therapy. Both of these approaches have the advantage that as medical decisions are made by computers, both the medical criteria and the procedures for dealing with missing or redundant data are made systematic and modular. As medical knowledge changes or as a particular decision rule is found inadequate, the knowledge or rule can be changed without a major reprogramming effort.

As data handling requirements become more diverse and complex, the need for more powerful methods for dealing with ambiguity and inaccuracy become apparent. One general approach to this problem is to separate the medical decision logic from the computer programs. This approach cannot relieve a kind of whimsical rigidity present in computer, as opposed to human, logic. Computerized interpretation can never totally encompass the myriad nuances and complexities involved in many medical decisions. Nor can computer algorithms easily remove the inaccuracies introduced at earlier stages. Yet computers can speed the maintenance and enhancement of knowledge within the ICU setting in well selected applications.

LIMITATIONS OF COMPUTER TECHNOLOGY

The historical limitations of computer technology have restricted the development of computerized monitoring. The computers that have been used for monitoring were first generation minicomputers or industrial process-control computers. The software, i.e., computer programs, available for these computers was relatively primitive by today's standards and compounded limitations imposed by small memory sizes and slow processor speeds. The lack of adequate software meant that ICU systems' developers spent inordinate effort in programming. As a result, today's systems have an enormous investment in software developed for currently obsolete computers. Future advances in computer hardware and software technology will accentuate this discrepancy. Programs usually cannot be simply transferred to other ICUs or even implemented on a new computer in the same ICU without a high reprogramming cost. Thus, while a particular system might be particularly good at monitoring the ECG and another at consultation in fluid balance, their strengths cannot easily be merged.

Many of the potential advantages of computerized data handling depend heavily upon having a computer of large enough capacity to support many simultaneous activities reliably and quickly. At present, probably no single computer used in monitoring is sufficiently large or reliable. These limitations will be circumvented both by distributing the computing load among several processors and by enlarging the memories of these processors. The use of multiple processors will add to the overall system reliability. Microprocessors, i.e., small, low-cost computers, will be used to preprocess data from one or more bedside instruments before transmission to a main ICU computer. This concept is now being employed by Glaeser.[6]

The requirements and emphases for data handling systems change with time. Unfortunately, because of the rigid structures imposed by older systems, these changes have frequently not been gracefully included. While the major applications in the past have been for signal processing, future applications are likely to stress data management and interpretation. Simple implementation of new applications will probably require the transition to newer computers with more powerful software.

CONCLUSIONS

Evaluation of the effectiveness of patient care in the ICU will require significant developments in information gathering and analysis. Some of the problems to be met are:

1. Improvement of instruments for physiologic monitoring, particularly inclusion of logic for detecting internal malfunction and for discarding signal artifact.

2. Easier methods of recording man-collected data.

3. Systems for reformatting collected information serving the user rather than requiring a compromise between display format and retrieval convenience.

4. Methods for elimination of redundant or non-information-bearing data, thus removing confusing information and permitting more efficient storage and retrieval of useful data.

5. Methods of long-term audit of care to evaluate the effectiveness of therapy. The audits should be fed back periodically to update methods of patient care.

The ICU record, like the general medical record, has become a disordered dumping ground for ever-increasing amounts of data. To date, little progress has been made in organizing this chaos other than the time-based 24-hour ICU record. The demands for logical analysis of ICU systems for implementation of automation may serve to provide additional structure. The early steps of automating ICU record keeping, however, have not led to vast improvements in information synthesis. On the technologic level, microcomputers can make bedside instruments smarter and more reliable; better entry and display devices can make the recording and retrieval functions more suitable for the clinical environment. Newer generations of minicomputers will remove many limitations of previous computers and will permit storage and analysis of larger data sets. If these technologic developments are to realize their potential, however, clinicians will have to analyze their methods of decision making, recognize the weaknesses in their logic, determine their criteria for success, and devise algorithms for more effective patient care.

REFERENCES

1. Almasi, J. J., and Schmitt, O.: Automated measurement of bioelectric impedance at very low frequencies. Comput. Biomed. Res., 7:449, 1974.
2. Bleich, H. L.: The computer as a consultant. N. Engl. J. Med., 28:141, 1971.
3. Committee of Medical Aspects of Automotive Safety: Rating the severity of tissue damage, J.A.M.A., 215:277, 1971.
4. Cox, J. R., Jr., Fozzard, H. A., Nolle, F. M., and Oliver, G. C.: Some data transformations useful in electrocardiography. In Stacy, R. W., and Waxman, B. D., (Eds.): Computers in Biomedical Research. Vol. III. New York, Academic Press, 1969, pp. 181–206.
5. Cox, J. R., Jr., Nolle, F. M., and Arthur, R. M.: Digital analysis of the electroencephalogram, the blood pressure wave, and the electrocardiogram. Proc. IEEE, 60:1137, 1972.
6. Glaeser, D. H., Trost, R. F., Brown, D. B., et al.: A hierarchical minicomputer system for continuous post-surgical monitoring. Comput. Biomed. Res., 8:336, 1975.
7. Hilberman, M., and Peters, R. M.: A data collection system for intensive care. Crit. Care Med., 3:27, 1975.
8. Kirklin, J. W.: Personal communication, 1976.
9. Komaroff, A. L., Reiffen, B., and Sherman, H.: Problem-oriented protocols for physician-extenders. In Walker, H. K., Hurst, J. W., and Woody, M. F., (Eds.): Applying the Problem-Oriented System. New York, Medcom Press, 1973, Chapter 17.
10. Osborn, J. J., Beaumont, J. O., Raison, J. C. A., et al.: Measurement and monitoring of acutely ill patients by digital computer. Surgery, 64:1057, 1969.
11. Osborn, J. J., Beaumont, J. O., Raison, J. C. A., and Abbott, R. P.: Computation for quantitative on-line measurements in an intensive care ward. In Stacy, R. W., and Waxman, B. D. (Eds.): Computers in Biomedical Research. Vol. III. New York, Academic Press, 1969, pp. 207–251.
12. Sacks, S. T., Palley, N. A., Afifi, A. A., and Shubin, H.: Concurrent statistical evaluation during patient monitoring. AFIPS Fall Joint Computer Conference Proceedings. Vol. 37. Montvale, New Jersey, AFIPS Press, 1970, p. 609.
13. Sheppard, L. C., Kouchoukos, N. T., Kurtts, M. A., and Kirklin, J. W.: Automated treatment of critically ill patients following operation. Ann. Surg., 168:596, 1968.
14. Shoemaker, W. C.: Algorithm for early recognition and management of cardiac tamponade. Crit. Care Med., 3:59, 1975.
15. Shortliffe, E. H., Davis, R., Axline, S. G., et al.: Computer-based consultations in clinical therapeutics: explanation and rule acquisition capabilities of the MYCIN system. Comput. Biomed. Res., 8:303, 1975.
16. Shubin, H., Palley, N., and Weil, M. H.: Computer surveillance of the seriously ill patient. J. Assoc. Adv. Med. Instrum., 6:48, 1972.
17. Shubin, H., Weil, M. H., Afifi, A. A., et al.: Selection of hemodynamic, respiratory and metabolic variables for evaluation of patients in shock. Crit. Care Med., 2:326, 1974.
18. Siegel, J. H., Farrell, E. J., Miller, M., et al.: Cardiorespiratory interaction as determinants of survival and the need for respiratory support in human shock states. J. Trauma, 13:602, 1973.
19. Siegel, J. H., Goldwyn, R. M., and Friedman, H. P.: Pattern and process in the evolution of human septic shock. Surgery, 70:232, 1971.
20. Siegel, J. H., and Strom, B. L.: An automated consultation system to aid the physician in the care of the desperately sick patient. In Stacy, R. W., and Waxman, B. D., (Eds.): Computers in Biomedical Research. Vol. IV. New York, Academic Press, 1974, pp. 115–134.
21. Stacy, R. W.: The comprehensive patient-monitoring concept. In Stacy, R. W., and Waxman, B. D., (Eds.): Computers in Biomedical Research. Vol. III. New York, Academic Press, 1969, pp. 253–276.
22. Taylor, D. E. M.: Computer-assisted patient monitoring systems. Biomed Eng., 6:560, 1971.
23. U.S. Department of Health, Education, and Welfare: Public Health Services and Mental Health Administration; National Center for Health Services Research and Development (Contract No. HSM 110–70–406). Evaluation of computer-based patient monitoring systems. Prepared by Arthur D. Little, Inc., Vol. I, Summary, Appendices A-E, 1973.

24. Warner, H. R., Gardner, R. M., and Toronto, A. F.: Computer-based monitoring of cardiovascular functions in postoperative patients. Circulation, *37* (Suppl. 2): 68, 1968.
25. Warner, H. R., Olmsted, C. M., and Rutherford, B. D.: HELP—a program for medical decision-making. Comput. Biomed. Res., *5*:65, 1972.
26. Weed, L. L.: Medical Records, Medical Education, and Patient Care: The Problem-Oriented Record as a Basic Tool. Cleveland, Case Western Reserve University Press, 1969.
27. Weil, M. H., Shubin, H., and Rand, W. M.: Experience with a digital computer for study and improved management of the critically ill. J.A.M.A., *198*:147, 1966.

CHAPTER 8

DETERMINANTS OF SURGICAL INTENSIVE CARE

JOSEPH M. CIVETTA, M.D.

Present-day utilization of intensive care illustrates the danger of combining anecdotal experience with quasi-statistical analysis to lead from an unwarranted assumption to a foregone conclusion. Everyone agrees that intensive care is very important, necessary, and effective. Hospitals either have a unit (or units), are in the process of constructing such a facility, or think that it is a necessary addition. But do objective data support the idea that intensive care units have reduced mortality and morbidity? The only published data[3,6] suggest that there may be no difference. Yet survival following disastrous complications is not uncommon in an Intensive Care Unit (ICU), and the mortality rates from major surgical procedures do decline, though improvements in technique obviously contribute to this. Is such anecdotal and unproven reliance on the ICU concept justifiable? Can it indeed be justified? In fact, need it be justified? Let us look at some of the real determinants of intensive care in an attempt to separate fact from fantasy as well as to establish prudent guidelines for the use of intensive care during this period of maturation of the concept.

Critical illness is certainly only a single factor determining the necessity for intensive care. Many other socioeconomic, practical, and financial factors actually determine the delivery of such care. There is an increasing number of pressing reasons why such critical appraisal of the delivery of intensive care is important at this time. It has been estimated that if maximum intensive care were used on all potential patients in the country, it would use up approximately 20 per cent of the gross national product or $200 billion/year. This is an expensive resource and we would be forced to evaluate its usage in terms of economic feasibility whether or not we wish to approach any of the more philosophical concepts. Furthermore, intensive care in our present context can provide a system that can prolong life without, unfortunately, the necessity for justification to continue such a course.

Objective data are also needed, therefore, to select the time, duration, and application of intensive care, as well as to answer the more fundamental question of whether intensive care accomplishes its goal of reducing morbidity and mortality from critical illness.

DETERMINANTS OF INTENSIVE CARE

Five major areas need to be considered in addition to the absolute medical diagnosis which renders a patient suitable for the delivery of intensive care. These include: the attitudes and personality characteristics of the medical personnel involved in decision making; the ethical considerations directed to the judgment process; the attitudes of the patient and his family toward the illness; financial questions; and, finally, the practical day-to-day determinants of the usual overcrowded and understaffed unit.

MEDICAL ATTITUDES

As one assumes the responsibility for patient care, he should rightly be willing to invest knowledge, time, and energy to bring the patient to full recovery. The motivations to achieve such a goal seem never greater than when dealing with an iatrogenic complication. Surgical training rightly emphasizes the necessity for continued, aggressive medical care. A successful outcome in another seemingly hopeless case reinforces the necessity to persist with aggressive management. A multitude of similar cases with a fatal outcome does not leave such a strong mental imprint or act as a stimulus in deciding how to proceed in the future. However, as has become increasingly evident in the last few years,[11] a certain pattern of complications and setbacks exists in individual patients to the extent that the ultimate outcome is usually obvious to all connected with that patient's care. It would appear that this "never say die" attitude should be tempered by early realization of the impossibility of achieving a successful outcome in every case.

Although surgical training dictates the necessity for personal investment to achieve ultimate success, the decision to embark on surgical therapy clearly may set the stage for an impossible postoperative situation. The conclusion that without surgery the patient's illness will be fatal, in and of itself, does not justify embarking on surgical therapy unless, considered in its own merits, an improved chance of survival will result. Diagnoses that are changed or added in the course of the illness may alter not only the surgical procedure contemplated but the postoperative care as well. A frequent and obvious example concerns the patient scheduled to undergo radical extirpative cancer surgery and who is expected to require intensive care postoperatively. If disease beyond the limits of surgical therapy is encountered, the original operative plan and the necessity for postoperative intensive care will quite reasonably be altered. Less obvious and perhaps more important, changes in plans should occur when, during the course of an illness, the constellation of complications achieves sufficient weight to preclude any reasonable hope for survival. Such changes may be subtle enough on a day-to-day basis to escape notice until considerable time, effort, and resources have been expended. It is at this time that withdrawal of intensive care, which may seem reasonable, will be most difficult.

Finally, though much is made of the necessity for a personal doctor-patient relationship, a certain abstract quality must be preserved toward the disease process. Thus, enthusiasm for a new surgical procedure, particularly in its developmental and evaluational period, may result in continued delivery of intensive care based on an understandable desire to develop a successful technique. Often, too, personal involvement in a difficult and lengthy postoperative course may cloud one's ability to be truly objective.

ETHICAL CONSIDERATIONS

The development of life-support systems has raised certain moral questions concerning the necessity to prolong life. While the traditional distinction between active and passive euthanasia is seemingly clear-cut,[9] in an intensive care situation such a distinction not only is blurred but may be subject to criticism. Positive actions with a passive intent—shutting off a respirator, for example—achieve a result (i.e., death) as rapidly as does an active injection of an overdose of morphine. The moral distinction between such actions as turning off the respirator and injection of an overdose of a narcotic may well be ideally real, but, practically, the individual performing such action may feel no difference. Withdrawal of active intervention has been supported by moral theologians[4, 8] whenever the medical judgment obviates any reasonable expectation of recovery. A separate question is whether active euthanasia is justifiable. The prolongation of suffering implicit in passive euthanasia may be viewed as discordant with human goals. Although this problem is thorny, it rarely applies to the intensive care setting where passive euthanasia usually has a very definite and immediate effect. However, should our ability to discriminate and predict outcome earlier in a patient's course improve, the implications of utilizing passive euthanasia may achieve greater importance.

THE PATIENT AND FAMILY

Although an increased sensitivity to and awareness of the importance of the wishes of the patient and his family to determine his course must be stressed, common intensive care situations may prove to be unintelligible to them. Thus the family member who stares in fear and bewilderment at the myriad of machines surrounding his loved one may assume that these are only harbingers of doom, when in fact the patient is making satisfactory progress. The extent of illness and prognosis with its attendant corollaries of the necessity for active intervention must be carefully explained to patients and their families. Familiarity with the environment rapidly removes the mysterious and magical qualities of such unknown mechanical contrivances for those who work on an ICU.

The converse is equally true: the patient with clearly untreatable disease may appear to be making satisfactory progress to the family. Communication of the factors that render the illness terminal may be extremely difficult. The distinction between appropriate wishes on the part of the family and appropriate intervention based on the medical diagnosis may be difficult to define. Our responsibility rests in the communication of the overall picture so that they may have the basis to make appropriate judgments rather than ones based on fear, bewilderment, and other emotions.

FINANCIAL FACTORS

Because the feeling that aggressive interventions should be made in patients with critical illness, costs for providing such care have skyrocketed without any critique of the effectiveness of such interventions. This clearly will not be the case in the future of intensive care or of medicine in general. Overall intensive care costs include laboratory utilization, equipment, blood products, and medications, all of which are used more frequently in intensive care patients. In most hospitals, the daily intensive care rate does take into account the increased personnel costs so that the rate is usually two to four times that of an ordinary hospital room. The magnitude of the ancillary charges can be seen in Figure 1. Although the Surgical Intensive Care Unit (SICU) rate was $210/day, patient charges/24-hour period exceeded $750/day. Characterization of the factors influencing these costs can be seen in Figure 2. In this study,[1] over half the hospital stay for patients who died was spent in the ICU, whereas only 17 per cent of the hospital stay was similarly utilized in those who lived. This difference related to post-ICU convalescence explains the tremendous difference in daily costs seen in Figure 1 for these two groups. At the present time, the most critically ill patients amass daily charges of between $1,200 and $1,500/day. Laboratory utilization ap-

PATIENTS COST-1971

DAILY ROOM CHARGE:	$ 96.00
DAILY SICU CHARGE:	$210.00
12 BED SICU BUDGET:	
PERSONNEL	$ 625,000.00
SUPPLIES	$ 637,000.00
TOTAL	$1,262,000.00
PER PATIENT	$ 1,440.00

TOTAL PATIENT COST	DIED	SURVIVED
TOTAL BILL:	$10,064.00	$9,259.00
AVERAGE DAILY COST:	$ 500.00	$286.00

| REAL SICU DAILY COST: | $761.00 |

Figure 1. Cost factors for patients in 1971 at Massachusetts General Hospital. Personnel and supplies alone resulted in a patient cost of $1,440. The real daily cost, including medications, laboratory tests, and blood products, exceeded $750/day.

Figure 2. Differentiation in daily costs of intensive care based on survival. Patients who died spent less time in the hospital and twice as long in intensive care, resulting in a much higher percentage of their total hospitalization being spent in the intensive care unit. It was for this reason that the average cost for patients who died was twice that of those who survived.

CHARACTERIZATION-SICU (1970)

	DIED	SURVIVED	DIFFERENCE
TOTAL HOSPITALIZATION	20.3 DAYS	32.3 DAYS	–12 DAYS
< 10 DAYS	41%	0	+ 41%
> 21 DAYS	41%	81%	– 41%
RANGE	2-121 DAYS	19-77 DAYS	—
SICU STAY	11 DAYS	5.6 DAYS	+ 5.5 DAYS
% HOSPITALIZATION	55%	17%	

proximates 50 per cent of this cost, and therein lies a major problem.[7] The distinction between appropriate and inappropriate laboratory utilization in critically ill patients has never been formalized. Extreme variations in blood gas tensions, serum electrolytes, and blood sugars occur commonly in critically ill patients within a 24-hour period. This alone necessitates and justifies obtaining frequent blood samples. Retrospectively, however, if such variations did not materialize, repetitious confirmation on normal values would appear. Further investigation into a prudent plan to determine what is an appropriate number of tests is certainly desirable though difficult to obtain.

The majority of patients who have been subject to intensive care find that they are required to make relatively small payments, since third-party coverage is usually nearly complete. An individual may well be proud of his $30,000 hospital bill if he had to pay only $100 or $200 out of pocket. The link between his insurance premium and his hospital bill is often tenuously grasped, if considered at all.

These financial factors, then, should be at least a suasive reason for examining the delivery of intensive care.

PRACTICAL CONSIDERATIONS

The most important factor limiting the delivery of intensive care appears to be personnel availability. Most large hospitals serving a population base in which delayed presentation of illness and penetrating trauma are common seem to require a greater number of intensive care beds than is available. In many institutions, the physical space necessary to render such care is already provided. Although paramedical personnel are utilized, an adequate number of experienced and educated nurses proves difficult to sustain. This leads commonly to the exchange of patients, a practice that determines that one of the basic criteria for admission is to be sicker than the "wellest" patient in the unit. Comparisons necessary because of the practical limitation of space make triage decisions somewhat easier, but the importance of developing a method to distribute this limited resource adequately should be applicable whether or not any other limitations exist.

Capital equipment and utilization of other hospital resources are, in fact, disproportionately expensive when compared with the rest of the hospital. It has been estimated[5] that the hospital in which 3 per cent of its total beds are dedicated to intensive care expends 20 per cent of its total resources in adequately supporting that facility. Despite personnel and economic limitations and without supporting objective data, most hospitals continue to expand these facilities. The principal reason would seem to be the number and percentage of successfully treated complications that have been documented in ICUs compared with the obvious impossibility of handling a similar episode on an ordinary patient floor.

PREDICTIVE UTILIZATION

Our goals, then, must be to identify those factors that have the greatest influence on mortality and morbidity; those patient groups at high risk for developing complications—especially when amenable to early intervention—and factors that may be related to overall success. Other factors to be considered include the patients' underlying age-related mortality and overall disease-related survival. Finally, decision points should be established so that planned reassessment will permit earlier discontinuation of extraordinary means of supporting life in situations in which no reasonable chance of survival is seen to exist.

METHODS TO OBTAIN PREDICTIVE UTILIZATION

Early attempts to obtain insight into utilization of intensive care resources came from retrospective analysis of mortality and morbidity. In Figure 3, data from the SICU at the Massachusetts General Hospital are presented. The fact that more than three-fourths of the patients suffered hypotension, respiratory complications, and cardiac complications while 90 per cent survived suggested the ICUs do indeed provide a milieu in which such complications can be dealt with successfully. Patients who died developed a significant number of complications, as displayed in Figure 4. However, a similar number and similar types of complications developed in patients who survived the same type of critical illness. Figure 5 displays patient discharges by day according to whether the patients were alive or had died. The great majority of survivors were discharged within the first

COMPLICATIONS IN SYSTEM
(% OF TOTAL GROUP)

CARDIAC	88	SEPSIS	35
RESISTANCE/SHOCK	75	G.I.	30
RESPIRATORY	78	BLEEDING	27
RENAL	57	C.N.S.	21

Figure 3. Analysis of patients' charts for development of specific system complications. Numbers displayed represent percentage of total group who developed complications in each major system.

Figure 4. Analysis of 70 patients who died during their intensive care stay. The number of complications averaged 7.4 per patient, with the distribution by systems as indicated.

COMPLICATIONS-SICU		
PATIENTS WHO DIED IN SICU:		
	N= 70	
TOTAL COMPLICATIONS:		518
AVERAGE NUMBER OF COMPLICATIONS:		7.4
CARDIAC 2.00	CNS 0.55	
RESPIRATORY 1.87	G.I. 0.44	
"SHOCK" 0.81	SEPSIS 0.39	
RENAL 0.85	HEMOSTASIS 0.36	
	OTHERS	0.10

week, whereas the number of deaths was reasonably constant throughout the entire period. However, at no time could the duration of stay be used to predict survival, since many patients lived adequately though they had undergone a very long period of intensive care.

A second approach comparing duration of illness and ultimate survival to system-related complications was then attempted. In Table 1 it can be seen that cardiac, resistance, and renal complications were found with greater frequency in the patients who died. In Table 2 certain complications were more common in patients whose intensive care stay was prolonged. Variance was so great that individual system complications could not be used as an overall determinant of survival. It became clear that a pattern of sequential organ system failure developed in patients who remained in the ICU for long periods of time, but that even in such cases a significant number of complications did not preclude overall chance of survival.

High-intensity, short-duration intensive care seems reasonable, since a significant number of patients may develop complications that can be treated successfully. Prolonged utilization of intensive care resources results in the development of an increasing number of complications related to both the underlying disease process and the appearance of iatrogenic and intensive care–related complications. These include nosocomial infections, stress-

Figure 5. Distribution of discharges by type: live vs. dead. Note that the majority of patients were discharged within the first week but that distribution was skewed to the right. The number of patients discharged living was approximately the same as those who died after the first week. At no time can a prediction of survival or death be made on length of intensive care stay.

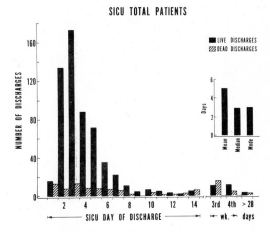

SICU TOTAL PATIENTS

Table 1. COMPLICATIONS BY SYSTEM, SURVIVAL-RELATED

	SHORT	LONG
Cardiac		
Live	55	93
Die	96	96
Resistance/Shock		
Live	45	67
Die	81	93
Renal		
Live	5	27
Die	66	97

induced gastrointestinal bleeding, various encephalopathies associated with metabolic imbalance, sleep deprivation and other psychoses, and coagulation disorders associated with multiple transfusions and sepsis. Patients who suffer these complications tend to utilize the highest levels of intensive care for long durations with low survival rates.[10] When combined with diseases of inherently high mortality rates and age-associated mortality in the elderly, it becomes clear that a geometric increase in resources invested is necessary to produce even a single surviving patient.

For example, the association of respiratory and renal failure in the elderly patient who has undergone emergency aneurysmectomy has an overall mortality approaching 95 to 98 per cent.[11] If only elderly patients with an inherent 5-year survival rate of 10 per cent are treated, one might anticipate treating 400 patients to achieve a single 1 to 2 year survivor. Since this group requires the most expensive care necessitating full-time ventilator support and hemodialysis, the daily bill might well exceed $1,500. If a hospital bill of $20,000 would result, the overall investment then would be approximately $8 million to achieve a single 1 to 2 year survivor. The magnitude of the problem and the urgency of a reasonable solution should be obvious from this single example.

Table 2. COMPLICATIONS BY SYSTEM, DURATION-RELATED

	SHORT	LONG
Sepsis		
Live	20	47
Die	12	62
Gastrointestinal		
Live	5	20
Die	30	50
Central Nervous System		
Live	5	20
Die	21	32
Bleeding		
Live	10	27
Die	21	47

Another retrospective approach has been utilized by Fairly and co-workers[2] based on achieving a larger and larger data base from patients treated. However, as soon as particular subgroups are distinguished, 95 per cent confidence limits become so large as to be of little value in predicting outcome in a single instance. Although complicated disease processes with extraordinarily high mortality rates can be culled out by this method, an extraordinarily large data base would be required to provide sufficient numbers in those subgroups to permit confident judgments.

Prediction based on multiple factor analysis theoretically should overcome many of the above limitations. If combined with repeated assessment during the patient's illness, the broad confidence limits inherent in the statistical analysis may well be narrowed by sound clinical judgment. In general terms, survival can be determined as a function of many factors. Using complications at various times in the illness and age, statistically significant correlations can be identified. In Figure 6 complications were reviewed before operation, after 48 hours of intensive care treatment, and at the end of the intensive care stay in terms of ability to predict survival. These numbers were significant at the probability level less than 0.001, but r^2 or variance again proved to cover with certainty only one-third of the group. Since individual system complications did reveal marked differences in survival, it was felt that this approach might be useful in a predictive fashion. Hence statistical manipulation based on observed patients' survival was then attempted. Patient discharge from the ICU is determined by medical recovery or when death occurs. If a sufficient number of patients are followed, eventually all those who were to die will have done so and those who remain will be surviving patients. Any patient who lives one day after the last death will be a survivor by definition. The multiple r technique using weighted coefficients for complications observed for each system was used, incorporating a constant such that solution of the equation would result in an absolute number. If this number was greater than the day of death of the last dying patient, the patient under consideration should survive. Using complications that developed preoperatively, intraoperatively, and during the first 48 hours of intensive care, such a number might be used to predict the ultimate outcome. The general survival equation can be seen in Figure 7, and coefficients A, B, C, . . . n are displayed in Figure 8. Prospective testing of this equation in a single ICU has shown that 95 per cent of patients who have a number greater than 30 survive, and no patient with a number of 15 or less has yet survived. Few patients fall into the 15 to 30 range. At the present

Figure 6. Multiple r analysis performed on 100 patients at Jackson Memorial Hospital, Miami, Florida. Life span as a function of complications and age was statistically significant at P < 0.001.

MULTIPLE r ANALYSIS

LIFESPAN AS A FUNCTION OF:

48 HOUR COMPS	$r = 0.52$	$r^2 = 0.27$
+ AGE	$r = 0.58$	$r^2 = 0.33$
+ TOTAL COMPS	$r = 0.58$	$r^2 = 0.34$
+ PREOP COMPS	$r = 0.58$	$r^2 = 0.34$

SURVIVAL =

A × RENAL + B × AGE + C × SEPSIS +
D × SHOCK + E × GI + F × BLEED +
G × FLUID + H × CARDIAC + I × RESP
+ CONSTANT

Figure 7. Survival equation based on weighted complications per system with the addition of a constant so that the absolute number might be considered in relation to observed patients' survivals. In practice, the coefficients A, B, C . . . are multiplied by the number of complications as specifically defined for each system.

time, this system in conjunction with repeated careful clinical assessment throughout the intensive care course distinguishes those patients likely to survive and those patients likely to die at 48 hours after admission in well over 90 per cent of the total admissions. This method is used not so much to predict survival or death in an individual case, but rather to identify groups of patients most likely to benefit from intensive care and those in whom utilization of this valuable resource is likely to be attended by an extremely low probability of survival. Further statistical manipulations will be used to determine whether resolution of early complications has a favorable effect when related to ultimate survival, and a prior weighting of individual complications within systems might improve this discriminatory ability.

PRESENT IMPLICATIONS

No system yet devised answers all questions as to the allocation of intensive care resources. Certain patterns have become more obvious. One need not continue unrestricted, aggressive intensive care till the moment of utter hopelessness. Rather, careful reassessment and appreciation of the interrelated effects of individual system complications should enable earlier judgments to be made in patients who ultimately have no chance of survival. Triage decisions should be made without relationship to the overall exigencies of the day. If further intensive care in a patient would be terminated because a younger, more "salvageable" patient presented, at a time of bed space limitations, the same decision to terminate active care ought to be made in the absence of any limitations. Qualitative improvement in the delivery of intensive care or understanding of pathophysiologic processes and availability of new treatments will always require reassessment and reestablishment of the limits of aggressive intervention. Quantitative changes in intervention must not be viewed in the same light. For example, if an increasing number of vasoactive substances is required to maintain a

RENAL	=	-10.2	BLEED	=	-2.6
AGE	=	-0.25	FLUID	=	1.1
SEPSIS	=	-5.6	CARDIAC	=	-0.75
SHOCK	=	-5.6	RESP	=	-0.45
GI	=	-3.4	CONSTANT	=	57.7

Figure 8. Coefficients corresponding to A, B, C . . . as described in the survival equation. Marked variation between the import of specific system complications can be seen by the magnitude of the constant. As long as the solution of the equation resulted in a number greater than 43, survival could be predicted. Numbers less than 15 have not been associated with survival.

diminishing level of cardiac function, a further increase in the dosage of existing medications cannot reasonably be expected to reverse what is seemingly an inexorable downhill trend. A new type of medication or assist device, on the other hand, should be tested aggressively as a qualitative improvement. Finally, the immediate effect (i.e., death) of withdrawal of active intervention has directed our feelings to require perfect accuracy in making such "life and death" judgments. We do not seem to require our other medical judgments to be so accurate, perhaps because there is no comparable immediate result. Statistical methods are not intended to supplant the thinking precesses that are inherent in any medical judgment, but rather to provide a framework of reason rather than emotion to enable such judgments to be made more easily.

Intensive care, then, has probably achieved a reasonable measure of success in its first phase of development. This, however, has created new problems previously unconsidered: since the resource is limited, its utilization depends upon which patients should be treated, for what reasons, and for how long.

REFERENCES

1. Civetta, J. M.: The inverse relationship between cost and survival. J. Surg. Res., *14*:265, 1973.
2. Fairley, H. B., Schlobohm, R. M., Singer, M. M., et al.: The appropriateness of intensive respiratory care. Crit. Care Med., *1*:115, 1973 (Abstract).
3. Griner, P. F.: Treatment of acute pulmonary edema: conventional or intensive care? Ann. Intern. Med., *77*:501, 1972.
4. Jakobovits, I.: Jewish Medical Ethics. New York, 1959, p. 123.
5. Martin, L. E.: Cost and management: problems of intensive care units. Mod. Hosp., *118*:97, 1972.
6. Mather, H. G., Pearson, N. G., Read, K. L. O., et al.: Acute myocardial infarction: home and hospital treatment. Br. Med. J., *3*:334, 1971.
7. Morgan, A., Daly, C. and Murawski, B. J.: Dollar and human costs of intensive care. J. Surg. Res., *14*:441, 1973.
8. Pope Pius XII: Am. Q. Papal Doc., *4*:393, 1958.
9. Rachels, J.: Active and passive euthanasia. N. Engl. J. Med., *292*:78, 1975.
10. Skillman, J.: Ethical dilemmas in the care of the critically ill. Lancet, *2*:634, 1974.
11. Tilney, N. L., Bailey, G. L., and Morgan, A. P.: Sequential system failure after rupture of abdominal aortic aneurysms: an unsolved problem in postoperative care. Ann. Surg., *187*:117, 1973.

Part II

GENERAL ASPECTS
OF SURGICAL INTENSIVE CARE

CHAPTER 9

FLUID AND ELECTROLYTE MANAGEMENT

Frank E. Gump, M.D.

Management of fluid and electrolyte problems in the critically ill patient constitutes one of the most important areas in intensive care medicine. Venipuncture provides access to the body fluids for both diagnosis and treatment and makes it possible for the physician to influence body composition in a very direct way. A thorough appreciation of the effects of injury on the metabolism of water, sodium, and the other electrolytes will prevent or minimize many of the fluid disorders seen in the intensive care unit. This is especially true in surgical patients who present unique problems because of the high fluid volumes often required for resuscitation.

In the present chapter, the body fluid compartments and the principles governing normal fluid exchange will be discussed first. This leads to the concept of balance, which is of great value in critically ill patients for both water and electrolytes. Finally, specific fluid and electrolyte abnormalities will be considered in terms of volume, tonicity, and composition. Although a general discussion of fluid management will be presented, every effort has been made to focus on the special problems seen in the intensive care unit.

FLUID COMPARTMENTS AND TONICITY

Although the concentration of ions in solution is readily determined with a flame photometer, it is well to remember that the *volumes* of the various fluid compartments are of even greater importance in surgical care. While the extent and distortions present in these fluid volumes are not readily determined by direct measurement, a knowledge of the various subdivisions of total body water is essential in both understanding and managing complex fluid and electrolyte problems. Definition of these compartments has been

DISTRIBUTION OF WATER
IN ADULT HUMAN BODY

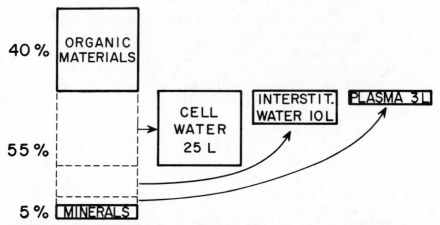

Figure 1. Total body water represents about 55 per cent of the body weight. Its three compartments are indicated in this figure. Interstitial water plus plasma composes extracellular water.

approached by isotope dilution techniques, but, with the possible exception of plasma volume, such measurements are not available to the clinician. However, normal values have been reported by a number of investigators.[7,8] The three compartments that compose total body water are shown in Figure 1 and represent average values for a 70 kg adult.

Total Body Water

Tritiated water has been utilized as the isotope to determine body water. Water represents 50 to 60 per cent of body weight, the amount being greater in lean people as opposed to the obese. Females have a lower percentage of total body water because of increased subcutaneous adipose tissue. Body water can be subdivided into compartments, intracellular fluid representing 40 per cent of body weight and extracellular fluid approximately 20 per cent of body weight. The extracellular portion is further partitioned into the plasma volume (approximately 5 per cent of body weight) and the extravascular extracellular or interstitial fluid. Interstitial fluid cannot be measured directly by any of the isotopes used in indicator dilution determinations, but represents the difference between the total extracellular fluid and the portion in the intravascular space (plasma volume).

In a clinical setting, blood volume is the only compartment that can be readily measured. While the red cell volume and the plasma volume may be determined separately, the complexities involved in the former measurement have led clinicians to approximate blood volume from the measured plasma volume and the large vessel hematocrit. Radioiodinated serum albumin (RISA) is used to mark the circulating plasma proteins, and modern instruments allow serial determinations to be made by automatically correcting for background counts. The results must be interpreted carefully in acute situations because the intravascular space may expand and contract. Under such circumstances a normal value may not reflect an important disparity between the measured volume and the vascular space that has to be filled.

The three compartments making up total body water also differ in composition. Potassium and magnesium represent the principal cations in intracellular water, and phosphates and proteins the primary anions. Sodium is largely excluded from this compartment by processes that require energy. On the other hand, sodium is the principal cation of extracellular fluid, while chloride and bicarbonate represent the principal anions. The importance of sodium relates to its control of the distribution of water throughout the body. The number of molecules of sodium per unit of water determines the osmolality of the extracellular fluid. If sodium is lost, water is excreted in an effort to maintain normal osmolality, and if sodium is retained, water must also be held in order to dilute it. The total amount of sodium in the body is approximately 4000 mEq, but much of this is in the skeleton. Fluid and electrolyte problems revolve around the exchangeable sodium, which totals 2800 mEq or 40 mEq/kg body weight. Control of this important substance is largely accomplished by the kidney, since it can regulate excretion. Fixed losses take place in the skin and stool, but they are small under normal circumstances. It is well to remember the high sodium concentration of biliary, pancreatic, and small intestinal secretions (130–150 mEq/liter), since unreplaced losses will have a marked effect on sodium balance.

The ionic composition of plasma and interstitial fluid can be considered identical for practical purposes, although small differences result from the difference in protein concentration. Plasma has a higher protein content, and these organic anions necessitate an increase in the total cation concentration. Also, the concentration of inorganic anions is somewhat lower in the plasma than in interstitial fluid. These relationships are set forth by the Gibbs-Donnan equilibrium.

Permeability and Tonicity

The differences in composition between intra- and extracellular fluid are actively maintained by the cell wall. This is a semipermeable membrane, since it is completely permeable to water but selectively permeable to other substances. Although the total number of osmols is equal on both sides of the cell wall, the *effective* osmotic pressure is determined by substances that cannot pass through the semipermeable membrane. This is well established in the capillary cell boundary between plasma and interstitial fluid. The limited passage of plasma proteins is responsible for the effective osmotic pressure, usually referred to as colloid osmotic pressure, of this compartment. Similarly, substances whose passage is limited by the cell wall, such as sodium, contribute the effective osmotic pressure in extracellular fluid. It is important to keep in mind that water can pass freely through all cell membranes. This implies that the movement of water across the cell membrane will always equalize the effective osmotic pressure inside and outside the cell. If effective osmotic pressure is altered in the extracellular fluid, it will result in a redistribution of water between the cellular and extracellular compartments. These shifts of body water result from changes in composition rather than changes in volume, so that intracellular water is far less affected by increases or decreases in extracellular fluid volume than in osmotic pressure.

The osmotic pressure of a solution is considered in terms of osmols or milliosmols and relates to the number of osmotically active particles present in solution. Therefore, one millimole of sodium chloride, which dissociates into sodium and chloride, contributes two milliosmoles. One millimole of an un-ionized substance, such as glucose or urea, will contribute one milliosmole. In considering fluid and electrolyte problems, terms such as osmol (or milliosmol) are not as frequently employed as are equivalents or milliequivalents. An equivalent of an ion is its atomic weight expressed in grams divided by the valence. When dealing with univalent ions, a milliequivalent is the same as a millimole. In the case of divalent ions, one millimole equals two milliequivalents. These concepts are important in body electrolyte balance, since in any solution the *total* cations, expressed as milliequivalents, must equal the total anions, also expressed in terms of milliequivalents.

NORMAL EXCHANGE OF FLUID AND ELECTROLYTES

WATER BALANCE

Body weight has become a critically important measurement in the intensive care unit because acute changes reflect increases or decreases in total body water. As noted previously, total body water represents 50 to 60 per cent of body weight. In a 70 kg adult this would be 35 to 42 liters of water, a wide range that is related to age, sex, and body compositional differences among normal adults. Thus, a single measurement of body weight is generally of little value in quantitating total body water. However, in the context of the intensive care unit, short-term weight changes are largely due to changes in total body water rather than to the gain or loss of body tissue. Thus, serial measurements of body weight are of great value in that they reflect increases or decreases in total body water. Even if the absolute value for total water remains uncertain, knowledge of the direction and amount of change of this parameter can assume great importance in the diagnosis and treatment of complex fluid and electrolyte disorders. When bed scales are not available or when reliable weights cannot be obtained because of the patient's condition, it becomes necessary to carry out water balance determinations. Daily water balance measurements, including an estimate of evaporative losses, can then be added or subtracted, and the resulting cumulative water balance reflects the changes in total body water.[4]

Water balance measurements have received limited clinical application because of difficulties in measuring the water content of solid food, water in the stool, and evaporative water losses. Certain of these problems are actually simplified in the intensive care unit in that almost all water intake is intravenous and readily measured. In view of the lack of oral intake stools are infrequent and urinary output is routinely measured. Evaporative losses are under 1000 ml/day in afebrile patients (Fig. 2), and even lower with full-heated humidification of a closed airway. Even in febrile patients, estimates (with wider deviation than with normal temperature) are available that make it possible to approximate losses.[5] In the air conditioned environment, most febrile patients will still lose less than 2 liters a day through the skin and airway. Hyperventilating patients with high fevers may go as high as 3 liters a day, but this is unusual. Major burns are an obvious exception, but except for this group of patients, reasonable approximations of evaporative water

INSENSIBLE WATER LOSS

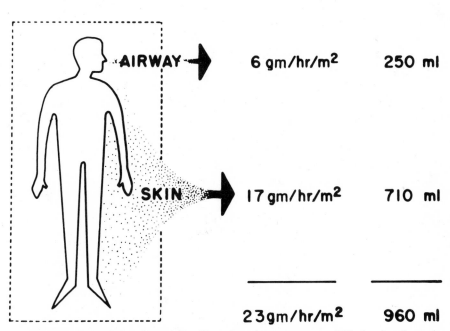

AIRWAY	6 gm/hr/m^2	250 ml
SKIN	17 gm/hr/m^2	710 ml
	23 gm/hr/m^2	960 ml

Figure 2. Water is lost through the skin and respiratory passages. This drawing shows the distribution of water loss between skin and lung under normal conditions. The right-hand column represents losses/24 hours in a 70 kg adult; the figures on the left are grams of water/hour/m^2 body surface area.

loss can be made and in turn make it possible to calculate daily and cumulative water balance from fluid intake and output records.

Since serial body weights or water balance measurements give information primarily about *changes* in total body water, other means are important in diagnosing an absolute volume deficit or excess. Plasma volume is the only clinically available measure of volume but may be of limited value, since predicted normal values vary considerably. Clinical examination of the patient is essential, and certain signs and symptoms point to the existence of abnormalities in body fluid volume. The cardiovascular system is the most sensitive indicator, and a central venous pressure below 3 cm of water, tachycardia, and even orthostatic hypotension all indicate a volume deficit. Excess volume is more common in the intensive care unit, since patients often arrive after resuscitation with large volumes of intravenous fluid. Increased venous pressure, increased cardiac output, a gallop or increased pulmonary second sound, pulmonary congestion, or sometimes even edema are all well recognized signs of fluid overload.

At times the central nervous system provides evidence of total body water deficits such as apathy, decreased deep tendon reflexes, stupor or coma, but isotonic excesses have little or no effect on central nervous system function. Tissue signs are traditionally used to gauge hydration, but are slow to develop. Decreased skin turgor, recessed eyes, or a shrunken tongue are late signs of fluid deficit just as subcutaneous edema is late evidence of overload.

Sodium Concentration

Sodium is the major osmotically active substance in extracellular fluid, and some of the basic facts about this cation are listed in Table 1. Osmolality can be measured directly, but unless glucose or urea levels are markedly increased, the serum sodium level represents a reliable index. Hyponatremia is far more common in the intensive care setting than the opposite condition.

Table 1.   Sodium Data (average values for a 70 kg male)

Body composition	
Total body sodium	4000 mEq
Exchangeable sodium	2800 mEq or 40 mEq/kg body weight
Intracellular	250 mEq or 3.5 mEq/kg body weight
Extracellular	1600 mEq or 23 mEq/kg body weight
Balance	
Intake	100 mEq/day (or 6 gm NaCl)
Output	80 mEq/day urine
	10 mEq/day stool
	10 mEq/day evaporation
Concentration	
Plasma	138–142 mEq/liter
Cell	8 mEq/liter
CSF	130 mEq/liter

Low serum sodium values may be due to sodium loss and depletion of the total exchangeable sodium, accumulation of water, or some combination of the two. The latter is more common in the critically ill patient unless there is a lesion of the gastrointestinal tract resulting in large losses of intestinal secretions. Dilutional hyponatremia will occur after any major injury or operation and corrects itself during the diuresis that accompanies recovery. While antidiuretic hormone (ADH) plays a physiologic role in this response, inappropriate secretion of ADH has also been described. However, its importance remains somewhat questionable except in patients with certain neoplasms.

Recent work has documented an internal shift of sodium into cells in low-energy states. This has long been an area of controversy, but there is little doubt that hyponatremic states in some depleted patients respond to improved nutritional support far better than to saline administration. In some instances, water retention due to cardiac, renal, or hepatic disease is responsible, and improvement requires proper treatment of the involved organ.

Finally, no surgeon should forget the importance of infusion therapy in the genesis of dilutional hyponatremia. This is of special concern in the intensive care setting, where large fluid volumes are commonly administered to support a failing circulation. Many of the solutions given to these patients are hypotonic in terms of their salt content. In the case of dextrose and water this is obvious, but the dilutional effect of protein hydrolysates, amino acids, mannitol, salt-free albumin, and even intravenous fat must be kept in mind.

While acute hypotonicity (serum sodium below 130 mEq/liter) will produce central nervous system symptoms due to edema, a more gradual fall in serum sodium concentration is difficult to recognize clinically unless there is progressive oliguria. Treatment requires intravenous saline at a rate that depends on the clinical situation, and replacement according to formulas that multiply the deficit by the estimated extracellular fluid volume is probably not as effective as close monitoring of blood pressure, mental state, urine output, body weight, and serum sodium concentration. Hypertonic saline represents a possible approach, but the extremely concentrated 3 or 5 per cent solutions are rarely necessary. Now that less hypertonic solutions are becoming available ($Na^+ = 220$ mEq/liter), the use of hypertonic saline may become more widespread.

Hypernatremia represents the opposite extreme and is usually iatrogenic. It can be readily corrected by administration of salt-free water. Although it is not a common condition, it is a dangerous one and requires vigorous treatment with dextrose and water.

POTASSIUM CONCENTRATION

There is a great deal of potassium in the body, but serum potassium determinations ''see'' only a small fraction of this total (Table 2). Such

Table 2. POTASSIUM DATA (AVERAGE VALUES FOR A 70 KG MALE)

Body composition	
Total body potassium	3800 mEq
Exchangeable potassium	3300 mEq or 46 mEq/kg
Intracellular	3240 mEq or 45 mEq/kg
Extracellular	60 mEq or 1 mEq/kg
Balance	
Intake	80 mEq/day
Output	70 mEq/day urine
	10 mEq/day stool
Concentration	
Plasma	3.6–5.0 mEq/liter
Cell	140 mEq/liter
CSF	3 mEq/liter

determinations reflect the extracellular potassium, which totals only about 60 mEq. Obviously, most of the almost 4000 mEq of potassium is intracellular, but the concentration of the small extracellular fraction is crucial to cardiac and skeletal muscle function. Extracellular potassium levels are affected not only by exogenous potassium that may be administered, but also by the release of potassium from the cells as the result of the catabolic response to injury. Acidosis has the same effect but to a lesser degree. Potassium is an important ion in acid-base abnormalities because it competes with hydrogen ion in the exchange with sodium that takes place in the renal tubule.[1] In the rest of the body, accelerated loss of potassium results in the movement of hydrogen ion into the cell to replace the lost potassium. This also plays a role in metabolic alkalosis, which requires potassium for successful treatment.

FLUID AND ELECTROLYTE ABNORMALITIES

ABNORMALITIES OF VOLUME

Patients coming to a surgical intensive care unit (ICU) usually arrive following operation, injury, or a severe septic complication. In many instances a period of hypotension antedated admission, so that high-volume intravenous fluid resuscitation can almost be said to be a common denominator in such patients. For that reason, an increased fluid volume is by far the most common abnormality seen in patients admitted to a surgical intensive care unit. Therefore, a review of the intake and output records prior to admission is essential, as is an effort to compare the body weight on admission to the ICU with the patient's preoperative or preinjury weight. The fluid therapy required during resuscitation is commonly associated with a gain in weight, reflecting a positive water balance. Similarly, efforts to maintain blood pressure and urine output during major operations in the face of the vasodilation associated with all anesthetic agents will inevitably result in a positive water balance.

In a series of patients whose injuries were associated with shock, resuscitation according to standard guidelines resulted in a positive water balance in all patients. The actual volume increases varied from 2.8 to 9.0 liters.[3] When such patients arrive in the ICU, it is important to ascertain how much of a volume increase was associated with their previous treatment. Plasma volume measurements may be helpful, but it is important to follow water balance in these patients carefully while they are under continuing treatment. Diuresis is expected, but studies show that it is not automatic. Failure to excrete these large fluid loads constitutes an important threat to the ICU patient.

Abnormalities in fluid volume can also develop in the ICU itself. The hormonal environment of the critically ill patient promotes water retention, and a further insidious gain in water is possible in these patients, especially when attention is directed to major problems in other areas. The concern that long-term mechanical ventilation might contribute to water retention by stimulating volume receptors in the right atrium has also been expressed.[10] For these reasons, daily weights or water balance calculations are essential.

The treatment of fluid overload may be simple or exceedingly complex. Fluid restriction represents the obvious starting point and can often be made more severe than is usually realized. As a rule, the need to preserve a minimal urine output represents the limiting factor. In most instances diuretics must be added. Furosemide and ethacrynic acid inhibit tubular reasorption of sodium and are sufficiently potent so that a diuresis can be stimulated even in the presence of renal hypoperfusion. Therefore, it is important to avoid the use of these potent agents in situations where the oliguria is due to unrecognized or inadequately treated hypovolemia. A single intravenous dose of 50 to 100 mg of furosemide or ethacrynic acid represents an adequate dose. While dosages have been pushed to high levels in oliguric patients, this is not necessary when dealing with fluid volume excess in patients who have maintained their renal function. The end point in these patients is simply to achieve a negative water balance. Weight loss greater than the 200 to 400 gm of tissue lost due to the combined effects of catabolism and a negative calorie-nitrogen balance serves to document the fact that the water load is being excreted.

The addition of albumin to accelerate mobilization of fluid has been recommended.[1] The rationale relates to the fact mentioned previously that much of the fluid excess is outside the vascular system. Increasing the colloid osmotic pressure in the plasma by infusion of salt-poor albumin will mobilize interstitial fluid into the vascular space, from which excretion via the kidneys should follow. While there is general agreement that albumin infusions are important in depleted patients with albumin levels below 3.0 gm/100 ml, it is not as certain that albumin will mobilize additional fluid in patients with higher serum albumin levels. Much of the interest in this area relates to the lung and efforts to mobilize interstitial fluid from that organ in patients with acute pulmonary failure. Difficulties in raising serum albumin levels by albumin infusion and uncertainty regarding the ability of capillaries in such patients to contain the infused albumin have limited the application of this method.

At times, the abnormality is a decrease rather than an excess of extracellular or total body water. It has, in fact, been pointed out that an extracellular fluid volume deficit is by far the most common disorder in the surgical patient.[8] This reflects the fact that surgical patients often appear in the emergency area with vomiting and diarrhea or blood loss, all of which may be coupled with a decreased fluid intake. However, resuscitation and operation usually precede admission to the intensive care unit, so that most patients arrive with these deficits either corrected or overcorrected. Still, there are volume deficits that can take place in the intensive care unit. Efforts to unload water with potent diuretics may actually overshoot the mark and lead to a dangerously low plasma volume. Evaporative losses are rarely large enough to result in significant fluid deficits except when there is destruction of the stratum corneum as is seen in third-degree burns and certain dermatologic conditions.

Continuous intestinal suction may also lead to volume deficits because the volume of intestinal secretions is large. The patient with gastrointestinal pathology must be closely monitored, for dangerous deficits may develop rapidly. While intestinal drainages are routinely measured, losses due to vomiting, diarrhea, or intestinal fistulas may be far more difficult to quantitate. Table 3 provides an estimate of secretion volumes from different parts of the gastrointestinal tract. When a clinical situation results in external losses of these secretions, it is obvious that hypovolemia can develop rapidly. The varying electrolyte content of the individual secretions should also be noted (Table 4). Losses of potassium, hydrogen, and chloride are of special importance since they may lead to severe metabolic alkalosis.

ABNORMALITIES OF SODIUM CONCENTRATION

The sodium ion is primarily responsible for the osmolarity of extracellular fluids, and therefore its concentration in serum is a very reliable guide to the tonicity of body fluids. While hypo- or hypernatremia does result in clinical signs, these signs have received little emphasis since the advent of the flame photometer, which provides a simple method of laboratory diagnosis. It is also worth noting that abnormalities of volume are more critical to body function in comparison with abnormalities of concentration, which are better tolerated. Unfortunately, a disproportionate amount of attention is placed on concentration simply because of the ease and availability of measurements as opposed to the difficulties in determining volume abnormalities.

A number of factors combine to determine the concentration of sodium in extracellular fluid. The major influences are shown in Figure 3, which depicts the pituitary adrenal axis, which acts directly and through the renal mechanisms to regulate the exchange of sodium, potassium, and water. The shift of sodium into cells and the addition of free water from oxidation of

Table 3. VOLUME OF GASTROINTESTINAL SECRETIONS

Gastric	2500 ml/day
Small intestine	3000 ml/day
Saliva	1500 ml/day
Pancreatic	700 ml/day
Bile	500 ml/day
Total	8200 ml/day

Table 4. COMPOSITION OF GASTROINTESTINAL SECRETION (mEq/LITER)

	Na	K	Cl
Gastric	60–80	8–10	80–100
Small intestine	100–110	4–6	80–120
Saliva	10–12	20–28	10–12
Pancreatic	135–145	4–6	60–80
Bile	140–150	4–6	80–110

FACTORS AFFECTING TONICITY

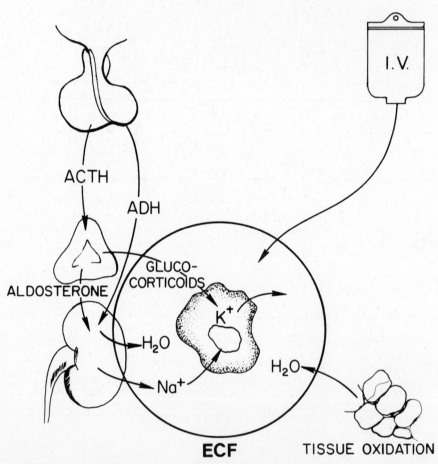

Figure 3. This figure depicts the factors that influence the tonicity of extracellular fluid (ECF). Sodium, potassium, and water exchanges are under the control of the pituitary-adrenal axis and are mediated via the kidneys. Shift of sodium into the cells and increased free water from tissue breakdown are thought to contribute to the hyponatremia seen in severe catabolism. Intravenous fluid management can obviously play a direct role.

body tissues are often neglected. However, decisions made by the surgeon regarding the volume and sodium concentration of intravenous fluids probably have the most direct effect on the tonicity of extracellular fluid.

In the intensive care unit, hyponatremia is commonplace, while hypernatremia is rare (and usually iatrogenic). This is consistent with previous statements regarding the tendency of critically ill patients to retain water, and it is generally accepted that low serum levels reflect an increase in water more than they do a decrease in total exchangeable sodium. However, the situation is somewhat more complex than it appears at first glance. Edelman and coworkers pointed out some time ago that body potassium is an important and predictable determinant of daily changes in serum sodium concentration.[2] They expressed the relationship between sodium, potassium, and body water in the following way:

$$\text{Serum Na}^+ = k \cdot \frac{\text{Total Na}^+ + \text{total K}^+}{\text{Total body water}}$$

This equation explains that the tendency of patients in an intensive care unit to show hyponatremia in the face of sodium retention is due not only to a positive water balance but also to potassium loss.

Efforts to raise serum sodium concentration have also led to the use of hypertonic saline. The original preparations were extremely hypertonic, containing either 500 or 833 mEq/liter, but recently the tonicity of these solutions has been greatly reduced and is in the neighborhood of 220 to 280 mEq/liter. Hypertonic solutions have been used extensively in the treatment of major burns in an effort to reduce the large positive water balance associated with treatment of these injuries by noncolloid therapy. Hypertonic saline has also been advocated in other varieties of shock. Despite the frequency of significant hyponatremia in the intensive care unit, hypertonic saline is rarely indicated. The ideal approach to this problem relates to prevention, which can usually be accomplished by limiting fluid administration, especially dextrose solutions without saline, and providing adequate amounts of potassium. Unless the hyponatremia is both severe and acute, it is probably better to avoid hypertonic saline, since these patients usually have an increased amount of body sodium. Gradual efforts to unload free water and replace body potassium probably represent more effective therapy.

Hypernatremia is rare in the intensive care unit and is often the result of overly zealous salt replacement. If the condition is severe enough, free water (dextrose and water) can be administered, but it is important to realize that an expansion of extracellular fluid will follow.

ABNORMALITIES OF POTASSIUM CONCENTRATION

Potassium has an intracellular concentration that is about 30 times greater than its plasma level. The differential is maintained by the activity of the cell membrane, and if there is injury to the cell, potassium will leave and sodium moves into the cell to preserve osmotic equilibrium. It is important to remember that there is little relationship in the concentration of potassium in the cell and in the plasma, so that a deficit of potassium may exist in one compartment without any evidence of this in the other. While the plasma potassium level tells us little about total body potassium, it may be important in itself if the value is very high or very low. High levels, about 7 mEq/liter, may result in cardiac arrest, while very low levels will have a profound effect on muscle function.

Since the presence of hypokalemia does not provide precise information about total exchangeable potassium, it is essential that the clinician evaluate the patient in regard to either a low intake or increased losses of potassium. Low intake may be associated with poor nutrition or alcoholism. In the ICU patient, this depletion may be aggravated by potassium-free intravenous infusions. Increased losses are usually associated with loss of gastrointestinal secretions, especially gastric juice, which is high in potassium. Diarrhea may also cause persistent loss of potassium. Losses via the kidneys are equally important. In the ICU setting, this is often associated with the use of diuretics or steroids but at times it reflects a form of renal failure.

Low serum potassium levels may also exist without any real loss of potassium from the body. This is especially common in alkalosis and is thought to reflect a shift of additional potassium into the cells. A similar situation may arise in the course of parenteral nutrition, where large amounts of administered glucose will take potassium along when moving into cells.

It is not always easy to diagnose a deficiency in total potassium. The surgeon must be alert to factors in the patient's history, such as nutritional depletion, alcoholism, or losses through the gastrointestinal tract or kidney. Besides determination of serum potassium concentration, it is important to follow electrocardiographic changes and collect urine to monitor loss via that route. The greatest danger of a low potassium state is its effect on the heart. When intracellular potassium falls, it results in bradycardia and eventually a fall in blood pressure. The electrocardiogram shows characteristic changes and is of great value, since it is thought to reflect intracellular potassium levels rather than the plasma concentration. Muscle weakness is also a characteristic feature, and actual paralysis may develop. Smooth muscle is also affected, and some instances of persistent paralytic ileus will not improve until potassium repletion has been accomplished.

Hyperkalemia, on the other hand, is not complicated by the need to differentiate between plasma levels and the amount of potassium in the body. Total body potassium is not easily increased, since even if an excess is administered, it is excreted by the kidney. Hyperkalemia may exist in the sense of an increased level in the plasma, and renal failure is far and away the most common cause. Metabolic acidosis will also raise serum potassium because the hydrogen ion displaces potassium from the cells. Once again, the main effect is on the heart, and the electrocardiogram shows changes that can readily be differentiated from hypokalemic states. Treatment requires correction of the underlying cause, but temporary measures may assume great importance when levels are dangerously high. The technique is to transport potassium into the cells until renal excretion or dialysis can catch up with the high serum potassium levels. Dextrose and insulin have been used for this purpose, but it is also important to remember that if acidosis is present, correction of this abnormality with sodium bicarbonate will result in a prompt drop in serum potassium levels.

ACID-BASE ABNORMALITIES

Disorders of acid-base balance are commonplace in the critically ill, and the classic clinical syndromes are often modified by special techniques used in treating organ failure. The intensive care physician not only must recognize these abnormalities but must understand the underlying disturbance if treatment is to be effective. Contemporary acid-base theory defines an acid as a substance that can donate a hydrogen ion, and the term pH represents the concentration of free hydrogen ions in solution. The actual pH value is inversely proportional to the concentration of hydrogen ions in solution. The addition of strong acid to water will obviously lower pH, but the presence of buffers will modify this effect. In vivo pH is held in the normal range primarily by maintaining plasma concentration of two substances: HCO_3^- at 24 millimoles/liter, and CO_2 near 1.2 millimoles/liter. This represents the normal 20:1 ratio of $HCO_3^-:CO_2$. While it might be arbitrary to focus on the concentrations of HCO_3^- and CO_2 when there are many other buffer pairs present in plasma, the important point is that the body exercises acid-base homeostasis by controlling arterial P_{CO_2} and HCO_3^- levels. Pulmonary control of P_{CO_2} and the renal bicarbonate mechanism determine survival except over very short time periods where other buffers may play a role. Probably the most important role played by the other buffers relates to the protection that they provide against sudden respiratory failure with abrupt rise in P_{CO_2}. Since renal compensation requires many hours to be effective, the buffering capacity of whole blood provides an important defense against sudden changes in plasma pH.

Regardless of the specific clinical problem, acid-base analysis depends on examination of the blood. The physician working in an intensive care unit will want to know three things: the pH of the blood, what role the lung is playing in the abnormality, and how much nonvolatile acid or base is present. Present-day electrodes provide rapid measurements of pH, making it possible to quantitate the abnormality existing in the extracellular fluid. Similarly, electrodes designed to measure P_{CO_2} provide information regarding the role of the lung. However, there is no way in which the nonrespiratory constituents in any abnormality of the acid-base composition of extracellular fluid can be evaluated directly and quantitatively in the way that the pulmonary constituent (P_{CO_2}) and the arterial pH can be. Because of the dominant role of the $HCO_3^-:CO_2$ system, the plasma bicarbonate concentration offers a useful index of the extent of accumulation of excess nonvolatile acid or base, but it does not represent a quantitative measure. For that reason, much work has been expended in an effort to combine with the evaluation of arterial pH and P_{CO_2} an accurate estimate of the nonrespiratory component.[6] One of the first of these derived variables was the CO_2 combining power, or CO_2 capacity, of Van Slyke. More recent variables based on CO_2 titration of whole blood have included the buffer base of Singer and Hastings, the standard bicarbonate of Jorgensen and Astrup, and the base excess of Astrup and Siggaard-Andersen. All of these derived measurements share a common objective, which is to compensate for errors that arise when one attempts to evaluate the accumulation of nonvolatile acid or base in the whole body from a blood sample that reflects only the vascular compartment.

Base excess is the derived variable in general use today, and it represents a calculation of the amount of acid or base needed to bring the HCO_3^- of the sample to 25 millimoles/liter. This calculation is carried out at a P_{CO_2} of 40 mm Hg, and since it is expressed in terms of milliequivalents per liter of blood, it is theoretically possible to estimate how much mineral acid or alkali has to be given to achieve neutrality. In practice, this makes little sense because CO_2 titration of blood in vitro is not the same as "whole body CO_2 titration," since in vivo exchanges of ions between multiple compartments cannot be reproduced by CO_2 titration of blood in a test tube. Therefore, base excess or deficit measurements should be regarded as an index rather than a measure of nonvolatile acid or base. It should be obvious that there are no effortless rules that can be applied in treatment; rather, application of the information made available by comprehensive acid-base analysis of blood must be applied in accordance with the clinical problems facing the patient.

In some clinical laboratories, CO_2 titration of the blood sample is not carried out. Instead, the P_{CO_2} and pH of the sample are measured, and bicarbonate is calculated. This neglects the influence of abnormal P_{CO_2} on the HCO_3^- of the sample, but studies show that the effect is usually less than 3 mEq/liter despite wide ranges of P_{CO_2} (25–60 mm Hg).

Acid-base problems have traditionally been considered in terms of metabolic, respiratory, and mixed disturbances. In the intensive care unit, metabolic acidosis is usually due to the gain of acid, such as is seen in diabetic acidosis, shock, renal failure, and even hyperalimentation when synthetic amino acid mixtures are employed. This is because of an excess of cationic amino acids whose metabolism results in a net excess of hydrogen ion. These problems are not encountered when protein hydrolysates are used.

The other general mechanism underlying the development of metabolic acidosis relates to loss of HCO_3^- from the extracellular space. Renal losses may be responsible, but this is more common in chronic renal disease than in the acute variety seen in the intensive care unit. Loss of small intestinal secretions may be an important factor, since the bicarbonate concentration is higher than in plasma.

Metabolic alkalosis results from the gain of HCO_3^- or the loss of acid from the extracellular fluid. While alkaline ingestion in patients with peptic ulcer is well known, different agents are involved in the ICU patients. Intravenous treatment with sodium bicarbonate is by far the most common problem, and it is not always easy for these patients to excrete the excess sodium. Transfusion alkalosis may result from the large amounts of sodium citrate in banked blood (17 mEq/unit).

Loss of acid from the stomach may result in alkalosis, and the role of potassium depletion in this syndrome has been mentioned previously. Renal alkalosis is in large part due to the loss of potassium from the kidney, and it is common in the ICU because of the widespread use of diuretics.

Respiratory acidosis is due to retention of CO_2 with an increase of Pco_2 and carbonic acid. CO_2 is almost entirely eliminated in the expired air, and its concentration in the body depends on the relationship between metabolic production and alveolar ventilation. A number of factors seen in the ICU setting can depress the respiratory center, or there may be physical problems limiting ventilation.

Finally, there is respiratory alkalosis, which is exceedingly common, since hyperventilation is associated with many stressful conditions. At times, hemorrhagic, cardiogenic, or septic shock produces complex abnormalities of acid-base regulation. Alkalemia is often seen in the early stages, and later on acidemia may predominate. Such patients make up the typical ICU population, and the complexity of these states as well as associated metabolic alterations produces mixtures of the four basic acid-base abnormalities described above.

The foregoing has been a very compressed tabulation of the more common acid-base problems encountered in the intensive care unit. In all instances, an understanding of the underlying physiologic or pathologic mechanisms is essential if treatment is to be effective. For that reason, proper evaluation of the patient's clinical state is necessary in order to interpret properly the information that is now available from a comprehensive analysis of the acid-base status of arterial blood.

REFERENCES

1. Berliner, R. W., Kennedy, T. J., Jr., and Orloff, J.: Relationship between acidification of the urine and potassium metabolism. Am. J. Med., *11*:274, 1951.
2. Edelman, I. S., Leibman, J., O'Meara, M. P., and Birkenfeld, L. W.: Interrelations between serum sodium concentration, serum osmolality and total exchangeable sodium, total exchangeable potassium and total body water. J. Clin. Invest., *37*:1236, 1958.
3. Gump, F. E., Kinney, J. M., Iles, M., and Long, C. L.: Duration and significance of large fluid loads administered for circulatory support. J. Trauma, *10*:431, 1970.
4. Gump, F. E., Kinney, J. M., Long, C. L., and Gelber, R.: Measurement of water balance—a guide to surgical care. Surgery, *64*:154, 1968.
5. Gump, F. E., Mashima, Y., and Kinney, J. M.: Water balance and extravascular lung water measurements in surgical patients. Am. J. Surg., *119*:515, 1970.

6. Hills, A. G.: Acid-base Balance. Baltimore, Williams and Wilkins Company, 1973.
7. Moore, F. D.: Body Cell Mass and Its Supporting Environment: Body Composition in Health and Disease. Philadelphia, W. B. Saunders Company, 1963.
8. Shires, G. T.: Fluid and electrolyte therapy. *In* Kinney, J. M., Egdahl, R. H., and Zuidema, G. D.: Manual of Preoperative and Postoperative Care. Philadelphia, W. B. Saunders Company, 1971, p. 42.
9. Skillman, J. J., Parikh, B. M., and Tanenbaum, B. J.: Pulmonary arteriovenous admixture: improvement with albumin and diureses. Am. J. Surg., *119*:440, 1970.
10. Sladen, A., Laver, M. B., and Pontoppidan, H.: Pulmonary complications and water retention in prolonged mechanical ventilation. N. Engl. J. Med., *279*:448, 1968.

CHAPTER 10

USE OF BLOOD AND BLOOD COMPONENTS

John A. Collins, M.D.

Of all the complex therapeutic agents used in the treatment of the seriously ill patient, blood and blood products are among the least understood. This reflects a common defect in undergraduate medical education, where little time is devoted to this lifesaving but dangerous category of treatment. Blood is simultaneously a drug, a fluid and electrolyte solution, a metabolic and endocrine challenge to the patient, and an organ transplant. Perhaps its many facets account for its ignored status in medical education—it is difficult to pigeonhole along traditional lines. It is, however, commonly if not familiarly or knowingly used, and has great potential for harm or good.

This chapter will consider what is available from the blood bank by considering the nonclotting components, the indications for transfusion including the clotting components, the risks of transfusion in three main categories (transmitted diseases, transfusion reactions, and massive transfusion), and finally current trends and future projections in transfusion practices. The references are few and broad and can be used to expand reading further along certain lines if so desired.

COMPONENTS

Table 1 lists the major nonclotting components, which are briefly discussed in this section. The clotting components are discussed in the section on indications for transfusion, and are listed in Table 2.

Red Cell Preparations. "Packed" red cell units (they are really sedimented) are units of whole blood with two-thirds of the plasma fraction removed. As use of packed cells becomes more common, more of the whole blood collected has the plasma removed at the time of collection. This has greatly aided the preparation of other components, especially the clotting

Table 1. Major Nonclotting Components

	Composition	Donors	Comments
Packed red cells	Rbc + ⅓ plasma	Single	Two-thirds plasma removed; otherwise same as whole blood.
"Washed" red cells	Rbc + electrolyte solution	Single	Most plasma, white blood cells, platelets removed. Various methods available.
Frozen red cells	Rbc + electrolyte solution	Single	Same advantages as washed red blood cells, plus preserved functional state, plus indefinite storage.
Plasma protein fraction	Plasma minus gamma globulin	Pooled	Various trade names. Pasteurized, very low risk of hepatitis.
Albumin	5% solution in saline	Pooled	Pasteurized, probably no risk of hepatitis.
Albumin	25% "salt poor"	Pooled	Pasteurized. Can rapidly expand plasma volume, especially in edematous patients.
Concentrated leukocytes	Varying numbers of granu-locytes in small volume	Single or multiple	Two methods in use; efficacy being evaluated.
Immune globulins	Various types for specific functions	Pooled	Apparently free of hepatitis.

components, and this may be the greatest single advantage to the use of packed red cells.

Many of the reasons for using packed red cells have been overstated by professional blood bankers in promoting the concept of component therapy. Packed cells are not a good example of component therapy at its best because they are rather "dirty." The amount of leukocyte and platelet antigens is reduced but not to very effective levels, the amount of debris is reduced, the potential metabolic effects of the stored citrated plasma are reduced, but none of these are eliminated. The risk of hepatitis is probably reduced very little if at all because it takes so little infected plasma to transmit the disease. Nevertheless, most transfusions are given for the red cell content, and a surprising amount of what is present in whole blood is potentially disadvantageous or even harmful to the patient, so for the recipient some gain from packed red cells is evident.

A far better form of red cell therapy involves the use of "washed" red cells or buffy coat poor red cells. These preparations come close enough to eliminating the plasma, leukocyte, and platelet components as to represent real advantages to the patient, as well as to the system through the preservation of components for specific needs. Recent simple advances, such as use of hydroxyethyl starch as the sedimenting agent, may make this an economically and practically realistic way to give a much cleaner form of red cells.

Frozen red cells are the "cleanest" form of red cells currently available because of the extensive washing necessary in the thawing and deglycerolizing process. In addition, frozen red cells are indefinitely storable, a feature that is ideal for the management of inventory of rare blood types on a regional basis, and for inventory control in general because of the cyclic variations in voluntary donations. Finally, the functional status of the red cells is preserved as it was at the time of freezing. The recent development of "rejuvenating" formulas can be nicely dovetailed with freezing technology to restore the functional capacity of red cells about to be lost through outdating to above normal levels, and to preserve them in this state until needed. This may prove to be the most advantageous use of freezing technology. The disadvantages of freezing red cells are the cost (probably at least double the cost of liquid storage), the fact that once thawed the cells must be used in 24 hours or be discarded, and the loss of about 10 per cent of the collected red cells during processing. Technical advances in all these areas are possible, even likely.

Plasma protein fraction is available under a variety of trade names. All are basically plasma minus the gamma globulin. Pasteurization (60° C for over 10 minutes) eliminates the risk of hepatitis, so these preparations are vastly preferable to whole plasma for volume expansion. There is no conceivable use for pooled whole plasma, which carries a very high risk of hepatitis, so it is not even listed here. Recent reports indicate that these fraction preparations may contain a vasodilating substance, but this may be apparent only when the lungs are bypassed or when rapidly infused.

Albumin is present in isosmotic (5 per cent in saline) and hyperoncotic forms (25 per cent). There is probably no risk of hepatitis. The 25 per cent form can draw a significant amount of interstitial fluid into the vascular space, especially in a hypoalbuminemic edematous patient, so it must be given cautiously with a watch for pulmonary edema. All albumin preparations have been used in increasing amounts in recent years, with a resultant sharp increase in price and threatened shortages.

Concentrated leukocyte preparations are used for providing the recipient with functioning granulocytes. These are harvested either by differential centrifugation or by filtering-contact trapping. There are differences in yield and perhaps in phagocytic and bactericidal function. These are now being investigated. This could become a significant new field of component therapy if the technical problems are mastered. There is a high incidence of febrile reactions in previously transfused patients.

Immune globulin preparations are very familiar to surgeons because of the development of human tetanus immune globulin. A number of other specific immune globulins are available, and more are being developed. It seems clear now that the varying results obtained in the use of pooled gamma globulin to prevent hepatitis after transfusion have been due to chance variations in specific antihepatitis activity.

INDICATIONS FOR TRANSFUSION

Anemia. Management of a red cell deficit is one of the commonest problems confronted by the surgeon. When to transfuse and how much? As usual, one must consider risk, benefit, and need. The significant risk of transfusion is discussed subsequently. As noted, it may be much lower with some types of red cell preparations.

The benefits of red cell transfusions are not as clear as they may seem. The red cell mass in any patient represents a dynamic equilibrium, the balance between production and loss. Any disorders of production and/or loss that can be corrected, should be. This will be far more effective than transfusing red cells, the effect of which will soon be lost in the dynamic turnover. If the hematocrit remains elevated after transfusion, it is because the balance between production and loss has changed favorably, not because the transfused cells are somehow persisting indefinitely.

Given the fact that transfusion represents only a temporary increase in red cell mass, and that at significant risk, are there situations where such temporary benefits outweigh the risks? Increasing the hematocrit increases oxygen delivery by increasing the oxygen content of blood. At the same time, increasing hematocrit tends to decrease oxygen delivery by increasing the intrinsic resistance of blood to flow. It is not possible to say where the optimal hematocrit lies, and it is likely that the hematocrit that is optimal for oxygen delivery will be different under different circumstances. The main deficit is in our very incomplete understanding of the flow properties of blood in vivo. Present methods of measurement in vitro emphasize such variables as hematocrit and plasma viscosity, but slight such variables as the elastic properties of red cells and the degree of interaction between red cells, and almost completely ignore such factors as pulsatile flow, turbulent flow, and the geometry of the vascular system. In addition, not enough is known about the velocity of flow in vivo in different locations and under different clinical circumstances.

There are, however, some consistent responses to anemia in intact animals and in humans. One of the most important is the proportional increase in cardiac output that accompanies acute lowering of red cell mass, if blood volume is preserved. This increased cardiac output is accompanied by an increase in left atrial pressure, although central venous pressure may remain unchanged. An important question is whether this increase in cardiac output represents increased work by the heart, presumably in response to peripheral signals resulting from the reduction in oxygen delivery, or whether this results solely from the fall in the resistance of blood to flow. If the latter is true, then the circulatory response to anemia represents a "free ride," that is, no new workload for the heart, and the effects of anemia are essentially self-correcting. There is evidence on both sides of this question, but the most compelling is that chronically anemic patients and animals develop left ventricular hypertrophy, which indicates that there probably is an increase in the workload of the heart.

The human heart occupies a central but vulnerable position in the response to blood loss. Oxygen requirements actually increase because of the need to maintain maximal output at lower filling pressures, while oxygen supply, which occurs during diastole, is adversely affected by the fall in diastolic pressure and the reduction in the time spent in diastole. The mixed venous oxygen tension is always near the minimal functional level for the heart, a peculiar situation that greatly increases its vulnerability. These circumstances point up the great importance of coronary vasodilatation in the response of the heart to stress. When coronary dilatation is limited, as by banding, myocardial function declines as hematocrit falls below normal, whereas the heart with normal coronary arteries can function quite well at significant degrees of anemia. This experimental observation has obvious clinical implications.

Studies in intact animals indicate that work performance and ability to survive various challenges, including hemorrhage, are best at normal hematocrit levels. Stress testing anemic patients, however, indicates little impairment of work performance down to hemoglobin or hematocrit levels half of normal. This discrepancy has been resolved by recent appreciation of the ability of the body to alter the function of hemoglobin by changing the affinity of hemoglobin for oxygen. In chronically anemic patients, the hemoglobin that remains is a much more efficient delivery agent for oxygen, accounting for much of the remarkably efficient compensation for chronic anemia. This change in the function of hemoglobin can be accomplished in a few days or less. This compensatory mechanism cannot offset the loss of more than half the red cell mass, however, and even that much only under optimum conditions. In addition, there are many factors that significantly alter the function of hemoglobin that may not be under the patient's immediate regulatory control, such as pH, temperature, osmolality, arterial oxygen tension, arteriovenous pH gradient, and others.

To try to summarize what is known about the optimal hematocrit, the most important point is that it will vary with the clinical circumstances. Actual or imminent threats to the oxygen delivery system, coronary artery disease, increased oxygen demands (especially sepsis and fever), and a fixed limit on the cardiac output are all factors that favor providing the anemic patient with a higher hematocrit. On the other hand, the patient whose blood loss is completed and who is recovering quietly and uneventfully can in many instances tolerate anemia down to half normal hemoglobin or hematocrit values, and in some cases even lower.

Among indications for red cell transfusion that are *not* legitimate we must rank wound healing. Wound healing is impaired by protein deficiency, not by anemia. *It is poor medicine to transfuse a patient with red cells solely to improve wound healing.*

The anemic patient who must be operated upon represents a difficult special problem. Unquestionably, the rigid guidelines often applied for general anesthesia (hemoglobin concentration above 10 gm/100 ml) at times work to the patient's detriment. The decision to transfuse a stable patient before operation should be based on the factors already cited. The most important are an evaluation of how the patient is tolerating his anemia (for example, what is the patient's exercise tolerance) plus the nature of the projected operation and the chances for extensive or sudden blood loss. Well compensated patients undergoing operations with little chance of major blood loss should not be transfused preoperatively. There is no arbitrary level of hemoglobin concentration required for anesthesia that can be applied across the board.

Hypoalbuminemia.   Unquestionably, albumin is one of the least rationally used blood products. There is widespread confusion about quantitative factors, persistence and fate after infusion, and indications for use.

The readily accessible albumin pool in most adults is about 140 gm in the intravascular space, but about 180 gm in extravascular "pools." The albumin space is thus over twice as large as that calculated from plasma volume and plasma concentration. In hypoalbuminemia, moreover, these relationships change in such a way that the intravascular pool sustains less decrease in albumin concentration than does the extravascular pool, so that the deficit in the readily accessible pool is significantly greater than twice that estimated from plasma concentrations and assumed plasma volumes. This source of error increases as the plasma albumin concentration falls.

In addition, administered albumin persists for different times in different patients, and at different times in the same patient as circumstances change. One key to duration is the nutritional status of the patient. Unfortunately, the typically severely ill, hypoalbuminemic patient is usually severely catabolic from starvation plus a variety of superimposed catabolic stimuli, especially wounds and sepsis. It is precisely this patient who uses the administered albumin for calories. In this setting, albumin is merely expensive and dirty (because of its nitrogen content) sugar that persists as albumin for only a short time after infusion.

The plasma albumin concentration represents a dynamic equilibrium, even more so than for the red cell concentration because the turnover rates are more rapid. In the normal state, there is a turnover of about 14 gm/day, but this can be greatly accelerated by disease. To a large extent, the plasma albumin concentration reflects the nutritional status of the patient. Supplying sufficient calories and amino acids will correct the problem more safely and far more effectively.

The indications for the use of albumin are also unclear. The most favorable circumstance would be one in which a sudden loss of albumin threatens to result in harmful body fluid distribution in a well nourished adult who is not severely catabolic. In these conditions the administered albumin will persist longer, and the patient will retain the elevated concentration through increased synthesis. Extensive hemorrhage treated by non-colloid-containing fluids would be an example. If pulmonary edema or hypovolemia is a threatened or actual problem, albumin administered in a concentrated form is rational therapy. Some circumstances may not be as favorable as they appear. It is clear that there is extensive loss of capillary integrity for large protein molecules early after a large burn. Albumin in such circumstances has no effect on plasma volume, and its use makes little sense. A difficult problem exists in the surgical patient with acute pulmonary insufficiency. In at least some of these patients, a similar loss of functional integrity probably exists in the pulmonary capillaries so that concentrated albumin will not be helpful in diminishing pulmonary edema, although if the lesion is patchy perhaps the albumin may help in the nonporous areas. This important problem urgently needs clarification. During the administration of concentrated albumin solutions, left atrial pressure may rise significantly, especially if the patient is edematous; pulmonary edema can be caused by the very therapy intended to prevent its occurrence.

Albumin is scarce. It is available only from human sources. The cost of albumin is rising alarmingly. It should be used carefully and intelligently. Too often, it is used as an inadequate, ineffective substitute for proper nutritional support.

Hypovolemia. Blood loss can be treated by a variety of fluids, but when it is rapid and extensive enough to threaten exsanguination, whole blood is the mainstay of replacement. If exsanguination is imminent, type-specific blood should be used until fully cross-matched blood is available. In most institutions, blood can be accurately typed within five to ten minutes of the arrival of the specimen at the blood bank. Most patients can be kept alive with simple salt solutions until then. The risk added by not waiting for a full cross match is relatively small, and is certainly acceptable under such circumstances.

Clotting Defects. Component therapy has significantly improved the treatment of various clotting disorders in recent years. Most patients with clotting disorders can now be carried through even extensive operations successfully. By far the best results are achieved if these patients are managed throughout the operative period in close cooperation with a physician experienced in the management of these problems and with the blood bank and coagulation laboratory. Prescheduling is often a great help in successful management.

Table 2 indicates the approximate compositions of some of the more common components. Factor VIII is measured in "units"; each unit equals the activity present in 1 ml normal fresh plasma. The formula for calculating unit requirements is:

$$\frac{\text{desired increase in activity } (\%) \times \text{plasma volume (ml)}}{100} = \text{units needed}$$

There is some question as to whether the use of fibrinogen is ever indicated. The risk of hepatitis is high, and hypofibrinogenemia is usually a manifestation of intravascular consumption. Replacement alone is usually futile; if the underlying process is interrupted, replacement soon becomes unnecessary if the liver is functioning. Fibrinogen levels are normal in stored blood, so replacement of blood loss provides sufficient activity. Similarly, Factor IX concentrate carries a very high risk of hepatitis and is a product that has very few specific indications for use.

The evaluation of the bleeding patient is the same in broad outline as for any patient: history, physical examination, and laboratory testing. The most important decision by far is to estimate if the bleeding is due to a mechanical problem or if there is a defect in the hemostatic mechanism. The commonest cause of postoperative bleeding is a large open blood vessel; the surgeon has been inadequate, not the patient. An honest, objective assessment will often lead to prompt reoperation and cure, while self-deceptive procrastinating will prolong the physiologic problem, increase the amount of sequestered blood, deplete the blood bank, and lead to breakdowns in the hemostatic mechanism where none existed.

A minority of bleeding patients will have a faulty hemostatic mechanism. Preexisting hemostatic defects may become evident from the family history, the patient's previous responses to injury (dental extractions and childbirth are especially helpful), a history of spontaneous bleeding, and a detailed history of drug ingestion. On physical examination one should look for evidence of bleeding from areas of minor injury or no injury, and signs of pertinent underlying diseases (e.g., liver, spleen, lymphoid). Simple, widely available laboratory tests can be very helpful: platelet count, prothrombin time (Factors VII, X, V, II, and fibrinogen-fibrin), partial thromboplastin time (Factors XII, XI, IX, VIII, X, V, II, and fibrinogen-fibrin), thrombin time (fibrinogen-fibrin), fibrinogen level. More sophisticated and specific laboratory tests may be available and can be helpful when indicated, espe-

Table 2. Components Available for Managing Clotting Disorders

	Clotting Factors	Amount (compared with one unit of normal blood)	Volume (ml)	Minimum desirable level of factor for surgical hemostasis	Source	Risk of hepatitis
Fresh frozen plasma	All except platelets	0.9	240	—	Single donor	Single donor
Cryoprecipitate	VIII I	0.5 0.25	10	30% 100 mg/100 ml	Single donor	Single donor
Factor VIII concentrate	VIII	(individually assayed, expressed as Factor VIII units)	10–30	30%	Pooled	Moderate to high
Multifactor complex (Konyne, Proplex)	II VII IX X	2 2 2 2	40	20% 20% 20% 10%	Pooled	High
Fibrinogen	I	(stated)	(lyophilized)	100 mg/100ml	Pooled	Very high
Platelet-rich plasma	Platelets All others	0.9 0.8–0.9	220	Not defined	Single donor	Single donor
Platelet concentrate	Platelets	0.6–0.8	25	Not defined	Single donor	Single donor
"Modified plasma" (residual after preparation of cryoprecipitate, when fresh)	II V VII IX X	0.8–0.9 0.8–0.9 0.8–0.9 0.8–0.9 0.8–0.9	220	20% 20% 20% 20% 10%	Single donor	Single donor

cially tests for fibrinolytic activity, but much information can be deduced from the above. Some results can be superficially misleading, and expert advice is always a good idea. For example, a circulating anticoagulant (heparin, or fibrin-fibrinogen complexes and breakdown products) will give abnormal results in all the clotting tests that measure a fibrin clot as the end point, including the most common methods for measuring fibrinogen. Differentiating the effects of extensive transfusion from those of disseminated intravascular coagulation can be tricky and will be discussed later.

Treatment is aimed at correcting the cause if possible, and replacing deficiencies only when necessary. The most rapid way to reverse the multiple factor deficits in patients who have been receiving vitamin K antagonists (Factors II, VII, IX, X) is by administering fresh frozen plasma, single donor plasma, or multifactor complex. Care must be taken to avoid volume overload with plasma. Fresh frozen plasma is also effective for the multiple deficiencies found in patients with liver disease (Factors II, V, VII, IX, and X), and provides both Factor V and Factor VIII for patients who have been massively transfused with old stored blood. For those blood banks that produce their own cryoprecipitate, the residual fresh or fresh frozen plasma is a good source of Factors II, V, VII, IX, and X, and therefore suitable for patients who have liver disease or who are receiving vitamin K antagonists. Cryoprecipitate as a grouped product from a few donors is a good alternate source of fibrinogen in the few circumstances in which fibrinogen may be needed.

Platelets are now available in concentrated form, which is the most sensible way to raise levels in the recipient. One unit of platelets refers to the number of platelets in a unit of normal blood. One unit of platelets will raise the platelet concentration of the usual adult at least $5,000/\mu L$, but the actual increment will be less in patients who are bleeding actively, or with fever or sepsis, and of course in patients with platelet-destructive disorders. In the latter, platelet infusions are often futile until the destructive disorder is at least modified. A desirable platelet level for elective operation has not been defined. It may be that evidence of spontaneous bleeding is more useful than actual platelet counts. We have performed uneventful splenectomies on patients with platelet counts of 10,000 but without evidence of spontaneous bleeding. Platelet preparations contain some red cells, so that typing is necessary. Platelets cannot be stored for much more than 24 hours, so that preplanning is necessary whenever possible. Ways of extending this preservation time are actively being sought.

There are several reports that document improvements in survival of transfused platelets when the donor and a previously transfused or multiparous recipient are matched for histocompatibility antigens (HL-A) as well as ABO group. In such a situation, consideration should be given to this extra effort if the methodology is available locally. It is now possible to harvest rather large numbers of platelets from a single donor at weekly intervals by a process known as plateletpheresis. The single donor strategy minimizes the chance for immunizing the recipient in situations where prolonged, repeated transfusions of circulating blood elements or transplantation of other tissues or organs is anticipated. These studies further emphasize the presence of broadly antigenic material in whole blood; in the case of platelets, moreover, there is absolutely no benefit to the recipient from having nonfunctional platelets in the transfusion, which is the situation in all but very fresh blood. Red cells do not contain HL-A antigens. Fresh blood contains all the labile clotting factors and most of the platelets of normal blood, but none in concentrated form. Collection of such blood imposes a great burden on most blood banks and requires an unusually available donor pool. The reasons for using fresh whole blood in preference to available components are often semimystical. They certainly remain undocumented.

RISKS OF TRANSFUSION

TRANSMISSION OF DISEASE

The most important disease transmitted by whole blood is hepatitis. This probably accounts for most of the deaths related to transfusion in the United States. The incidence of hepatitis following transfusion is very difficult to define because of the difficulty in following patients adequately. The most important variable in determining the incidence of hepatitis appears to be the source of the blood. Blood obtained from commercial sources that rely on paid donors from the lowest socioeconomic groups is the most likely to cause hepatitis, while the safest blood is that obtained from a donor (paid or unpaid) who has an established record of safety in prior recipients. A generally accepted rule of thumb is that there is one death per 1,000 units of blood, one case of clinical hepatitis per 100 units, and one case of deranged liver chemistries within six months for every 10 units of blood. This incidence varies considerably between regions, largely reflecting the source of blood for the areas involved.

Efforts to control this disease have progressed in recent years. Federally licensed blood banks are required to screen all donations for hepatitis-associated antigen (HAA) and to discard all HAA-positive donations. The Red Cross has adopted a more sensitive radioimmunoassay for detection of HAA. Elimination of HAA-positive blood may reduce the incidence of hepatitis from transfusion by 25 per cent, although the more sensitive assay methods are still being evaluated. The second major approach has been legislation at state levels requiring the labeling of blood as to whether from a voluntary or paid donor. An implied legal liability all but excludes use of blood from paid donors. This appears to have been of considerable benefit in previously high risk areas, as Chicago, which relied heavily on commercial paid donor operations. The legislation is imperfect, because it is not the act of payment that is at fault, and some of the safest donors are professional donors with established records. Also, there are forms of economic incentive that do not involve direct payment. In addition, there must be a concomitant rise in "voluntary" donations if the system is to succeed. The third approach to limiting the risk of hepatitis is to use the least amount of plasma possible. This means using plasma products only when necessary and using the lowest risk forms. A corollary of this would be to use effectively "washed" red cells when only red cells are needed.

Passive immunization with pooled gamma globulin has had very uneven effect, undoubtedly due to the chance variation in antihepatitis activity among different batches of pooled gamma globulin. Even if specifically identified batches were available, there would not be nearly enough to cover all those at risk.

The ultimate answer to hepatitis control lies in active immunization. Until then, thoroughly "washed" red cells are probably the most effective alternate, but even this remains to be documented.

Cytomegalovirus (CMV) is now the second most important agent transmitted by blood transfusion. Again the incidence is not clear, but is less than that for hepatitis, and the clinical manifestations are less severe. Some of the hepatitis now attributed to the hepatitis B virus may be due to CMV. Epstein-Barr virus is also transmitted by transfusion, but apparently much less frequently; again it may account for an occasional instance of hepatitis. Many other diseases have been transmitted by transfusion, but none with the consistency of the viral diseases. Unquestionably, many more diseases are transmitted than we now recognize and this list will lengthen considerably. Again, it is certain that using only the fraction of blood required will minimize the chance for transmitting disease, as various infectious agents are associated primarily with certain components.

TRANSFUSION REACTIONS

The most lethal immediate transfusion reaction is that caused by bacterial contamination of the stored blood (Table 3). The onset is usually very soon after beginning the transfusion and may be catastrophic, with severe vascular collapse. The mortality is very high. The essential step in treatment is to stop the transfusion at the first sign of trouble, followed by the usual methods for the treatment of severe gram-negative sepsis, including bactericidal antibiotics covering a wide range of gram-negative organisms. This should be done on suspicion alone. The diagnosis can often be rapidly confirmed by gently centrifuging an aliquot from the remaining blood and gram-staining the supernatant. Abundant gram-negative organisms can often be seen. A sample of the remaining blood should also be cultured, but sometimes no growth is obtained either because the organisms are no longer viable, or because they will grow only at low temperatures. For this reason, in addition, the immediate examination of a gram-stained sample is advantageous. This complication should be very rare in a modern blood bank, but accidents do happen.

Table 3. MORE IMPORTANT TRANSFUSION REACTIONS

TYPE OR CAUSE	ONSET	MANIFESTATIONS	COMPLICATIONS	TREATMENT	DIAGNOSIS
Contaminated blood	Rapid	Septic shock	High mortality	*Stop the blood,* treat sepsis	Gram stain, blood cultures (patient and transfusion)
Immediate hemolysis	Rapid	Chills, fever, back pain, oliguria, anemia	Renal failure, DIC	*Stop the blood,* diuresis and fluid loading	Hemoglobinuria, hemoglobinemia, re–cross match, clinical check
Delayed hemolysis	Days to weeks	Anemia, perhaps icterus	Anemia; occasionally renal failure	Nonspecific, maintain hydration	Re–cross match against same donor
Antibodies to transfused plasma proteins	Rapid	Anaphylaxis, pulmonary edema	Pulmonary edema, anaphylactic shock	*Stop the blood,* treat the complications	Requires sophisticated immunologic investigation
Antibodies to leukocyte antigens	Variable	Initially urticaria, more serious as repeated	Initially none, later may be vascular collapse	Antihistamine for urticaria	Requires sophisticated immunologic investigation; can be minimized by using washed red cells; HL-A typing may help
Antibodies to platelet antigens	Early (? urticaria) Late (purpura)	Occasionally late and persisting severe thrombocytopenia	Late severe thrombocytopenia; short or no duration for transfused platelets	Induced thrombocytopenia may require exchange transfusion or plasmapheresis	Requires sophisticated immunologic investigation; can be minimized by using washed red cells; HL-A typing may help

Hemolytic transfusion reactions are probably the next most serious, and are more common than those due to contaminated blood. The onset again is often soon after beginning the transfusion. Chills and fever often predominate at first; in the anesthetized, paralyzed patient the sudden onset of abnormal generalized bleeding should make the clinician investigate the possibility of a hemolytic transfusion reaction. Hemoglobinemia, hemoglobinuria, and a rapid fall in hemoglobin concentration are found in immediate hemolysis. Once again, it is important to stop the transfusion immediately. The identification of the patient and of the blood should be rechecked. A fresh, anticoagulated blood specimen should be drawn carefully and sent to the blood bank along with the remnant of the transfusion. Sometimes free hemoglobin can be identified in the patient's plasma by the gross color change alone. Urine output should be monitored closely and a centrifuged specimen of urine tested for hemoglobin. The blood bank should carefully recheck the records to see if the blood was given to the proper patient, and a retyping and cross match procedure should be performed along with a direct Coombs' test. If the patient has received multiple transfusions at about this time, all the transfused blood samples should be checked as above, and, if possible, intertransfusion incompatibility should be sought.

The two dreaded complications of hemolytic reactions are acute renal failure and diffuse bleeding. Prompt, full hydration and an induced diuresis will probably lessen the chance for developing renal failure. Alkalinization is usually advocated, but it may be very difficult to alkalinize the patient's urine, and the pathogenesis of the renal failure may have little to do with what is in the renal tubular lumen. Pathologic bleeding may be controlled with the judicious use of heparin, but usually satisfactory recovery occurs spontaneously and various forms of treatment only further complicate the situation. Some hemolytic reactions occur in a delayed manner, with little in the way of symptoms, except for unexplained anemia and perhaps an elevated bilirubin. Such reactions are less frequently followed by renal failure. Any patient who is discovered to be receiving the wrong blood should, if possible, have a diuresis induced and be followed closely as outlined above, even if there are not overt manifestations of trouble.

The commonest cause of hemolytic transfusion reactions is probably an error in labeling, typing, cross-matching, or administering the blood. In a well run blood bank, most such errors occur outside the blood bank and reflect either the rush of an emergency situation or the all too superficial attention many clinicians apply to the complex series of acts required to successfully transfuse a patient. The series of checks and the paperwork involved are not useless red tape, and each year patients are killed because blood banking practices are equated with bothersome bureaucracy.

Reactions against IgA are well documented but rare. They occur early after the start of the transfusion and resemble anaphylaxis. Reactions to other plasma proteins probably also occur, and as a group these reactions may account for the occasional appearance of pulmonary edema during transfusion due to altered pulmonary capillary permeability.

Urticarial reactions are the commonest clinically observed form of transfusion reactions; fortunately they are usually benign and limited. Antihistaminics usually control the symptoms. At least some of these reactions are due to incompatibility to leukocyte antigens. These become progressively more severe with succeeding transfusions, extending to febrile and vascular manifestations. Reactions against platelet antigens are now being documented. An unusual manifestation is prolonged thrombocytopenia in the recipient. It is especially important to use only the fraction of blood required, and that as scrupulously "clean" as possible, in the patient who faces the possibility of a continuing requirement for transfusions. This in fact is good policy for any patient receiving any blood product, but currently can be applied only at significantly added cost.

Circulatory overload as a transfusion "reaction" should be detectable by the observant clinician. Air embolism has fortunately become rare since plastic bags have replaced glass bottles for blood storage.

In case of doubt regarding whether or not a transfusion reaction is occurring, it is always safest to stop the transfusion and consult with the blood bank about the safest course to pursue.

MASSIVE TRANSFUSION

Some of the recognized problems that may result from the massive transfusion of liquid-stored blood are indicated in Table 4. The term "massive transfusion" should indicate at least one blood volume as a continuous

Table 4.   DELETERIOUS EFFECTS OF MASSIVE TRANSFUSION

Increased transmission of disease

Increased chance for immunologic mishap

Metabolic:
    Citrate toxicity
    Coagulation abnormalities
    Hemoglobin dysfunction
    Acid-base imbalance
    Hypothermia
    Hyperkalemia

Miscellaneous:
    Microembolization
    Plasticizer toxicity
    Impaired red blood cell deformability
    Infusion of denatured proteins
    Impaired antibacterial defenses
    Infusion of vasoactive substances
    Infusion of thromboplastic debris
    Elevated ammonia, phosphate levels
    Graft versus host reaction

transfusion in less than 12 hours. Often under such circumstances the rate of transfusion will at times be the maximum that can be obtained clinically, and it is at such times that the metabolic problems of transfusion become of great concern. These problems represent the current shortcomings in our ability to store human blood in a readily available form.

In analyzing the potential for harm to the patient from any of these shortcomings, one must be aware of the arithmetic of exchange transfusion. Table 5 gives the calculated percentage of the patient's original blood volume remaining after the transfusion of the indicated amounts. The "best" situation indicates perfect replacement; as each drop of blood is lost from the patient it is replaced simultaneously and in equal amount by bank blood. The "worst" situation indicates a patient who has acutely lost half of his blood volume, then hemorrhages and is transfused at half a blood volume until the hemorrhage stops. His blood volume is then returned to normal by continuing transfusion. The "best" situation, of course, never occurs, while the "worst" is incompatible with life. Massively transfused patients fall in between, probably closer to the best than to the worst. Despite these uncertainties, one can roughly estimate the degree of exchange in relation to the amount of blood transfused; it is less than most clinicians assume. Thus, hemorrhage and transfusion of one blood volume is not a complete exchange by any means; at least 25 per cent of the patient's original blood elements remain, and this will be added to by any new synthesis or release from stores during and after transfusion. These considerations become important in evaluating the development of such complications as generalized bleeding.

Citrate Toxicity. Probably the highest lethal potential of any of the metabolic problems of massive transfusion resides in the binding of the recipient's ionized calcium by the transfused citrate. If blood were simply calcium-free, there would be little problem, but transfusion represents an infusion of free citrate ions. Citrate exists in a planned excess in liquid-stored blood to ensure complete binding of calcium and therefore complete anticoagulation. The patient's defenses against citrate are twofold:

Table 5. PER CENT OF ORIGINAL BLOOD VOLUME REMAINING
AFTER EXCHANGE TRANSFUSION*

| | MAGNITUDE OF HEMORRHAGE AND TRANSFUSION | | |
SITUATION	1 Blood Volume	2 Blood Volumes	3 Blood Volumes
Best	37	14	5
Usual	30	11	4
Worst	18	3	1

*In the "best" situation, the patient remains normovolemic throughout; in the "worst" situation, bleeding and transfusion take place at a half normal blood volume, which is returned to normal only after the bleeding stops. The "usual" situation represents initial loss of half the blood volume, which is then rapidly replaced, with subsequent hemorrhage and transfusion occurring at a normal blood volume. (For details see Collins, J. A.: Problems associated with the massive transfusion of stored blood. Surgery, 75:274, 1974.)

metabolic removal of the citrate, and mobilization of more ionized calcium. Citrate is a normal intermediary metabolite, part of the tricarboxylic acid cycle, and is being metabolized constantly in almost every nucleated cell in the body. It is very rapidly metabolized after infusion, but there is considerable ignorance of the effects of hypoperfusion and hypothermia on the rate of removal. Calcium is mobilized in two steps: the release of parathyroid hormone, which occurs very rapidly after beginning a transfusion of citrated blood, and the mobilization of calcium from bone by the effect of the newly released hormone. The latter step requires skeletal perfusion, and there is good evidence that this falls significantly in response to blood loss, but again the quantitative relationships during transfusion are not known.

Further complicating the problem is the fact that the treatment, the infusion of ionized calcium, is potentially as lethal as the disease, and that the situation can change from minute to minute because of the varying rates of transfusion and the rapidity with which citrate can be removed.

The recent development of calcium ion-specific electrodes is allowing a more realistic evaluation of this potentially serious problem in animals and in patients. It is already clear that ionized calcium levels fall significantly during rapid transfusion, but the importance of these declines in terms of cardiac function is not known. A rule of thumb, based on considerable clinical experience, is that an adult of average size who has a reasonably intact circulation can tolerate a sustained rate of transfusion of one unit of blood every five minutes. The uncertainties regarding the effects of hypoperfusion and hypothermia on the patient's defenses are enough to make careful clinical investigation of this problem a high priority, aiming for the development of practical, effective, and safe guidelines for the use of supplemental calcium. For the moment, it is probably safest not to give calcium to the transfused patient unless there is unexplained cardiovascular impairment. If calcium is thought necessary, it must be given in the ionized form (calcium chloride) and must not be mixed with the citrated blood.

Coagulation Abnormalities. The development of generalized abnormal bleeding in the massively transfused patient is particularly distressing because it greatly diminishes the chances for controlling the life-threatening hemorrhage. Traditionally this impairment of clotting function has been blamed on the bank blood, but analysis does not support such a simple interpretation.

Bank blood is, indeed, deficient in a number of clotting elements. After the first day of storage the platelet count should be considered to be nil. By three weeks, levels of activity of Factor V and Factor VIII are no better than 10 per cent, perhaps less. Ionized calcium of course is lacking, but this is rapidly reversed and the cardiovascular effects occur before clotting effects. Factor XI falls to 20 per cent normal activity by the third week of storage, but this seems to be relatively inconsequential.

There are a number of observations against a simple dilutional cause for abnormal bleeding. On quantitative grounds, the degree of depression of platelet counts and, when measured, Factor V and Factor VIII is often well below what should be expected, considering the mathematics of exchange transfusion. In addition, fibrinogen levels are often below normal in these patients, while fibrinogen levels in stored blood are normal. Finally, many of the very severely injured casualties studied prospectively in Vietnam showed serious clotting impairments before transfusion began, with actual improvement during transfusion and reversion to the markedly abnormal pattern when transfusion was stopped. All of this evidence favors a pathologic consumption of clotting factors in these patients, disseminated intravascular coagulation (DIC).

Bank blood is hardly blameless, however, in the development of these abnormal bleeding states. There is a dilutional effect when old stored blood is used. It is conceivable that stored blood may make the patient more susceptible to the development of DIC through its content of thromboplastic cell debris and the partial activation of some clotting factors during storage. A hemolytic transfusion reaction is of course a well recognized and powerful trigger for DIC. Recently, a question has been raised of platelet functional impairment in heavily transfused patients. If confirmed, this finding should lead to earlier use of platelet supplementation, and to a search for and removal of the cause of the induced functional defect.

The treatment of these pathologic bleeding states is by no means clear or satisfactory. Replacement of depleted clotting factors by use of blood components is needed when the level of depletion becomes great, but it is likely that the key to management lies in removing the bulk of dead tissue and above all in preserving perfusion (cardiac output) as well as is possible. Sustained normal perfusion appears to be essential to breaking the vicious circle of DIC. The use of heparin has not been very helpful and has lost some of its former support.

Hemoglobin Function.   Prolonged storage in citrate leads to depletion of 2,3,-diphosphoglyceric acid (2,3-DPG) and increased affinity of hemoglobin for oxygen. This makes hemoglobin a less effective delivering agent for oxygen at physiologic gas tensions. In effect, the functional amount of hemoglobin is reduced by replacement with stored red cells at the very time the patient's life is threatened by insufficiency of the oxygen-delivery system. This has led to considerable concern about the functional value of liquid-stored red cells. The exact importance of hemoglobin function within the ranges determined by the loss of 2,3-DPG has not been established, however, despite its theoretical importance. A fair amount of sometimes contradictory data can be summarized as follows: at normal hemoglobin concentrations the change of hemoglobin function within this range produces corresponding changes in mixed venous oxygen tension and in cardiac output, but the ability to perform work and to survive hemorrhage (in animals) is not markedly impaired. With reduced hemoglobin concentrations, however, the ability of animals to perform work and to survive hemorrhage has been related to hemoglobin function. If this pattern of findings holds, we can conclude that the effect of the depletion of 2,3-DPG is less important if hemoglobin concentration and blood volume are maintained near normal.

Moreover, 2,3-DPG is regenerated after transfusion and can be back to normal levels by as soon as 24 hours.

There may be special circumstances in which hemoglobin function becomes critical, such as coronary insufficiency, or a relatively low fixed limit on cardiac output. The question really is one of how much price is worth paying for improved levels of 2,3-DPG in stored blood and under what circumstances this is important. Only further research can answer that.

Acid-Base Imbalance. Stored blood is quite acidotic owing largely to the free citric acid in the anticoagulant and to the formation of lactic acid during storage. The base deficit of stored blood can be 40 mEq/liter. The massively bleeding patient may also be acidotic owing to the formation of lactic acid. Paradoxically, transfusing the stored blood into the acidotic recipient usually restores acid-base balance to normal, or even produces a metabolic alkalosis in the recipient because there are 15 mEq of sodium citrate in each unit of blood that become converted to sodium bicarbonate as the citrate is consumed. The reason for the paradox is that the acids involved are normal intermediary metabolites that are rapidly removed as perfusion is restored. There is no need for adding alkalinizing agents to the management of the heavily transfused patient unless the patient remains seriously hypoperfused. In such a patient, calcium is probably needed as well or even more. Whenever possible, acid-base manipulations should be based on objective measurements. Blood gas analysis should be readily available wherever these patients are cared for.

Hypothermia. In order to raise 10 units of blood from 4° C (the temperature of storage) to 37° C, the body must generate an additional 145 kcal, which represents a requirement for an additional 30 liters of oxygen plus the carbohydrate and fatty substrate. The result is that most heavily transfused patients become cold, a tendency intensified by an air conditioned environment, open body cavities, and paralysis, all of which often pertain during an operation. There is some evidence that cold impairs the metabolism of citrate and lactate, making hypocalcemia and acidosis more likely to occur. The acidosis plus the cold itself may be additive with the transfused blood in producing hyperkalemia. Cold shifts the affinity of hemoglobin for oxygen even further in the direction of impaired function. Hypothermia has a number of other disadvantages not related to massive transfusion.

The technical problem in heating blood is that red cells may lyse at 41° C or above, so that the blood must be rapidly raised from 4° C to 37° C, but the heating surface cannot safely exceed 41° C. This requires either slow flow, which is unacceptable, or a large surface for contact. Several heating devices now available seem to combine effectiveness and safety and should be used during massive transfusion. Hypothermia is an avoidable complication that is unique in that it may worsen many other potential complications of transfusion.

Hyperkalemia. The potassium concentration of old stored blood averages about 30 mEq/liter. This is an impressive number, but this is an excess (above normal) of about 25 mEq/liter of *plasma*. Thus the "excess" potassium in 10 units of blood is about 75 mEq. Since this takes at least an hour to infuse, it is not such an alarming number. The potassium excess, moreover, is "reversible." Most of this extra potassium has leaked out of viable red cells because of inhibition of the sodium-potassium exchange mechanism at 4° C. Upon warming (transfusion) this process reverses, and the transfused stored red cells take up most of the extra potassium within several hours. Heavily transfused patients tend to be hypokalemic, probably as a result of the metabolic and respiratory alkalosis common in these patients. Transient hyperkalemia, however, may increase citrate toxicity.

Microembolization.   Simple observation of the standard filter used for transfusion after the passage of several units of blood will impress upon the observer how much solid debris is present in stored blood. These filters are relatively coarse. Use of finer filters reveals even more debris, of a size large enough to be trapped in the pulmonary microvasculature.

Such material cannot be harmless, but it has been difficult to show significant impairment from this material in transfused primates. Indeed, it has been hard to find the material in the lungs after transfusion. Although some reported that arterial hypoxemia was related to the amount of blood transfused in combat casualties in Vietnam, we could find no such relationship when the type of injury was taken into account. Some experimental models showing considerable benefit from the use of fine filters have had too many artefacts to be convincing. On the other hand, both the primates and the combat casualties had normal pulmonary vascular beds and could have tolerated significant embolization without impairment.

Some currently available fine filters do not seem to impede the rate of transfusion, and therefore can be recommended for use during massive transfusion; but if the clinician finds that using such filters slows the rate of transfusion in an exsanguinating patient, it would be best not to use them until the obtainable rate of transfusion becomes compatible with the patient's needs.

Others.   The other problems in Table 4 have been even less well studied than those discussed, but some may be important. Considerable interest revolves around the possible toxicity of the plasticizers used in the plastic bags in which blood is stored. These devices represent a great practical improvement over the glass bottles in use until less than 20 years ago. The plasticizer, however, leaches into protein-containing fluids at a steady rate, and can be found in the fluids and tissues of transfused patients. The ubiquity of plastics in our culture is such that significant amounts are also found in people who have never been transfused. It is hoped that investigations now under way will answer this very real, practical problem.

TRENDS AND PROJECTIONS

The history of blood banking and of transfusion practices has been one of steadily increasing effectiveness at lower risk to the patient. While the direction of progress is reassuring, the rate of progress is not. Citrate-stored blood is still the mainstay of transfusion therapy. Even the significant improvements resulting from the relatively small modifications represented by CPD took an inordinate amount of time to "reach the bedside." Much of the delay has been at the Federal regulatory level. Some of this has clearly been for the benefit of the patient, but some of it has been difficult to understand.

Given the uncertainties, there are several clear trends in transfusion practice. Component therapy is just beginning to gain wide acceptance, yet is an eminently reasonable way to treat the patient and at the same time make better use of a precious national resource. Sporadically and on a regional basis, but inevitably, most red cell transfusion will soon be given as primarily red cell transfusions, with the unneeded and at times potentially harmful other fractions removed. The use of platelet concentrates has risen markedly in recent years, in part because of the better availability allowed by the use of red cell concentrates. Special plasma fractions and concentrates, particularly for the replacement of specific clotting fractions, have also been used with increasing frequency. Not all of these uses have been rational. Unquestionably the use of albumin remains one of the least scientifically based aspects of transfusion practice, and one that urgently demands more and better data on which to make recommendations.

Much current attention is being devoted to the red cell, to prolong storage in both the liquid and nonliquid states and to tailor hemoglobin function to certain specifications. Some "rejuvenation" formulas are particularly attractive because they combine the salvage of red cells about to be outdated with the production of altered functional states for special purposes. The freezing of red cells has opened new vistas for special purposes, because frozen red cells have an almost indefinite shelf life. Cost factors are such, however, that freezing is not likely to become the standard method for red cell preservation unless some dramatic technical advances are made. Various additives produce specific benefits in liquid-stored red cells, but cost benefit analyses are only beginning to be made and much more evaluation of potential toxicity is needed. Relatively untapped fractions of blood, such as the various classes of leukocytes, are now being harvested, and methods of preservation are being developed.

In all, blood banking appears to be moving at an accelerated rate toward the goal of being able to give the patient what he needs, when he needs it, but the problems in all aspects are still very real. Of all the problems listed, the most important remains the one of having enough blood available when and where it is needed.

SELECTED REFERENCES

Chaplin, H., Beutler, E., Collins, J. A., et al.: Current status of red-cell preservation and availability in relation to the developing national blood policy. N. Engl. J. Med., *291*:68, 1974.

Collins, J. A.: Problems associated with the massive transfusion of stored blood. Surgery, 75:274, 1974.

Greenwalt, T. J., Finch, C. A., Pennell, R. B., et al. (Eds.) General Principles of Blood Transfusion. Chicago, Ill., American Medical Association, 1973.

Jamieson, G. A., and Greenwalt, T. J. (Eds.): Transmissible Disease and Blood Transfusion, National Red Cross Symposium, May 1974, Washington, D.C., New York, Grune and Stratton, 1975.

Mollison, P. L.: Blood Transfusion in Clinical Medicine. 5th Ed. London, Blackwell Scientific Publications, 1972.

National Heart and Lung Institute, Blood Resource Studies: Supply and Use of the Nation's Blood Resource. Vol. 1. Washington, D.C., Department of Health, Education and Welfare Publication No. (NIH) 73–417, June 30, 1972.

Rothschild, M. A., Oratz, M., and Schreiber, S. S.: Albumin metabolism, N. Engl. J. Med., 286:748; 816, 1972.

CHAPTER 11

LABORATORY SERVICES FOR INTENSIVE CARE UNITS

S. R. GAMBINO, M.D.

Laboratory tests are an extension of physical diagnosis. Therefore, it should not be surprising that patients in intensive care units require a multiplicity of laboratory tests.

Laboratory tests amplify and expand the physician's senses, enabling him to "see," "hear," or "feel" things he could not with unaided senses. He cannot, for example, "see," "hear," or "smell" oxygen at toxic levels or at borderline low levels. If he waits until a patient is blue, injury may already have occurred. In monitoring oxygen therapy, therefore, there is no substitute for the laboratory measurement of the partial pressure of oxygen (Po_2).

If we deny a physician a laboratory test, we are in effect cutting off his senses. If, for example, we deny a nephrologist ready access to creatinine measurements, we might just as well deny him physical access to his patients.

In addition to amplifying and expanding the physician's senses, laboratory tests provide feedback information that is essential for correct diagnosis and therapy. Peter Drucker, in his book *Management*,[1] stresses the importance of feedback information if one is to obtain reliable results in any endeavor. Drucker recognized the critical role played by the introduction of the routine autopsy in medical practice 150 years ago. The autopsy served to provide (and should still provide) reliable and essential feedback information to the physician, thereby improving his diagnostic and therapeutic skills. Drucker attributed the rise of modern medical practice to the introduction of the autopsy.

Laboratory testing plays the same essential role as the autopsy does. Laboratory testing provides critical feedback. It is difficult, if not impossi-

143

ble, to control and to correct performance unless feedback is provided. The feedback information required, however, must be timely, relevant, and operational.

Feedback can be immediate, rapid, or delayed. For some laboratory tests, such as blood gases, very rapid feedback is essential. For others, such as tests of thyroid function, feedback can usually be delayed for days.

CLASSES OF LABORATORY SERVICE

From a practical point of view, it is convenient to divide laboratory testing into four classes. On the bases of turn-around time from test to result, the four classes include those tests for which:

1. Immediate feedback is often essential (e.g., blood gases, electrolytes, coagulation studies).

2. Less than one-hour turn-around time is often essential and a 15-minute turn-around is preferable (e.g., glucose, electrolytes, coagulation studies, spinal fluid studies, hematology studies).

3. Same-shift turn-around is highly desirable (e.g., cardiac enzymes and isoenzymes, admission profiles, hematology studies, microbiologic studies, levels of therapeutic drugs).

4. Several-day turn-around is acceptable (e.g., many hormone assays, some trace elements, general screening tests).

These four different turn-around times may require four different types of laboratory service. Immediate feedback is best achieved in a bedside laboratory. One-hour turn-around is best achieved in a stat laboratory. Same-shift turn-around is best achieved in a central laboratory within walking or short riding distance. Several-day turn-around permits regional centralization. There is much confusion in regard to planning and staffing laboratory facilities because these critical turn-around times are forgotten. This confusion can lead to incorrect planning and improper solutions.

Each of these four different types of laboratories can perform some of the functions of the laboratory "above" or "below" it. A bedside laboratory, for example, can perform many stat functions. A stat laboratory can perform some bedside functions and some central laboratory functions. A regional laboratory can perform some central laboratory functions, but it cannot, in most cases, perform any stat or bedside testing. Thus, no single laboratory facility can serve all of the disparate needs of medical practice.

Patients in surgical intensive care units require laboratory services from all four types of laboratories. It is essential, therefore, that the Director of Laboratories and the Chief of Surgery develop a plan for handling bedside, stat, and central testing in a coordinated fashion.

As a minimum standard, every hospital with a surgical intensive care unit should provide 24-hour, 7-day stat testing, with an optimum turn-around time of 15 minutes for some tests, and a maximum turn-around time of one hour for the remainder.

Stat tests to be provided in 1977 would include:

Amylase	Partial thromboplastin time
Bicarbonate	P_{CO_2}
Bilirubin	pH
Chloride	P_{O_2}
Creatinine	Potassium
Fibrinogen	Prothrombin time
Fibrinogen split products	Smear for platelet estimation
Glucose	Sodium
Gram stain of a smear	Spinal fluid for cells, bacteria,
Hemoglobin or hematocrit	glucose, and protein
Leuokocyte count and scan of	Urea
a stained differential smear	Urine examination, qualitative and
Osmolality, urine and serum	micro

A multiplicity of factors affect the quality of patient care in intensive care units. One of these factors is the time it takes to obtain critical laboratory data. If the time it takes for feedback information to arrive is too long, then the information is useless or even misleading. The laboratory should never be the limiting factor that determines the success of treatment. If the acquisition of laboratory data becomes *the* limiting factor, then something is wrong with the system. In order to avoid making the laboratory *the* limiting factor, it is essential that hospital administrators recognize the need to allocate money and resources for special laboratory services.

Where should these tests be carried out, by whom, and under whose direction?

Direction. It is best if the Director of Laboratories for the hospital assumed overall responsibility for all stat laboratory services, no matter where they were performed. The Director of Laboratories should be in charge for several reasons, including licensing requirements of regulatory agencies, broader laboratory experience of the director, greater efficiency in overall use of personnel and equipment in the hospital, and, finally, maintenance in supplying the stat needs of *all* sick patients coming to the hospital.

Since the Director of Laboratories will usually be too busy with many other matters to take personal charge of stat laboratory functions, he should see to it that responsibility for this function is delegated to one of his associates or to an interested and concerned member of the surgical or medical staff. A medical technology supervisor of stat laboratory functions should also be appointed.

Where. Where should the stat laboratory be located? This will depend on the particular design of the hospital. If the central laboratory is close to the surgical ICU, the stat laboratory can be located in a section of the central laboratory. If, on the other hand, distance is too great, then serious consideration should be given to the establishment of a separate stat laboratory within or near the surgical areas that care for critically ill patients.

Ideally, of course, in a well designed hospital, all critical care areas as well as the emergency room, the operating room, and the recovery room will be located close to the central laboratory and the radiology department. Few hospitals, however, are blessed with such good fortune.

Departments of pathology, surgery, medicine, and anesthesiology need to develop *interactive* rather than exclusive laboratory systems. It is not healthy, for example, for an institution to have a *completely separate* central laboratory run by a Director of Laboratories and a *completely separate* stat laboratory run by a Director of Anesthesiology. Such a situation indicates that the Director of Laboratories has not fulfilled his responsibility to the surgical staff and vice versa.

A useful mechanism for bridging the potential gap between the central laboratory and the intensive care unit laboratory is to work under the following guidelines:

1. The principle that *some* laboratory testing is required in the intensive care unit *must* be accepted by all.

2. The equipment that is to be used in the peripheral location is bought, owned, and maintained by the central laboratory.

3. The central laboratory provides training, quality control, and maintenance programs for the peripheral laboratory.

4. The Director of Laboratories will delegate to one of the laboratory supervisors the responsibility for maintaining liaison with the peripheral unit.

5. The Director of Surgery or Anesthesiology will likewise appoint a single responsible individual in the peripheral unit to be responsible for maintaining liaison with the central laboratory. The system will not work unless it is clear *who* is responsible at each end. The *who* can be almost any responsible person (nurse, inhalation therapist, doctor, aide) who works in the unit full-time and is expected to be there for at least a year.

Who.   If a separate stat laboratory is established, or if a section of the central laboratory is devoted to stat work, then the facility is best staffed by laboratory technologists. The minimum number of people required to run a stat laboratory 24 hours a day, 7 days a week is easy to calculate. If at least one technologist is on duty at all times, 8760 hours of technologist time is required per year (24 hours × 365 days). Since the average technologist is productive for no more than 7 hours a day, 10 months per year (considering vacation, holiday, and sick time, as well as the time needed to replace a person who leaves), each technologist will be productive for approximately 1500 hours per year. This means a minimum of six technologists are needed to do the work and one supervisor is required to oversee the operation. Thus, the *minimum* skeleton staff for a stat laboratory requires funding for seven positions.

It should be obvious that a multiplicity of separate stat laboratories, in or near each intensive care unit and staffed by laboratory technologists, is a costly solution to the problem. Even if cost is not a factor, there is still the problem of "adequacy of service." Each of the separate laboratories, with only one technologist on duty at any one time, is incapable of providing more than the "bare bones" essentials. How, then, does that laboratory expand its services? How does the laboratory, for example, introduce new services such as therapeutic drug level monitoring? If the staff for the stat laboratory comes out of a larger central pool under the direction of a single responsible head, then it is easier to provide expanded services.

For laboratory work performed within intensive care units we require a new cadre of *nurse-technicians*. Who, for example, should draw blood from a patient in the emergency room? Should it be a laboratory technologist who must spend 15 minutes traveling to and fro, only to find the patient in the bathroom, or should it be a member of the nursing staff assigned to the emergency room? Who, for example, should taken an emergency electrocardiogram? An ECG technologist who spends about 30 minutes going to and fro, only to find the patient has gone to an x-ray examination, or a member of the nursing staff on duty in the ICU who is with the patient most of the time? Who, for example, should collect blood from an artery or an arterial line, and perform an analysis by pushing a button on a completely automated blood-gas machine? Who should take readings on pressure monitors? Who should tweak the dials of respirators?

In 1977, the care of the acutely ill patient requires more than backrubs, smiles, starched uniforms, and clean sheets. It is impossible to separate the care of the sick patient from the monitoring of therapy, and monitoring always requires measurement.

Those measurements that are required immediately should be performed by members of the nursing staff assigned to the unit. Directors of nursing should support the development of nurse-technicians. These nurse-technicians already exist in many institutions. They have arisen de novo in order to fill a pressing need, and they can be found under many guises in most special-care units.

Diagnostic Gluttony.   Should a physician be permitted to order *any* test at any time? I think not. Considering that the laboratory is simply an extension of physical diagnosis allows understanding of why laboratory testing must be limited.

Can a physician examine any patient at any time, and perform any diagnostic maneuver he wishes? Of course not. To begin with, patients and relatives would call a halt if they thought there was unneeded hurt or abuse. Patients or family would also question the physician if the physical examination failed to cover areas of the body from which the patients' complaints arose. Furthermore, and most important, the physician is acutely aware of finite resources. The physician has only so much time for each patient and only a limited number of examinations can be performed in that finite time. Moreover, the physician selects those diagnostic procedures that training and experience have taught him are most effective in resolving diagnostic and therapeutic problems. In short, the examining physician does not do everything possible.

When it comes to laboratory tests, however, a physician may act as if he were a glutton for diagnostic input. This physician tends to experience the laboratory in the same way he experiences air and water—as an infinite resource. Air, water, and the laboratory are always there when needed and apparently inexhaustible. A simple, effortless, painless stroke of the pen is all that is needed to command the resources of the laboratory. It is not the physician's money that is used to pay for the test. It is not the physician's aides who perform the work to supply the test results. The laboratory is not experienced directly (which is still another reason for supporting direct involvement in laboratory testing by members of the ICU team). The laboratory is too often out of sight and therefore out of mind.

Today, over two billion laboratory tests are performed each year in the United States, and triple that volume is predicted by 1980. But will this projected tripling mean a tripling of benefits to be derived from laboratory testing? Probably not. Too often laboratory studies are neither carefully planned nor thoughtfully evaluated. Laboratory directors and clinicians must work together to improve the rational use of laboratory resources. The central laboratory is often overburdened with too much routine and unnecessary testing and is thereby unable to provide the full range of services required for the care of the acutely ill patient.

How, then, can a physician decide whether a laboratory test is worth ordering? Or in other words, how good should a laboratory test be? If a laboratory test is to be more useful than a good history and physical examination are, then it should have greater sensitivity and specificity than the history and physical examination have. Dr. Marc Silverstein, while on an elective in our laboratory, searched the medical literature for data on the sensitivity and specificity of a variety of procedures. Sensitivity is defined as the percentage positivity of a test in diseased subjects. A test with 100 per cent sensitivity would be positive in *all* patients with the disease. Specificity is defined as the percentage negativity in the absence of a specific disease. A test with 100 per cent specificity would be negative in *all* subjects free of a specific disease. Dr. Silverstein's findings are as follows:

Test or Function	Sensitivity (%)	Specificity (%)	Sum
Rectal examination for prostatic carcinoma	24	94	118
Physical examination for splenomegaly	28	98	126
Physical examination for hepatomegaly	71	62	133
Blood alcohol for alcoholic liver disease	40	100	140
History and physical examination for chronic obstructive lung disease	64	81	145
Film mammography vs. biopsy	72	75	147
Physical examination in breast cancer detected by x-ray study	68	81	149
History of smoking in cancer of lung	100	67	167
Blood test for lactose intolerance	76	96	172
History of drinking for alcoholic liver disease	76	100	176
History of diarrhea after lactose	100	88	188
Immunologic test for pregnancy (excluding ectopic, third trimester, and menopause)	100	96	196

These data indicate why many laboratory tests are replacing the physical examination. The laboratory test is superior to the physical examination. But these data also show that the history may often be better than the average laboratory test. If a laboratory test is to be better than the history, and if it is to be effective and efficient, then the laboratory test should have a combined sensitivity and specificity greater than 190 per cent.

The predictive value of a test, that is, the percentage of positive results that are true positives, will vary greatly with sensitivity, specificity, and prevalence. Prevalence is the single most important, but most neglected, factor affecting the predictive value of a test. For example, if you have a test with a sensitivity of 95 per cent and a specificity of 95 per cent, the predictive value varies with prevalence thus:[3]

PREVALENCE(%)	PREDICTIVE VALUE (%)
1	16.1
2	27.9
5	50.0
50	95.0

The experienced clinician has always known that a good physical examination and an excellent history are essential components of good medical care. The history and the physical examination increase the prevalence of disease in the population selected for testing, and thereby increase the predictive value of any test procedure applied to this selected population.

Finally, the laboratory is not a substitute for clinical judgment. As Alvan Feinstein has said, "Because contemporary clinicians have become preoccupied with the technology available for pathologic diagnosis, the 'science' produced by the technology has often obscured the difference between precise function in a machine and in a human mind."[2]

REFERENCES

1. Drucker, P. F.: Management. New York, Harper and Row, 1974, p. 268.
2. Feinstein, A. R.: Clinical Judgment. Baltimore, Williams and Wilkins Company, 1967, p. 362.
3. Galen, R. S., and Gambino, S. R.: Beyond Normality. New York, John Wiley, 1975.

CHAPTER 12

INFECTION HAZARD OF SURGICAL INTENSIVE CARE: Isolation Procedures in the Surgical Intensive Care Unit

STANLEY M. LEVENSON, M.D.

HAROLD LAUFMAN, M.D.

The hazard in intensive care units of nosocomial infection, i.e., one that develops during hospitalization and is not present or incubating at the time of admission to the hospital, has been acknowledged almost since the inception of such units. However, it has not been until recently that the scope of this problem has been appreciated and efforts have been made to cope with it. A number of reasons for this delay are apparent. In the original concept of intensive care, visual surveillance took precedence over many other aspects of care. This led to the development of the open ward type of unit, or, more accurately, a reversion back to the Florence Nightingale open ward with only token recognition of the need for isolation of a few patients. Another reason for delay in coping with the infection hazard of intensive care units is the relative paucity of good quantitative data on the extent of this hazard.

DEFINING THE PROBLEM

The problem of nosocomial infection in the surgical intensive care unit appears to be epitomized by a vulnerable host in a hostile environment. What are the chances of a patient in such a unit acquiring an infection? How

Supported in part by NIH Grant No. 5 K06 GM14208 (S.M.L., Rearch Career Award) and Department of the Army Contract No. DADA 17–70–C to the Albert Einstein College of Medicine.

long must a patient be in a surgical intensive care unit (ICU) before his or her chance of getting an infection is statistically greater than the chance of not getting an infection? What preventive measures have been proved, or are likely to be proved, valid? What is the cost/effectiveness ratio of such preventive measures?

INCIDENCE OF NOSOCOMIAL INFECTIONS

Cross-contamination leading to nosocomial infections is an important problem in all hospitals, and nowhere are these problems likely to be more frequent and severe than in surgical intensive care units. There are, however, surprisingly few hard data on the incidence and consequences of cross-contamination and cross-infection in surgical intensive care units.

The overall incidence of nosocomial infections in hospitals in the United States has been estimated to be about 6 per cent of all admissions; the incidence of such infections in surgical ICUs is acknowledged to be substantially higher, but just how much higher is not known, and it probably varies considerably from hospital to hospital, just as the incidence of postoperative wound infection does. It is not surprising that acquisition of infection by patients in surgical ICUs is unusually high, since the sickest surgical patients—and these are often the sickest patients in the entire hospital—are cared for in the surgical intensive care unit. Many of these patients have incipient or existing infections, and thus represent a threat to both other patients and the staff.

Whether or not a nosocomial infection develops depends, at the very least, on the following: (1) contamination of the patient with a potentially pathogenic microbe not present in the patient at the time of admission; (2) the nature, virulence, and numbers of the contaminating pathogen and of competing microorganisms already being harbored by the patient; and (3) the resistance of the host, that is, the status of the defense systems of the patient, immunologic (humoral and cellular) and nonimmunologic, local and systemic, and inherited and acquired.

The host-microbe interactions, and therefore the clinical consequences, including the occurrence of infection and its severity, are affected by a variety of factors, high on the list of which are various metabolic, nutritional, and therapeutic factors, some of which precede, accompany, and follow the host-microbe confrontation. Surgical patients, especially those in the ICU, differ from most nonsurgical patients, including those in the medical ICU, in that the surgical patients generally have traumatic or operative wounds, factors which increase enormously their vulnerability to infection.

One of the more definitive studies of microbial surveillance in a surgical ICU was published in 1974 by Northey and associates,[43] who carried out a prospective study of patients in an open ward type of surgical ICU. This unit was typical of such units in many hospitals in that it was crowded, had poor ventilation, and the patients in it seemed to have a high incidence of infections.

Northey and her colleagues found that the risk of colonization and infection increased significantly with length of stay of the patient in the surgical ICU. For example, after 3 days, the risk of unit-acquired colonization was 50 per cent, and the risk of infection was 23 per cent. At 10 days, the risk of colonization was over 90 per cent, and that of infection was 72 per cent. Colonization was most frequent in the upper respiratory and urinary tracts, while infection occurred most frequently in the urinary tract. Klebsiella species and Enterobacter most frequently colonized the throat, whereas *Pseudomonas aeruginosa* and Klebsiella species most frequently colonized tracheostomy wounds. *Pseudomonas aeruginosa* and *Escherichia coli* were the most frequent colonizers of the urinary tract. Among infected patients, the most common organism was *Pseudomonas aeruginosa,* followed by *E. coli,* Klebsiella, and Enterobacter species.

Thus, from this study and reports of others,[20] it appears that the most common nosocomial infections in surgical intensive care units are urinary tract infections, just as in other patient areas of the hospital. The next most common are pulmonary infections,[27] followed by surgical-wound infections, and septic phlebitis, often with bacteremia. The majority of these infections are ordinarily associated with some type of procedure or manipulation, as will be discussed later in this chapter.

The data of Northey also are consistent with those of many investigators[5,8,17,28] who have described the changing nature of the microorganisms of hospital-acquired infections. The last 15 years have seen a substantial decrease in the isolation of *Staphylococcus aureus* as the causative bacterial species, concomitant with a significant increase in gram-negative bacilli, including certain microorganisms which in the past had been considered "nonpathogens," such as *Serratia marcescens*. The reasons for this phenomenon have been discussed at length by a number of investigators,[5,8,28] who cite the fact that the early antibiotics were much more effective against gram-positive than against gram-negative bacteria. This is not meant to imply that staphylococcal infections have disappeared. On the contrary, *Staphylococcus aureus* persists, and we must be on guard to prevent its arising in the next decade or so in altered form to cause even greater problems than in the past.[18,19] Rosendal,[51] for example, reports from Denmark that more than 40 per cent of the *Staphylococcus aureus* organisms isolated from blood of patients are now resistant to the semisynthetic penicillins as exemplified by methicillin. Feingold[19] has expressed the fear that if penicillinase-resistant penicillins lose their effect in combating a staphylococcal infection, dire problems will result.

Fungal infections, especially due to *Candida albicans,* are increasing in frequency and pose difficult prophylactic and therapeutic problems.[9,48]

VECTORS OF MICROBES LEADING TO NOSOCOMIAL INFECTIONS

The sources of intensive care unit–acquired infection can be traced largely to other patients and personnel in the unit, to respiratory equipment, to intravenous and urinary catheters, and endotracheal and tracheal tubes, and to wash sinks and utility areas. Other causes, such as contaminated medications and solutions and contaminated shaving equipment, are much less frequent.

Contact and *fomitic* spread of virulent organisms to patients is more important than *air-borne spread*. It is generally agreed, and reconfirmed by the Northey study[43] and by studies by Laufman and associates[33] and others,[40] that the *prime vectors in the transmission of microbial contamination are the personnel who work in these units, and that the main route of contamination is direct contact.*

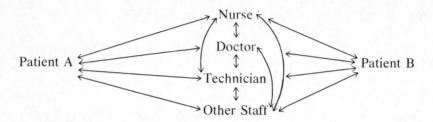

Failure of the staff to observe proper aseptic and hygienic practices, including hand washing, the wearing of gloves, and other precautions, is the primary factor. Human errors and breaks in technique occur all too frequently, with resultant microbial cross-contamination.

Fomitic spread from staff, patients, beds, dressings, and nebulizers is another important factor. For example, a reservoir of contamination discovered by Laufman and his associates is the hair of personnel working in the ICU. They found clear evidence that the hair of the personnel acquired bacteria from the environment in the course of a day's work, and that the bacteria were shed with motion of the head.

As a result of these observations, the recommendation was made that all ICU personnel routinely wear some type of head covering, or snood, which contains the hair. Similarly, all available evidence indicates that the personnel should wear clean scrub apparel similar to that worn in an operating room. Visiting professional and nonprofessional people should don clean gowns before entering a surgical ICU.

Group A streptococcus, *E. coli,* and most other enteric bacteria are spread almost exclusively by direct contact and fomites.[22] *Pseudomonas aeruginosa* is often spread by contaminated fluids, e.g., from nebulizers, sinks, and medications.[55]

Microbial cross-contamination by the *air-borne* route occurs, but less frequently than by the contact or fomitic routes. Numerous studies of the air-borne route of microbial spread have been carried out, and it appears that pneumococci, staphylococci, tubercle bacilli, and certain fungi and viruses are among the microorganisms commonly spread by this route.[54,64,65]

A number of agencies have issued guidelines for the design of intensive care units that require a window to be adjacent to every bed. These guidelines were originally drawn up for cardiac intensive care units and, unfortunately, were carried over to surgical intensive care units. Windows were considered an amenity to help orient a bedridden patient to the outside environment as a psychological lift. Certainly, this point cannot be faulted, except for the fact that when windows are present, the tendency to open them always exists, especially in the summertime and in the absence of appropriate air conditioning. Laufman[32] has shown cultures of bacteria, fungi, and yeasts among a heavy bacterial growth on culture plates exposed in intensive care rooms when the windows were open. Such contaminants may pose a serious threat to patients when open wounds are dressed or other invasive procedures are carried out.

Nor are window air conditioners necessarily an appropriate method of air handling in ICUs. An unusual source of pneumonitis was reported as being due to contamination of a window air conditioner.[7] Twenty-seven people developed symptoms interpreted to be those of hypersensitivity pneumonitis. Examination of the environment revealed contamination of the air conditioning system with a thermophilic actinomycete known to cause hypersensitivity pneumonitis, such as farmer's lung. Other defective air conditioning systems have been shown to deliver high concentrations of Aspergillus spores into operating rooms.[21]

NOSOCOMIAL AND MICROBIAL CONTAMINATION AND INFECTIONS CONSEQUENT TO OR CONDITIONED BY CERTAIN PROCEDURES

The presence of foreign bodies (e.g., intravenous catheters, urinary catheters, endotracheal tubes, tracheostomy tubes) all place the patient at increased risk to infection.

One of the procedures that has been studied sufficiently to define traceable reasons for reduction of infection is bladder catheterization. Andriole and associates[6] showed that institution of a sterile, closed system, or a sterile three-lumen system employing bladder rinses with antimicrobial solutions, resulted in a striking reduction in bacteremias over the use of the Foley catheter. Documented gram-negative rod bacteremias fell by 24 per cent, and those occurring within 10 days of indwelling bladder catheter insertion fell by 77 per cent.

The long-term continuous parenteral feeding of critically ill and injured patients carries certain risks of contamination and consequent infections, bacterial and fungal.[12,16,52] Bacteremia and local septic thrombosis and phlebitis are perhaps the most common complications of central venous catheterization, and the longer the plastic catheter is left in place, the more these septic complications are apt to occur. Special aseptic precautions in the insertion and follow-up care of indwelling venous catheters and in the preparation of the infusates lessen the hazards.

Respiratory tract contamination is most frequently due to breaks in technique by personnel or by improperly decontaminated and sterilized equipment. The vulnerability of the patient with an endotracheal tube or tracheostomy tube to cross-infection resulting from failure of the staff to use strict aseptic and atraumatic techniques in suctioning, changing tubes and tubing, and the like is well documented. Ventilatory assist apparatus and nebulizing equipment have been shown to be the cause of gram-negative bacillary necrotizing pneumonia.[49] Pierce and associates[45] demonstrated that when proper decontamination of nebulization equipment is carried out, the incidence of necrotizing pneumonitis is reduced.

PREVENTION OF SURGICAL INTENSIVE CARE UNIT–ACQUIRED INFECTION

Three approaches to prevention of infections in the ICU become apparent: protecting patients from pathogens; strengthening the resistance of the host; and treating established infections better. The following discussions will be limited to the first of these approaches; the other two are discussed in other chapters of this volume, and elsewhere.[1,4]

About a year ago, one of the authors wrote to about 50 directors of surgical departments, inquiring about the measures taken on their surgical intensive care units for the prevention and control of cross-contamination and asking for some assessment of the effectiveness of these measures. The replies ranged from very brief statements of one or two paragraphs which included statements that the problem was under complete control or completely out of control, to very long descriptions (in some cases up to 50 pages) of very detailed instructions, generally identical with those published by the Center for Disease Control, U.S. Department of Health, Education, and Welfare. In only a very few of the replies was there any suggestion that some critical prospective or retrospective assessments of the extent and level of competence of the prescribed policies and practices were being carried out, or how effective the measures were in the prevention and control of intensive care unit–acquired infections.

Intensive Care Unit Utilization.   It was apparent also from the replies that in most hospitals, seriously ill patients are generally transferred postoperatively from a recovery unit to an ICU. Other patients may bypass the recovery ward and be sent directly to the ICU. In some hospitals, the recovery unit and the surgical ICU are one and the same. When a recovery unit is run on a part-time basis, patients operated on in the afternoon or evening are taken directly to an ICU, usually located some distance from the operating room, and, like its recovery room counterpart, designed with virtually no isolation of patients, thus exposing the vulnerable postoperative patient to patients with established or potential infections. Some recovery rooms and ICUs have rules under which a patient with a serious infection cannot be admitted to the surgical intensive care unit, and is then sent directly to a general nursing floor, at times with inadequate attention to the patient's physiologic status or to isolation precautions. It is unjust, in our view, that a seriously ill patient should be deprived of optimal care simply because he harbors an infection. It is apparent that if every bed in a recovery room or in an intensive care unit were potentially an "isolation" bed (that is, the unit was so designed as to permit control of cross-contamination), all critically ill patients, with or without infections, could be given the same high quality of care in the ICU.

Architectural Configuration. Almost regardless of the source of pathogens in an ICU (the patients themselves are the single largest source), it is generally agreed, as mentioned, that the prime vectors of transmission of cross-infection are the personnel who work in these units. Therefore, it is obvious that every effort should be made to train all personnel in preventive hygienic measures, and to create an environment in which such measures can be carried out expeditiously. Unfortunately, the majority of current surgical intensive care units are poorly programed, with minimal architectural modifications of previously existing ward space. Most existing units are of the open ward type; others may consist of several rooms rather than one large room, and the number of patients in a given room may be limited to two to four. The beds in many such existing ICUs are often as close as two or three feet from one another, sometimes separated by cloth curtains, sometimes not. Traffic of professional personnel and visitors, as well as housekeeping and food employees, is almost constant. The air is often poorly circulated, stagnant, and occasionally odoriferous. Because sinks are inconveniently located and generally there is only one in a room, attendants, nurses, and physicians all too frequently go from patient to patient, examining and treating them, without washing their own hands.

In a typical current ICU, draw-curtains are available, ostensibly to provide privacy. It is obvious that when the curtains are open, patients are exposed to the disturbances of noise and activity in the ward in addition to cross-infection. When the curtains are drawn, patients are not protected against either noise or cross-contamination, but surveillance is limited. Generally, the room must be illuminated at all hours of the day and night for one or more of the patients, often with great disturbance to the other patients. If one patient requires cardiopulmonary resuscitation, all other patients are fully aware of it.

Many ICUs have one or two "isolation" rooms for the care and containment of patients with certain severe infections or for the care and protection of patients particularly susceptible to infection. However, such rooms, when available, are usually remote from the nurse's desk in a distant part of the ICU, thus limiting surveillance. The time-consuming use of caps, gowns, masks, boots, gloves, and the like, when enforced, often limits the number of visits as well as the time the physicians spend with the patients.

The paucity of hard data on prevention measures against nosocomial infection is the result of difficulties in evaluating new procedures in a complex clinical situation. Variations in the causative agents, the types of patient, and the work ethic of personnel are only some samples of factors that make evaluation difficult. A number of epidemiologic studies of nosocomial infections of patients on general wards have been carried out, however, from time to time, and many of these have shown, according to Williams,[65] that many of the procedures commonly employed in hospitals are more ritual than helpful.

A major aim of the architectural design of the surgical ICU should be to make the control of nosocomial infections possible and practical. We believe two complementary approaches will go a long way toward meeting this aim: (1) single bed cubicles and rooms with controlled air flow and filtration and convenient wash sinks are important architectural requirements; the judicious use of ultraviolet light may prove valuable, and (2) the use of whole or partial body isolators and transfer isolators.

It must be understood, however, that *architectural changes* alone cannot be expected to be a solution to the nosocomial infection problem. A sine qua non to success is the diligence with which special care personnel *adhere to known principles and techniques of preventive hygiene*. The cubicle and single-room design and the use of isolators will make it easier for them to do so.

SINGLE BED CUBICLES AND ROOMS.   We believe each bed in special care areas should be in an individual cubicle or room with windowed walls, or in an isolator. The windows between cubicles can be placed high enough so that one patient cannot see another from his position in bed. A minimum of 150 square feet should be provided for every cubicle. This would give adequate space around the bed for virtually any type of emergency care, including the use of large-size equipment. A fold-away front enhances space but is not mandatory if the door is wide enough to permit passage of a bed with ease. These cubicles should be arranged so that a wash sink is accessible near the entrance of each cubicle. The sink can be placed either just inside the entrance to each cubicle or between every two such cubicles. Over the entrance to each cubicle, an ultraviolet light may be installed to help provide microbiologically cleaner air where the ultraviolet rays strike. Typical ICU rooms or cubicles are now available with relatively low-cost prefabricated walls, closely resembling the cubicles of coronary care units as recommended by the Intersociety Commission on Heart Disease Resources. A number of surgical ICUs built with this design are already in use, and more are being planned.

Although as far as we are aware no studies have been published comparing the infection pattern in an open ICU with that in a compartmentalized unit, a number of studies have been published on comparison of an open ward with that of a subdivided ward for general hospital patients. Perhaps the most definitive of such studies was that by Whyte, Howie, and Eakin,[63] in which the rate of nasal acquisition of new strains of *Staphylococcus aureus* was compared for patients in a subdivided hospital ward that had controlled ventilation with two open wards that had natural ventilation. They found that the rate of acquisition of new nasal *Staphylococcus aureus* strains by patients who stayed two weeks or less was somewhat lower in the partitioned ward than in the open ward. However, there was no corresponding reduction in the rate of acquisition of tetracycline-resistant staphylococci or in the proportion of patients who became carriers of resistant strains. Nor was there evidence that the risk of postoperative wound sepsis due to *Staphylococcus aureus* was less in the compartmentalized ward. The study loses much of its applicability to the question of design of the intensive care unit for the prevention of cross-contamination when one realizes that there were no sinks between the compartments for hand washing, and no data are presented on the hygienic practices of personnel, both integral parts of the compartment design.

In previous studies, Williams[64] and Lindwell and coworkers[39] showed that in subdivided wards, the acquisition of *Staphylococcus aureus* by patients occurred at a lower rate than had been previously observed in open wards. Parker and coworkers[44] studied some aspects of cross-contamination on an infectious disease ward where patients were barrier-nursed in separate cubicles that opened onto a veranda; there was little, if any, transference of *Staphylococcus aureus* from patient to patient.

None of these studies was carried out in an intensive care unit in which personnel would have access to a wash sink located between patient cubicles, and where hand washing by personnel between patients would be mandatory. A comparative study is now in progress in which this type of configuration and monitored hygienic activity is being compared with the situation in an open ICU with respect to nosocomial colonization and infection.[33] At the time of this writing, results are not yet available, but there are indications that the advantages of the single cubicle and room construction will prove significantly more effective.

Air Handling.   The air-borne route of contamination is statistically less critical than the contact and fomitic routes, but, of course, that does not mean that the air-borne route is to be overlooked. Studies by many investigators have repeatedly reconfirmed the fact that the greater the air interchange or the better the ventilation in a room, the lower the bacterial count in the air. Modular ventilation systems, including so-called laminar airflow systems, were designed in the 1950s and 1960s to provide high-speed unidirectional airflow. Their value is still unproved. Lowbury[40] and later Shooter[53] demonstrated that when burn dressings were changed, or when operations were performed in well ventilated rooms, cross-contamination and infection rates were lower than when the same procedures were performed under poorly ventilated conditions. However, the correlation between types of bacteria found in the air and those found in infected wounds was poor,[26] except in unusual situations of massive contamination of the environment.[21,61]

The first requisite of air handling in a surgical ICU is that it provide good ventilation. This implies an exchange of at least 12 to 15 air changes per hour for every bed area. If the beds are in cubicles or rooms, it is important that the exhaust air from the rooms not be directed to the center of the nurses' work area in order not to endanger personnel with contaminated air. Where this configuration exists, the exhausted air should be filtered as it leaves such rooms. In large common wards containing many beds, good air circulation is more difficult to achieve. Much of the success or failure of the air handling in such units depends on directionality of air flow, temperature, humidity, and the maintenance of the equipment. For example, the air should enter the room from the center of the ceiling, not from the walls where it may flow across one patient before it reaches another. Air should be exhausted at the walls no higher than four feet off the floor. Exhaust grilles should be large, and the exhaust ducts should be outfitted with air pumps to provide active directionality to the exhausted air and to prevent backflow. Temperature should be adjustable between 68 and 76° F. Humidity should be stabilized between 50 and 55 per cent. Filtration of incoming air need not be of the high-efficiency (HEPA) type, but it should be effective and in conformity with code requirements. Up to 80 per cent may be recirculated with appropriate air handling capability.

STANDARD ISOLATION TECHNIQUES

We will not detail in this chapter the indications and recommendations for the isolation of certain patients, the degree of isolation required (e.g., strict, respiratory, protective, enteric, or wound and skin), and the descriptions of standard isolation techniques. These have been published in extensive form in a readable and clear monograph by the National Communicable Disease Center of the U.S. Department of Health, Education and Welfare, Public Health Service.[11] This monograph is readily available by writing to the agency. In addition, these isolation techniques have been described in a very recent book dealing with surgical infections prepared by the Pre- and Postoperative Care Committee of the American College of Surgeons.[4]

The main point we would like to emphasize is that the problem generally is not so much lack of knowledge of what to do on the part of the hospital staff, but, rather, failure to carry out the recommended aseptic and hygienic measures, even so simple a matter as hand washing in between patients and the wearing of gloves. Unfortunately, this failure often begins at the senior attending level and then filters down through junior attending physicians, the house staff, the nursing staff, the technicians, and the housekeeping staff. The net result is that the personnel become the chief vectors of the microorganisms, leading to cross-contamination and cross-infection, the spread being by direct contact as already mentioned. *An ambience must be developed whereby appropriate practices are "second nature" to all, and human errors are minimized.*

ISOLATORS

The use of mechanical means to isolate individuals (or parts of individuals) from exogenous microbial contamination by all routes or for the containment of the microbial pathogens of an infected patient offers a degree of reliability substantially greater than that provided by any of the other methods so far described. Thus, the usual current techniques of isolation employed in hospitals are not altogether satisfactory; when strictly applied, they may interfere with patient care by inhibiting frequent physician visits, they are expensive, and they are of limited effectiveness. They require an inordinate degree of physician and nurse cooperation, care, and attention to detail. Almost always, they are only partially applied, and their effectiveness is thereby diminished.

Laminar airflow is a fairly effective means of reducing air-borne contamination, but as already pointed out, by itself it cannot control contact or fomitic contamination, routes which are of major importance in the spread of infection. For control of the latter, the laminar airflow technique must be supplemented by the type of conventional isolation techniques (gowns, masks, gloves, boots) currently used in hospitals, techniques known to be fraught with difficulties and deficiencies.

Conceptually, mechanical barrier isolation is a logical solution to the problem of cross-contamination by exogenous microorganisms. Effective barrier isolation can prevent bacterial transfer from the environment to the patient, whether the contamination is air-borne, by direct contact, or fomitic. Isolators have been shown to be effective by work with a wide variety of experimental animals which have been maintained free of known bacteria, parasites, and fungi for many years in laboratories all over the world. The underlying principle making this possible is the absolute separation of the animals from the outside environment by a mechanical barrier and the provision of sterile air, food, and water. It matters little whether the mechanical barrier or isolator is made of heavy stainless steel or thin flexible plastic film so long as it prevents the transfer of microorganisms. It is this fact, namely the effectiveness of the thin plastic barrier, which has made possible the application of the techniques of the germ-free laboratory to problems of patient care, including intensive patient care.

An advantage of the isolator system is its intellectual simplicity; the impermeable but transparent plastic barrier between the patient and the environment permits necessary medical and nursing care, and minimizes accidental contamination by human error. Further, there is evidence that the environmental temperature and humidity within an enclosure affect to an important degree many metabolic and physiologic functions of seriously injured and ill patients, and thereby affect the resistance of such patients to infection. The isolator technique offers the ready control of environmental temperature and humidity. Another advantage of isolators over conventional isolation techniques is a saving of nurses' and physicians' time. Isolators also are likely to become more economical as designs improve and their use increases.

A series of isolators has been developed, generally made of flexible plastic film based on principles established in the germ-free laboratory. These include surgical,[34] whole-body, partial-body, and transfer isolators for use in the operating rooms, on the wards, and in the surgical intensive care unit.[14,30,35,36,42,50,56-58]

Complicated surgical operations can be carried out effectively by the isolator technique. Sick patients with severe injuries can be provided with microbial protection by being cared for in isolators on the wards for long periods. The use of isolators is readily integrated into the total care program for the patients. Various types of isolators may be used in conjunction with one another to provide a system for patient care in controlled environments throughout the critical periods of hospitalization.

The isolators for the bed-care of patients differ from those used in operating rooms in that the patient may be housed either entirely or in part inside the isolator, and the isolation may be maintained for comparatively long periods of time up to many months or years.

Available isolators vary in design, depending upon the specific clinical application, including the observational and manipulative requirements posed by a patient's illness or injury. The isolators range from simple gloved "bags" to protect anatomic areas of limited extent, to whole-body bed isolators and to room isolators in which patients may be maintained and treated for long periods. Some of the whole-body bed isolators are completely sealed units;[35,36] others are open at the bottom, but microbial contamination from below is prevented[14,58] by means of special design features and the use of vertical directional airflow.

A group of representative isolators is based upon the model originally described by Levenson, Trexler and associates.[35] This type of isolator has been used for the care of seriously ill surgical patients, i.e., those with very extensive deep burns, who require maximum medical and nursing care.

This type of isolator provides microbial security by means of a physical barrier that requires a minimum of changes in the pattern of movements necessary for medical and nursing care. Spatial requirements are also kept to a minimum so that the isolator can be used on a ward or in a room without structural modifications of the room. The body of this isolator is supported by a traction frame attached to the bed. The clear PVC film is approximately 0.1 to 0.2 mm thick, 200 cm high, and the length of a hospital bed. The framework attaches to the bed itself, and the framework can be folded readily so that the isolator can pass through hospital doors. The sides of the isolator usually extend 30 cm beyond the edge of the bed in order to provide room for the attendants in half-suits, but the sides are close enough to the patient to make gauntlet positions serviceable. If the patient can get out of bed, one side of the isolator may be extended an additional 30 cm or more to provide the necessary space (Fig. 1).

Because the plastic envelope is supported by a metal frame, it requires minimal internal air pressure to maintain its shape. Air entering the isolator is sterilized by mechanical filtration, and air leaving the isolator can be sterilized by a small incinerator, a chemical germicidal trap, or mechanical filtration. Sterilizing the outgoing air is important to prevent egress of microorganisms into the room air when patients with infections or carriers of virulent pathogens are housed in the isolators. An air pressure–flow sensor alarm system warns of any failure in air flow into and out of the isolator. The partial pressure of CO_2 in the isolator may also be monitored, but is not required. For patients with severe infections, a slightly negative pressure can be maintained within the envelope.

One or more half-suits and one or more gauntlet positions are attached to each side of the isolator. The half-suits permit physicians and nurses to reach everywhere within the isolator and to provide nursing and medical procedures no matter how complicated (Fig. 2). Gloves are attached to the half-suits at the wrists by means of rigid cuffs so that the gloves may be changed from the inside without contamination. The half-suits are usually attached to the side walls of the isolator. It is also possible to attach a half-suit to the patient entry port at the head of the isolator if necessary for special procedures, such as repeated bronchoscopies on a burned patient with serious respiratory tract injury.

The medical and nursing staff have felt that the half-suits allowed them to care for very sick patients and to have closer physical contact with the patient, much better than gauntlets alone, thus giving the patient a greater sense of security. This is particularly important in caring for children. The half-suits make it possible for the nurse to cuddle and mother a child in the isolator. Ventilation with controlled temperature and air flow is supplied to each half-suit.

The half-suits provide almost unrestricted mobility, but many nursing procedures demand a number of short-work sequences that do not require a great deal of mobility. For these functions, modified gauntlet positions are provided (Fig. 3). These are short truncated cones, made of frosty PVC or flexible polyurethane film attached at the large end to the isolator wall, and to standard gloves at the other end by the same sort of specially formed plastic cuff as used in the half-suits. These gloves can be changed without fear of contamination of the inside of the isolator in a manner similar to that used for surgical isolators. Moderately heavy rubber gloves are used for many procedures, but standard surgical gloves are used for more complicated and delicate procedures, such as venous cut-downs.

The modified gauntlet positions also have rigid curved face-pieces, which are bonded to the isolator wall and provide good visibility. Headbands maintain the position of the face-pieces away from the nurses' or doctors' faces.

The low air pressure in the envelope allows the nurses and doctors using the gauntlets to move in readily against the wall of the isolators. This gives quite substantial movement but requires a built-in ventilation strip at each position.

The patient is introduced through an entry port at one end of the bed. Depending on the nature of the patient's injury or illness, pre-entry washing of the patient to a varying degree is carried out. The use of the patient entry port makes it possible to move the patient without the risk of contamination either to another whole-body isolator or to a transfer isolator for transfer to other areas within the hospital.

Materials are introduced into the isolators by means of a sterile airflow

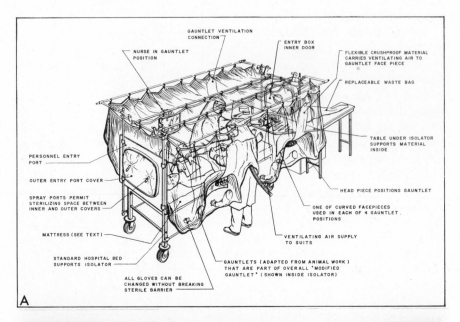

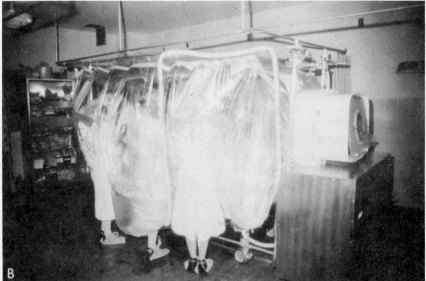

Figure 1. *A*, Diagram of a whole-body bed isolator with entry box attached. *B*, Side view of whole-body isolator diagrammed in Figure 1*A*. Nurses and doctors are in the half suits, three on each side; entry box is on the right. *C* and *D*, Severely burned patient in isolator. Nurses are in half suits with helmets with clear plastic face-pieces. Note mobility of nurse in Figure 1*D*.

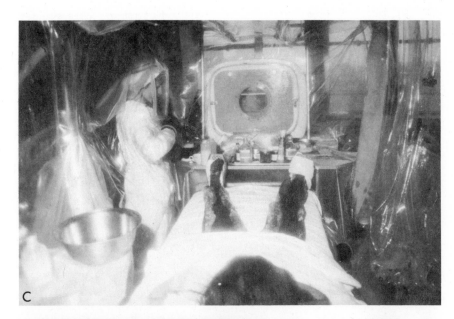

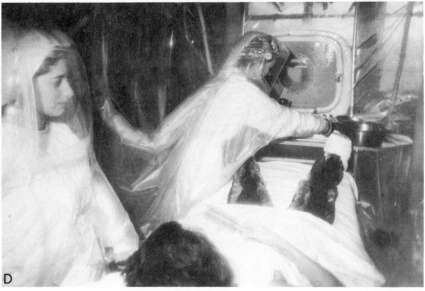

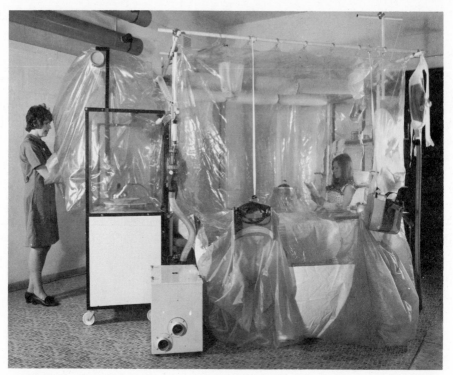

Figure 2.   Side view of another whole-body bed isolator with a volunteer subject. At left is a supply isolator and entry port. Two half suits for the medical and nursing personnel are shown suspended from the isolator supporting framework.

lock, an ultraviolet lock, a germicidal bath, or a downflow port. The sterile airflow lock consists of a double-doored chamber in the wall of the isolator, with a flow of sterile air that both flushes the interior of the chamber and maintains a positive pressure to prevent the entrance of contaminated air when the outer door is opened. The sterile supplies are doubly wrapped; the outer wrap is removed aseptically as the outer door is opened, and the inner bag is extracted with sterile tongs within the envelope of the sterile airstream. The outer door is closed, and the air wash is continued with both doors shut, and air exiting through an absolute filter. The inner door is then opened and the materials are brought in. This lock may be equipped with ultraviolet lights to kill any microorganisms that may have fallen on the materials to be entered while they were being unwrapped.

A liquid germicidal trap may also be used with the bed isolator. The trap contains a nonvolatile germicide, such as an iodophor preparation containing a wetting agent. Articles introduced are presterilized in double plastic bags or have an easily cleaned sterilizing surface (such as glass ampules) so that the trap serves as a liquid door, primarily to exclude possible air-borne contamination. Glass ampules are treated with hydrochlorite solutions prior to passage through the germicidal trap.

For the removal of supplies, equipment, dressings, excreta, and the like, a series of waste chutes may be attached to the sides of the isolator, or one of the double-door ultraviolet locks can be used. The waste chutes can be changed from the inside without breaking the sterile barrier. The waste chute technique has the added attribute that the removed material is automatically packaged in a closed bag, so contamination from that source is eliminated. A germicidal exit trap can also be used.

Storage of materials within the isolator is a problem not completely solved, particularly with isolators in which a great deal of manipulation is required for the treatment and care of patients. The wall space available for storage is limited by (1) the movement of personnel caring for the patient, and (2) the requirement for access to and visibility of the patient from all possible positions, especially for seriously ill or injured patients. Where free wall area is available, storage pockets can be inserted with supporting shelving outside the isolator. In addition, a small supply isolator can be attached

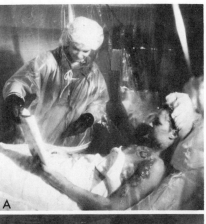

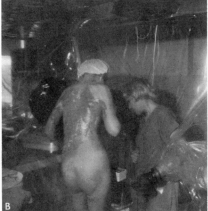

Figure 3. *A*, Severely burned patient in whole body bed isolator. Nurse in half suit and helmet with clear plastic face-piece. *B*, Patient standing up to be weighed; the balance is outside the isolator. The nurse is outside the isolator with left arm in gauntlet. Note the clarity of the isolator wall and room for patient.

to the whole-body bed isolator to provide a useful work space and storage unit.

The mattress is placed in a pocket over the bedsprings so that it remains outside the isolator envelope; sheets and blankets can be tucked underneath the edges. Tables, either at the side of or over the bed, are placed in pockets so they remain outside of the isolators. Plastic sleeves attached to the roof are used to elevate bottles or bags for intravenous infusions; monitoring leads, tubes, and the like can readily be passed through the isolator wall as needed.

A telephone, television set, and radio may be available to the patient through sleeves.

The isolators as received from the manufacturer are clean, but not sterile. The isolator, either new or cleaned for reuse, is hung from the framework and then leak-tested, using a halogen (Freon) gas. Any needed repairs are made. The inside of the bubble is then washed with soap and water, rinsed with water, and dried. It is then sterilized with a 2 per cent solution of peracetic acid, which is effective in both liquid and gas phases. Air is circulated through the bubble for 24 hours to remove the last trace of vapor, because this is irritating to the patients and personnel. The exiting peracetic acid is absorbed in a chemical trap containing weak alkali or charcoal to prevent the escape of irritating vapor.

The temperature of the air inside the isolator is close to that of the room air, and can be controlled most readily by controlling the room air. By contrast, the humidity inside the isolator is independent of room air, and can be regulated readily within a wide range by controlling the humidity of the air supply.

One often thinks of the isolator as primarily a device to limit influx of microorganisms from the outside. In fact, the communication of microbial agents works both ways, so that care must be taken with all material leaving the isolator, since if the patient within is infected, or is a carrier, large numbers of pathogenic microorganisms may be carried to the outside. This is prevented by the use of incinerators, filters, or germicidal traps for the exiting air, and the use of waste chutes, ultraviolet locks, and germicidal traps for exiting materials, as described.

OTHER TYPES OF WHOLE-BODY ISOLATORS

In addition to isolators built around standard hospital beds, they may be built around Stryker or Foster frames, Circo-matic beds, or other types of special beds to meet the particular needs of certain patients. Isolators designed especially for infants and children have been used for the maintenance of immunologically deficient patients for periods up to several years! As the children have grown, the isolators have been modified and enlarged so play equipment, such as climbing gyms or swings, can be housed within the isolators.

Transfer Whole-Body Isolators

Levenson, Trexler and associates[35] have designed a gauntlet whole-body "transfer" isolator supported on a wheeled stretcher. It is used for the transfer of patients from the admitting room to the ward isolator, and for the transfer of patients from the ward to other parts of the hospital, such as the operating room. A battery powered blower is mounted on the stretcher, along with the usual air hoses and air filters. At one end of the isolator is a 30-inch port, which matches that of the regular whole-body bed isolator to permit transfer of the patient.

Partial-Body Isolators

Partial-body isolators have certain advantages over whole-body bed isolators. (1) They exclude many endogenous organisms. Thus, when partial-body isolators are used for the extremities, the patient's endogenous organisms in the respiratory and gastrointestinal tract are excluded, along with exogenous microorganisms. (2) They are less of a psychological burden to the patient than whole-body isolators. (3) They are smaller and more easily managed. (4) Service to the patient, including serving food, and communication is no less efficient than for the normal patient. (5) The ventilation problems are also much simpler, with positive pressure supplied by air forced through a filter by a small blower. (6) Because partial isolators are smaller and simpler, they are also less expensive. This applies to both the plastic bubble cost and the supporting hardware. (7) Less hospital space is required.

The partial body isolators are normally ethylene oxide–sterilized.

Evaluation of Isolators

The use of whole- and partial-body isolators has been evaluated in a number of centers. As pointed out by Trexler,[57] "An isolator is really a device for automating sterile technique and as such can relieve personnel of much of the burden of maintaining sterility in addition to improving the microbial environment within the hospital."

One of the largest experiences with surgical patients is that of Burke and his coworkers[14] with severely burned children, using a gauntlet type whole-body isolator with vertical laminar airflow and open bottom. Their data indicate effective control of cross-contamination, minimal interference with medical and nursing care, and little evidence of any adverse psychological disturbances attributable to the isolator environment. Our own experience with adults—some suffering from very severe burns, some undergoing renal transplants, some with drug-induced agranulocytosis—cared for in whole-body and/or partial-body isolators also indicates that the ingress of exogenous microorganisms can be prevented, and that the medical and nursing care can be carried out with little difficulty, including such procedures as hemodialyses, complicated dressings, debridements, diagnostic x-rays, and inhalation analgesia.[35,36]

The patients have been able to watch television and read books and magazines (which were autoclaved), and have more visitors than would have been possible in the open isolator environment as usually practiced in hospitals. Some of the adult patients have had moderate psychological reactions during their stays in a whole-body isolator. What roles the patient's primary illness or injury and the care in an isolator played in these psychological factors are uncertain.

Hummel and his associates[24] working with burn patients in whole-body isolators also found that " . . . complete elimination of exogenous bacteria is possible. . . . Patient acceptance of the isolators has been good to excellent, and complete care of the moderately burned patient can be accomplished with few problems within these units. Considerable support from nursing service, dietary service, and central supply is necessary. . . . The chief source of contamination of the burns treated in reverse isolation seems to be from the patients' gastrointestinal tract," a view previously advanced by Haynes and Hench.[23] This latter point is discussed in the following section.

The possibility of buildup of microorganisms within an isolator has been raised. This can be prevented by appropriate ventilation and washing of the interior of the isolator. Also, for certain patients, such as those with extensive deep burns, who are kept in isolation for many weeks or months, periodic transfer of the patient to another isolator is practical.

Simple but effective isolators, we believe, will become an important element in many forms of patient care. The form of patient isolators is determined by the patient, his illness or injury, and the areas involved.

SOME ANCILLARY METHODS FOR PREVENTION OF NOSOCOMIAL INFECTION

Attempts to decontaminate patients totally (of all bacteria and fungi) in order to minimize the possibility of infection from microorganisms the patients already harbor have been made during the past ten years. Essential components of these attempts are the use of various chemotherapeutic agents and antibiotics; the maintenance of the patients in protected environments, either whole-body isolators, or a laminar airflow room with masking, gowning, gloving, and boots, or some combination of the two; and the feeding of a sterile diet. The feasibility of such decontamination was demonstrated first by van der Waaij and his associates with laboratory animals.[59] Most of the human attempts have been made in patients with leukemia.[29,37,38,60,66] Oral antifungal and antibacterial agents were used along with external washing and instillation of antibiotic and other chemo-therapeutic agents intranasally and intrapharyngeally. The data indicate that the antifungal agents must be begun first in order to "eliminate" the fungi. In general, the numbers and variety of bacteria were reduced remark-ably in the gut, and often, as far as determined, "eliminated." Less success-ful was the reduction of microorganisms on the skin and nasal passages, but the numbers were reduced substantially. There has been one preliminary report by Larkin, Moylan and Balish[31] in which this sort of effort has been carried out with 15 burn patients (average burn size, 40 per cent total body surface; range, 22–76 per cent). They found that while burned surfaces were free of pathogenic bacteria for approximately 20 days in all patients, five individuals had no pathogens at any time. Deep wounds did not become contaminated until five days after the surface areas. The most common pathogen isolated was *Streptococcus faecalis* (enterococcus), which ap-peared in the stool prior to wound colonization. All blood cultures were sterile, and the incidence of pneumonia was zero in spite of an inhalation injury rate over 40 per cent. There were no deaths in this series.

Because a patient free or almost free of microorganisms is very suscep-tible to chance contamination and to infection if the contaminant is pathogenic, van der Waaij and his associates have been attempting to define a gut bacterial flora that could be purposefully introduced into such indi-viduals and confer "colonization resistance."[59] Their animal experiments and preliminary studies with patients suggest that this may well be feasible.

Polk and coworkers[46] reported on an immunologic approach to the problem of respiratory-caused respiratory infections in the ICU. Their method consisted of active *immunization* of intensive care unit patients with heptavalent Pseudomonas vaccine. They found that vaccinated patients were less prone to death due to *Pseudomonas aeruginosa* infections than were placebo-treated controls. Alexander and his associates[2] had reported effectiveness of such vaccine for the prevention of *Pseudomonas aeruginosa* sepsis in burned patients.

Patients with granulocytopenia may not be able to benefit from this type of immunotherapy, since elaboration of opsonins and subsequent ingestion and killing of the bacteria by neutrophils are critical. In such patients, *white blood cell transfusions* may be useful. Infusions of *fresh, fresh frozen, or cryoprecipitated plasma* may provide certain humoral factors important for microbial defense, e.g., complement, which may be deficient in seriously ill and injured patients.

It is generally agreed that the *prophylactic use of antibiotics* for the prevention of urinary and respiratory tract infections is ineffective and should not be used for these purposes except in a few exceptional circum-stances, such as immediately after aspiration. The use of short-term broad spectrum antibiotics for the prevention of postoperative wound infections in patients undergoing so-called clean-contaminated operations is useful; in this case, the antibiotic is begun a few hours before operation, and is con-tinued intraoperatively and for 12 to 24 hours postoperatively.[13,47]

CONCLUSIONS

The needs of seriously ill surgical patients are such that the patients are benefited by being cared for in locations where skillful personnel and specialized equipment and facilities are available. Many of these patients are particularly prone to infections because of their underlying disease or injury and/or their therapy. The hospital environment in which they are placed, such as the surgical ICU, is one in which virulent and often antibiotic-resistant pathogenic microorganisms are prevalent. Some patients enter the surgical ICU with infections, some of which are overt, and some developing but not yet clinically apparent. Such patients represent a considerable threat to each other and to all the others on the unit. Further, the patients in surgical intensive care units are subjected to a variety of procedures, such as tracheal intubations, suctioning, and bladder and intravenous catheterizations, which expose them to microbial contamination and infections. The intensity and complexity of routine activity and the high incidence of urgent and emergency problems requiring rapid medical and nursing responses in the surgical ICU increase the likelihood of cross-contamination and cross-infection.

When nosocomial infections occur, they complicate the patients' courses, prolonging convalescence and increasing morbidity, economic cost, and mortality. It is likely that these problems will become even more pressing in the future. Patients with severe injury are particularly vulnerable to infections, and the continuing, alarming number of automobile and industrial accidents underscores this problem. Further, increasingly complex surgery, organ replacement, and the increasing use of immunosuppressive and cytotoxic drugs and radiation therapy tend to decrease host resistance and will place an even greater number of infection-prone patients in surgical ICUs for even greater periods of time than at present. Indwelling vascular catheters and catheters in other orifices both enhance the patient's chances for recovery and potentially lead to infection.

As the enormity of the problems of cross-contamination and cross-infection in special care units becomes more widely understood, a variety of architectural and equipmental solutions are being suggested. *In our opinion, the time has come for an infection safety code for special care areas just as there is an electrical safety code.* The known high cost of nosocomial infection to the patients, the hospitals, and society justifies the cost of adequate structural protection against cross-contamination and cross-infection.

In determining a system for the prevention and control of nosocomial infections on a surgical ICU, certain features emerge as important:

1. *An on-site leader* concerned about the problems of nosocomial infections who has the authority, charisma, personnel, equipment, supplies, and so on to determine, promulgate, and carry out necessary policies and procedures; we think this person should be a surgeon with special training and interest in intensive care, but an anesthesiologist or internist with such training and interest could function in this leadership role.

2. *An ambience* prevailing on the unit, encompassing an awareness and concern for the prevention and control of cross-contamination. Good practices with minimal lapses and errors must be second nature to all the staff, who, in turn, must educate and supervise visitors and other transients. *A feeling of pride, based on solid achievement, must emanate from all.*

3. Hard-hitting, responsible, *continuing surveillance record-keeping and reporting;* Socrates' admonition "know thyself" may be paraphrased to "know thy problem."

4. *A properly ventilated physical setup (designed to permit and facilitate)* optimal patient care and, at the same time, to permit and facilitate appropriate practices and measures for the prevention and control of cross-contamination. If recovery rooms and ICUs are designed using *the cubicle or single-room principle* and *the use of isolators,* we believe that a patient who must be kept in a recovery or intensive care area will have less chance of his tracheostomy becoming infected with his neighbor's microorganisms, and his own draining wound have less chance of endangering other patients, provided, of course, that all personnel use the facility appropriately and do not abuse the epidemiologic principles of hygiene in patient care.

5. *Strict control of traffic.* A "need to know, that is, need to be there" philosophy should prevail regarding the presence of anyone on the ICU.

6. An outstanding, knowledgeable *housekeeping staff,* aware of the problems of cross-contamination. Mead,[41] in 1720 (cited by Wangensteen[62]), had this to say about avoiding "pestilential contagion": "Nastiness is a great source of infection, so cleanliness is the greatest preservative."

7. A continuing *educational and orientation program.* Instruction must be given to attending physicians, house staff, nurses, dietitians, physiotherapists, students, technicians, maintenance and janitorial people, engineers, clergy, administrators, messengers, visitors, and anyone else who has reason to come into the intensive care unit.

8. An *active personnel health program* to detect any potential infectious threat. An awareness and concern of each individual connected with the ICU about this very important matter is paramount.

REFERENCES

1. Alexander, J. W.: Immunological considerations in burn injury and the role of vaccination. *In* Stone, H., and Polk, H. C., Jr. (Eds.): Contemporary Burn Management. Boston, Little, Brown and Company, 1971, p. 265.
2. Alexander, J. W.: Nosocomial infections. Curr. Prob. Surg., August 1973, p. 1.
3. Alpert, S., Salzman, T., Sullivan, C., Palmer, C., and Levenson, S. M.: Use of a surgical isolator for major surgery: influence on wound contamination and postoperative wound infection. *In* Heneghan, J. B. (Ed.): Germfree Research: Biological Effect of Gnotobiotic Environments. New York, Academic Press, 1973, pp. 87–95.
4. Altemeier, W. A. (Ed.): Manual on Surgical Infections, Pre- and Postoperative Care. Committee of the American College of Surgeons. Philadelphia, W. B. Saunders Company (in press).
5. Altemeier, W. A., Hummel, P. P., Hill, E. O., and Lewis, S.: Changing patterns in surgical infections. Ann. Surg., *178*:436, 1973.

6. Andriole, V. T., Stamey, T. A., Kunin, C. M., et al.: Preventing catheter-induced urinary tract infections. Hosp. Practice, *3*:61, 1968.

7. Banaszak, E. F., Thiede, W. H., and Fink, J. N.: Hypersenitivity pneumonitis due to contamination of an air-conditioner. N. Engl. J. Med., *283*:271, 1970.

8. Barrett, F. F., Casey, J. I., and Finland, M.: Infections and antibiotic use among patients at Boston City Hospital. N. Engl. J. Med., *278*:5, 1967.

9. Bernhardt, H. E., Orlando, J. C., Benfield, J. R., Hirose, F. M., and Foos, R. Y.: Disseminated candidiasis in surgical patients. Surg. Gynecol. Obstet., *134*:819, 1972.

10. Bodey, G. P., and Johnston, D.: Microbiological evaluation of protected environments during patient occupancy. Appl. Microbiol., *22*:828, 1971.

11. Brahman, P. S. (Ed.): Isolation Techniques for Use in Hospitals. U.S. Department of Health, Education and Welfare, Public Health Service, Public Health Service Publication No. 2054. Washington, D.C., U.S. Government Printing Office, 1970.

12. Brennan, M. F., Goldman, M. H., O'Connell, R. C., Kundsin, R. B., and Moore, F. D.: Prolonged parenteral alimentation. Ann. Surg., *176*:265, 1972.

13. Burke, J. F.: The effective period of preventive antibiotic action in experimental incisions in dermal lesions. Surgery, *50*:161, 1961.

14. Burke, J. F., Quinby, W. C., Bondoc, C. C., Cosini, A. B., and Syzfelbein, S. K.: Immunosuppression and temporary skin transplantation in the treatment of massive third degree burns. Ann. Surg., *182*:183, 1975.

15. Dietrich, M., Fliedmer, T. M., and Krieger, D.: Germfree technology in clinical medicine: production and maintenance of gnotobiotic states in man. *In* Heneghan, J. B., (Ed.): Germfree Research, Biological Effect of Gnotobiotic Environments. New York, Academic Press, 1973, pp. 21–30.

16. Duke, J. H., Jr., and Dudrick, S. J.: Parenteral feeding. *In* Ballinger, W. F., Collins, J. A., Drucker, W. R., Dudrick, S. J., and Zeppa, R. (Eds.): Manual of Surgical Nutrition. Committee on Pre- and Postoperative Care, American College of Surgeons. Philadelphia, W. B. Saunders, 1975, pp. 285–317.

17. Eickhoff, T. C.: Hospital Infections. Disease-a-Month, September 1972, p. 3.

18. Feingold, D. S.: The serum bactericidal reaction. IV. Phenotypic conversion of *Escherichia coli* from serum-resistance to serum-sensitivity by Diphenylamine. J. Infect. Dis., *120*:437, 1969.

19. Feingold, D. S.: Hospital-acquired infections. N. Engl. J. Med., *283*:1384, 1970.

20. Findlay, C. W., Jr.: Sepsis in the surgical intensive care unit. Med. Clin. North Am., *55*:1331, 1971.

21. Gage, A. A., Dean, D. C., Schimert, A., and Minsley, N.: Aspergillus infection after cardiac surgery. Arch. Surg., *101*:284, 1970.

22. Gardner, P., and Smith, D. H.: Studies on the epidemiology of resistance (R) factors.I. Analysis of Klebsiella isolates in a general hospital. II. A prospective study of R factor transfer in the host. Ann. Intern. Med., *71*:1, 1969.

23. Haynes, B. W. Jr., and Hench, M. E.: Hospital isolation system for preventing cross-contamination by staphylococcal and Pseudomonas organisms in burn wounds. Ann. Surg., *162*:641, 1965.

24. Hummel, R. P., MacMillan, B. G., Maley, M., and Altemeier, W. A.: Reverse isolation in the treatment of burns. J. Trauma, *10*:450, 1970.

25. Hummel, R. P., MacMillan, B. G., Maley, M., and Altemeier, W. A.: Comparison of complete barrier isolation and unidirectional air flow in the treatment of burn wounds. Ann. Surg., *176*:742, 1972.

26. Irvine, R., Johnson, B. L., Jr., and Amstutz, H.: The relationship of genitourinary tract procedures to deep sepsis in total hip replacements. Surg. Gynecol. Obstet., *139*:701, 1974.

27. Jackson, A. E., Southern, P. M., Pierce, A. K., et al.: Pulmonary clearance of gram-negative bacilli. J. Lab. Clin. Med., *69*:833, 1967.

28. Kislak, J. W., Eickhoff, T. C., and Finland, M.: Hospital-acquired infections, and antibiotic usage in the Boston City Hospital. N. Engl. J. Med., *271*:834, 1964.

29. Kohle, K., Simons, C., Dietrich, M., and Durner, A.: Investigation of behavior of leukemia patients treated in germfree isolators. *In* Heneghan, J. B. (Ed.): Germfree Research: Biological Effect of Gnotobiotic Environment. New York, Academic Press, 1973, pp. 71–77.

30. Kranz, P., Levenson, S. M., and LaDuke, M.: Designing for germfree environments. ASHRAE J., *3*:37, 1965.

31. Larkin, J., Moylan, J., and Balish, E.: Total reverse isolation in burn care. Seventh Annual

Meeting of the American Burn Association, Denver, Colorado, March 20–22, 1975, Abstract #23, p. 27.

32. Laufman, H.: The infection hazard of intensive care. Surg. Gynecol. Obstet., *139*:413, 1974.

33. Laufman, H., and Vandernoot, A.: Unpublished data.

34. Levenson, S. M., Trexler, P. C., Malm, O. J., LaConte, M., Horowitz, R. E., and Moncrief, W. H.: A plastic isolator for operating in a sterile environment. Am. J. Surg., *104*:891, 1962.

35. Levenson, S. M., Trexler, P. C., LaConte, M., and Pulaski, E. J.: Application of the technology of the germfree laboratory to special problems of patient care. Am. J. Surg., *107*:710, 1964.

36. Levenson, S. M., Del Guercio, L. R. M., LaDuke, M., Kranz, P., Johnston, J., Alpert, S., and Salzman, T.: Plastic isolators for special problems of patient care. *In* Research in Burns. London, E. & S. Livingstone, Ltd., 1966, pp. 563–685.

37. Levitan, A. A., and Perry, S.: Infectious complications of chemotherapy in a protected environment. N. Engl. J. Med., *276*:881, 1967.

38. Levitan, A. A., and Perry S.: The use of an isolator system in cancer chemotherapy. Am. J. Med., *44*:234, 1968.

39. Lindwell, O. M., Polakoff, S. J., Parker, M. T., Shooter, R. A., and Dunkerley, D. R.: Staphylococcal infection in thoracic surgery: experience in a subdivided ward. J. Hyg. *64*:321, 1966.

40. Lowbury, E. J. L.: Evaluation of patient isolators. *In* Proceedings of the Intl. Conf. on Nosocomial Infections, Center for Disease Control, August 3 to 6, 1970. Baltimore, Waverley Press, 1971, pp. 220–224.

41. Mead, R.: A Short Discourse Concerning Pestilential Contagion and the Methods Used to Prevent It. 5th Ed. London, Buckely and Smith, 1720, p. 48.

42. Morgan, A. P., and Kundsim, R.: Absolute isolation in burn care. Surg. Clin. North Am., *50*:1267, 1970.

43. Northey, D., Adess, M. L., Hartsuck, J. M., and Rhoades, E. R.: Microbial surveillance in a surgical intensive care unit. Surg. Gynecol. Obstet., *139*:321, 1974.

44. Parker, M. T., et al.: Staphylococci endemic in hospitals. Brit. Med. J., *1*:1101, 1965.

45. Pierce, A. K., Sanford, J. P., Thomas, G. D., et al.: Long-term evaluation of decontamination of inhalation-therapy equipment and the occurrence of necrotizing pneumonia. N. Engl. J. Med., *282*:531, 1970.

46. Polk, H. C., Jr., Borden, S., and Aldrete, J. A.: Prevention of pseudomonas respiratory infection in a surgical intensive care unit. Ann. Surg., *177*:607, 1973.

47. Polk, H. C. Jr., and Lopez-Mayor, J. F.: Postoperative wound infection in a prospective study of determinant factors and prevention. Surgery, *66*:97, 1969.

48. Pruitt, B.: Multidisciplinary Care and research for burn injury. J. Trauma, *17*:263, 1977.

49. Reinarz, J. A., Pierce, A. K., Mays, B. B., et al.: The potential role of inhalation therapy equipment in nosocomial pulmonary infection. J. Clin. Invest., *44*:831, 1965.

50. Robertson, A. C., Lynch, J., Kay, H. E. M., Jameson, B., Guyer, R. J., and Evans, I. L.: Design and use of plastic tents for isolation of patients prone to infection. Lancet, *2*:1376, 1968.

51. Rosendal, K.: Cited by Feingold, D. S.: Hospital-acquired infections. N. Engl. J. Med., *283*:1384, 1970.

52. Rubio, T., and Riley, H. D., Jr.: Serious systemic infection associated with the use of indwelling intravenous catheters. South. Med. J., *66*:633, 1973.

53. Shooter, R. A., Taylor, G. W., Ellis, G., and Ross, J. P.: Postoperative wound infection. Surg. Gynecol. Obstet., *103*:257, 1956.

54. Smylie, H. G., Davidson, A. I. G., MacDonald, A., and Smith, G.: Mechanical control of hospital ventilation and Aspergillus infections. Am. Rev. Resp. Dis., *105*:306, 1972.

55. Teres, D., Bushnell, L. S., Schweers, P., Hedley-Whyte, J., and Feingold, D. S.: Sources of *Ps. aeruginosa* infection in a respiratory/surgical intensive therapy unit. Lancet, *1*:415, 1973.

56. Trexler, P. C.: An isolator system for the maintenance of aseptic environment. Lancet, *1*:91, 1973.

57. Trexler, P. C.: Microbial isolators for use in the hospital. Biomed. Eng., *10*:63, 1975.

58. van der Waaij, D., Vossen, J. M., and Altes, C. K.: Patient isolators designed in The Netherlands. *In* Heneghan, J. B. (Ed.): Germfree Research: Biological Effect of Gnotobiotic Environment. New York, Academic Press, 1973, pp. 31–36.

59. van der Waaij, D.: Similarities between germ-free mice and mice with an antibiotic decon-

taminated digestive tract. *In* Minand, E. A., and Back, N., (Eds.): Germ-free biology, experimental and clinical aspects. Adv. Exper. Med. & Biol., Vol. 3. New York, Plenum Press, 1969.

60. Vossen, J. M., Dooren, L. J., and van der Waaij, D.: Clinical experience with the control of the microflora. *In* Heneghan, J. B. (Ed.): Germfree Research: Biological Effect of Gnotobiotic Environment. New York, Academic Press, 1973, pp. 97–106.

61. Walter, C. W., Kundsin, R. B., and Brubaker, M. M.: The incidence of airborne infection during operation. J.A.M.A., *186*:908, 1963.

62. Wangensteen, O. H., Wangensteen, S. D., and Klinger, C. F.: Surgical cleanliness, hospital salubrity, and surgical statistics, historically considered. Surgery, *71*:477, 1972.

63. Whyte, W., Howie, J. G. R., and Eakin, J. E.: Bacteriological observations in a mechanically ventilated experimental ward and in two open-plan wards. J. Med. Microbiol., *2*:335, 1969.

64. Williams, R. E. O.: Airborne staphylococci in the surgical ward. J. Hyg. *65*:207, 1967.

65. Williams, R. E. O., Blowers, R., Garrod, L. P., et al.: Hospital Infection: Causes and Prevention. 2nd Ed. London, Lloyd-Luke Medical Books, Ltd., 1966.

66. Yates, J. W., and Holland, J. E.: Controlled trial of prophylaxis of infections from exogenous and endogenous microorganisms. *In* Heneghan, J. B. (Ed.): Germfree Research: Biological Effect of Gnotobiotic Environment. New York, Academic Press, 1973, pp. 107–114.

CHAPTER 13

PSYCHIATRIC CONSIDERATIONS IN THE INTENSIVE CARE UNIT

DONALD S. KORNFELD, M.D.

During the last ten years, intensive care units (ICUs) have become an essential part of most general hospitals. Their value in the treatment of the critically ill has been clearly demonstrated, which is a tribute to our ability to apply modern electronic technology to the observation and treatment of patients. However, as we became more proficient in the use of the technical aspects of this environment, we also became more aware of the emotional impact of this experience. This concern should not be seen as a casual afterthought, since the physiological and behavioral manifestations of emotional states can introduce serious life-threatening complications into already tenuous situations. For example, anxiety can produce arrhythmias, and severe agitation can pose a threat to important catheters and cables.

In 1966, in reviewing the literature describing the psychiatric problems of open heart surgery patients in the recovery room, McKegney[12] used the term "ICU syndrome." Unfortunately, this became a catchall phrase used by some to describe and explain all such problems occurring in ICUs, an oversimplification with dangerous implications. In the past ten years we have come to realize that not all ICUs are the same, and certainly not all psychiatric problems occurring therein are the same. Therefore, it is essential that we take a much broader view of the ICU setting when we set out to review "psychological considerations in the ICU."

It is probably best to divide our review into four separate categories: (1) psychiatric reactions existing in association with the serious medical and surgical illnesses that bring patients to the ICU; (2) psychiatric reactions that are actually produced by the unique setting of the ICU itself; (3) emotional problems related to the transfer or discharge of patients out of the ICU; and (4) problems of the staff working in such units.

PSYCHIATRIC PROBLEMS ASSOCIATED WITH CRITICAL ILLNESS

Within the intensive care unit can exist all the psychiatric complications that accompany serious medical-surgical illness. Since the patients in the intensive care unit are, by definition, critically ill, it is likely that there is an even higher incidence of psychiatric complications in such a setting. The major problem is the acute organic brain syndrome, or delirium, a reversible state related to organic factors such as cerebral anoxia, metabolic disturbances, and toxic drug reactions. The symptoms vary, but typically include disorientation, memory loss, fluctuating states of consciousness, and perceptual distortions such as hallucinations and illusions. These symptoms, when accompanied by anxiety or agitations, can pose a serious threat to the life of a critically ill patient.

The clinical picture can resemble a schizophrenic psychosis, but the differential diagnosis must be made, since the acute organic brain syndrome is produced by an organic disturbance that is affecting the brain. The treating physician who mistakes these symptoms for a purely psychological reaction may delay the diagnosis and treatment of a serious underlying medical problem. The presence of disorientation and memory loss most likely indicates the presence of acute organic brain syndrome and not schizophrenia. When in doubt, an underlying organic basis should be sought, since the symptomatic treatment for both conditions is the use of phenothiazines.

First, the patient's physical status must be carefully reviewed. Are there any neurological signs? Is the electroencephalogram abnormal? What new drugs has the patient been given? How are the electrolytes? hemoglobin? oxygenation? What has happened to the blood urea nitrogen? Prior to hospitalization, had the patient been drinking alcohol or taking some sleeping pill or tranquilizer that has abruptly been withdrawn?

While this diagnostic work-up is in progress, symptomatic treatment can begin. The drug of choice is a phenothiazine or haloperidol; we use chlorpromazine (Thorazine). Unfortunately, the fear of cardiovascular complications has caused some physicians to refrain from using phenothiazines. When judiciously used, there is no significant danger, especially in the setting of the intensive care unit where the patient's vital functions can be monitored. In most cases, the patient's agitation is a more serious threat to his well-being than any drug side-effect.

It is our policy to initiate treatment with chlorpromazine, 25 mg intramuscularly, never using larger single doses initially; a very elderly or debilitated patient might first be given a test dose of 12.5 mg. A regimen of repeated doses, such as 25 mg intramuscularly four times a day while awake, is then established for each patient. This regular dosage schedule, based on the patient's physical status and response, is used until the psychosis is cleared. This is preferable to the exclusive use of doses given as necessary, which can produce a more labile and extended course. Additional 25 mg doses, when needed, can be used to supplement the basic regimen during the initial acute phase. The patient should be shifted to oral doses as soon as possible, using approximately double the intramuscular dose. (If fear of cardiovascular side-effects precludes the use of phenothiazines, haloperidol [Haldol] can be more safely used. One-half to 1 mg can be given intramuscularly instead of chlorpromazine.) In those cases in which it is established that the patient is suffering from drug or alcohol withdrawal, the appropriate treatment for these conditions should be instituted.

PSYCHIATRIC REACTIONS ASSOCIATED WITH INTENSIVE CARE

There are psychiatric problems that appear to be related to the unique environment of the intensive care unit itself. The nature and extent of these problems can vary, which may reflect differences in the construction and atmosphere of the individual intensive care units. The "intensive care unit" may refer to a small four-bed room, converted from a semiprivate room. The beds are separated only by curtains, and the patients, surrounded by monitoring equipment, are all within view of each other. On the other hand, the intensive care unit may be a newly constructed eight-bed unit with patients in individual cubicles and monitoring equipment judiciously concealed.

Obviously, the environment in each of these intensive care units is quite different from the other, and one may, therefore, expect differences in emotional responses. However, in either setting it is possible for a busy medical staff to become so involved with the monitoring devices that they do lose sight of the patients to whom they are attached. Similarly, the staff working in such an environment on a daily basis quickly accepts it as a routine work setting. They can forget that for the patient it is a new, unique, and often terrifying experience to be sick in such a setting.

The concept of the *intensive care unit syndrome* developed out of reports of the high incidence (38 to 70 per cent) of delirium following open heart surgery.[2,5,10] The delirium developed in the open heart surgery recovery room after a lucid postoperative interval. While a variety of operative factors appeared to contribute to the delirium, some felt that the environment of these rooms played a major contributory role.[5,10]

The typical open heart recovery room was a large open area with four to six beds separated by a movable curtain. Attached to the patients were electrocardiogram cables, intravenous tubing, and a bladder catheter. Although movement was possible, most patients remained relatively immobile as a result of pain and the implied limitation of motion caused by the cables and catheters. An electronic monitor with an oscilloscope was placed next to the bedside and flashed constantly. The patient was placed in a plastic oxygen tent that produced a constant background humming and hissing noise. Nurses and house officers arrived at frequent intervals to perform their chores. The room's overhead light was constantly on. There was always the possibility of an emergency with its associated activity. Thus, for the four to six days that most patients were there, they were subjected to an experience that combined the elements of a sensory monotony experiment with sleep deprivation.

Since they possibly had their cerebral function partially compromised by the cardiac bypass procedure, it was not surprising that these patients had a high incidence of delirium. The typical patient would appear lucid for the first three to four days. He would then experience an illusion; for example, sound arising from an air conditioning vent might begin to sound like someone calling him. This might then progress to auditory and visual hallucinations and frank paranoid delusions. Disorientation to time, place, and person could occur. In a typical case, the delirium would clear within 24 to 48 hours after the patient was transferred to a standard hospital environment where he could have a sound sleep.

Most of the patients interviewed in one study[10] looked back on their stay in the open heart recovery room as a disturbing experience. They noted the frightening atmosphere, the unusual sounds, and the sense of being chained. They said that uninterrupted sleep was virtually impossible. The average patient was glad to leave and return to the relative tranquillity of the hospital proper. It was, therefore, the conclusion of the investigators[10] that this recovery room delirium was the result of the impact of sleep and sensory deprivation on patients whose capacity to handle such stress was already impaired by chronic illness and the physical effects of surgery.

On the basis of these findings, it was suggested that certain modifications in nursing procedures and the design of these rooms might reduce the incidence of delirium:

1. Nursing procedures should be modified to allow the maximum number of uninterrupted sleep periods. The usual day-awake, night-sleep cycle should be maintained whenever possible.

2. Patients should be placed in individual cubicles. There they would not be awakened or made more anxious by activity occurring around other patients.

3. Monitoring equipment should be maintained, wherever possible, outside the patient's room. Bedside monitors should be turned on only when needed. This would reduce anxiety in those patients who are aware of the significance of these signaling devices and the danger implicit with any change in their pattern.

4. Patients should be allowed increased mobility by removing as many wires and cables as possible. Telemetry equipment would achieve increased mobility and allow the use of remote monitors.

5. The constant noise of oxygen and cooling tents should be modified or removed whenever possible.

6. An outside window should be visible to the patient to allow orientation.

In addition to restructuring the room, alerting the staff to the possible development of these psychiatric symptoms can also help prevent the development of the more florid forms of the psychosis. The recovery room nurse now visits each patient before the operation and describes the room in as much detail as seems appropriate. Patients are told about the postoperative delirium and are encouraged to report it to the nurses as soon as it begins. The relationship established prior to surgery can be useful in reducing anxiety postoperatively. More frequent bedside visits by nursing staff can also do much to reduce anxiety and to provide meaningful stimulation. If delirium does develop, patients can be allowed more sleep or transferred out of the room. If this is not possible, then chlorpromazine in small doses of 12.5 and 25 mg, intramuscularly, can be used effectively in controlling the symptoms.

Lazarus and Hagens[11] found that modifications in the open heart recovery room, designed to lessen anxiety, sensory monotony, and sleep deprivation, did produce a lower incidence of delirium after open heart surgery. In a similar study, Wilson[16] compared the incidence of postoperative delirium in 50 patients treated in an ICU without windows with 50 similar patients in an ICU with windows. He found over twice as many episodes of delirium in the ICU without windows. Heller and coworkers[8] have reported a reduction in the incidence of this delirium in recent years. They suggest that diminished time required on the heart-lung machine and modifications in the environment of the open heart recovery room may both have played a role.

The incidence of such reactions is lower in the coronary care unit than in the open heart recovery room.[6] Most patients appear, superficially, to tolerate the coronary care unit experience reasonably well, and the sophisticated equipment is seen as quite reassuring. Bruhn,[3] however, does report a significant increase in blood pressure and heart rate in a group of patients who were known to have witnessed the death of another patient. The higher delirium incidence in the open heart recovery room may reflect the role of operative factors in the production of delirium. The open heart recovery room environment also differs from the coronary care unit in a number of ways. The routines of the open heart recovery room are much more likely to produce sleep deprivation because of the multiple nursing procedures; the postoperative patient is likely to have more problems with pain for a longer period of time, which contributes to sleep deprivation and anxiety; and the many catheters and cables produce greater immobilization.

RESPIRATOR PROBLEMS

The surgical intensive care unit often has patients on some type of device to assist respiration. What does it mean to be totally dependent upon such a machine for life? It has become increasingly common for patients to be dependent on cardiac pacemakers and dialysis machines. Adapting to a respirator, however, is particularly difficult psychologically, since nothing is more anxiety-provoking than acute dyspnea. Therefore, to be dependent upon a machine for each and every breath is extremely stressful. You cannot "forget" about the device as you can with a pacemaker, or a dialysis machine when you are not on it. The respirator is constantly there and constantly needed.

In addition, some patients placed on respirators may be given a curare-like drug to allow smoother operation of the respirator. These patients, therefore, are totally dependent on others for all their needs, and an accompanying tracheostomy makes even speech impossible. Therefore, we have created an extremely stressful situation, the patient totally dependent upon others for all his bodily needs and unable to communicate effectively. Certainly it is a tribute to the adaptability of man that patients, for the most part, survive the situation psychologically, but the question remains of what can be done to lighten their burden and reduce the psychological price that they may later pay.

Viederman's[15] work with dialysis patients has demonstrated that the patient's relationship with the machine may reflect his early experience with total dependence. Certainly some patients "fight" their respirator as some patients "fight" dialysis. Unfortunately, our treatment for "fighting the respirator" can be total paralysis with a curare-like drug, which does temporarily relieve the respiratory crisis but can add to the psychological problems. Of course, in these critical medical situations, one does not have the time to work through the conflicts regarding dependency. Therefore, we must consider ways of diminishing the stress of the situation while the patient is experiencing it and learn how to deal with the unavoidable aftereffects.

Under ideal circumstances, we would want to be able to prepare our patients for this psychologically traumatizing experience. Obviously, for patients who are admitted directly to a surgical ICU following a severe accident or after an untoward complication during surgery, this cannot be done. I would suggest that in situations where the staff feels there is a possibility that following surgery a patient may require a period of assisted respiration, the patient be told that this possibility exists. I believe most patients can deal with that possibility when appropriately presented, and it is far better to awaken to find that this device is not necessary than to awaken and, without warning, find that you cannot breathe for yourself.

Most patients on respiratory devices live in fear of the machine failing or of people failing them. Patients who are unable to speak are dependent on the people about them to anticipate their needs. We must, therefore, provide such patients with alternative methods of communication. The first basic need is a device to call for help. It must be simple, and the patient must have absolute confidence in it. The obvious way to achieve this is to have someone respond as rapidly as possible when the device is sounded. Many patients undoubtedly will overuse it, making what seem to be unnecessary demands. However, in most instances, this is a way of testing to be certain that someone is available should some more serious problem arise. Another communication system should be devised so that the patient can make his special needs known. Some patients will be able to write, and intravenous infusions should, therefore, not be put in the writing arm. Other patients may have to use an alphabet board or a word board. Ideally, if members of the staff were trained to lip-read, this could be quite helpful. For some patients, partial deflation of the tracheostomy cuff would be possible to permit speech. The phonating tracheostomy tube probably is not going to be useful in patients who will not be on the respiratory device long enough to learn how to use it.

The staff should also be aware that suctioning can cause a frightening choking sensation; therefore, preoxygenating the patient and limiting suctioning to a maximum of 15 seconds should help reduce this particular frightening experience.[1]

An interesting psychological phenomenon can occur with tracheostomized patients: a tendency to react to the patient who cannot speak as though he were not there. A patient told me he felt it was very important to continue to write notes while he was on the respirator so that the staff would "know I'm here." The tendency, however, is to talk over and around such patients as though they were, in fact, not present. We should be aware that even sedated patients may not be totally oblivious to their surroundings. Therefore, the staff must be particularly careful not to discuss the patient at the bedside in a way that would cause anxiety. However, communicating with the patient about his situation is important. While he may not be able to ask detailed questions, we should make an effort to anticipate his concerns and provide as many reassuring answers as is realistically possible.

Weaning patients off a respiratory device can be especially difficult when a patient has been on a machine for a prolonged period of time. It has been said that approximately 30 per cent of the patients who have been on such a device for more than ten days may have such problems. Since the end-point for a patient's tolerance off the machine is dyspnea, a subjective phenomenon, it becomes extremely difficult sometimes to determine at what point the patient's anxiety is the major factor.

Bendixen[1] has suggestions regarding weaning in a variety of situations. In most instances, a patient, reassuring approach by the staff is adequate to accomplish the task. For more difficult problems, a psychiatric consultant may be needed. The psychiatrist can use psychotherapy to explore the basis for the persistent anxiety. Drugs and relaxation techniques may also be helpful.

PSYCHIATRIC REACTIONS AFTER INTENSIVE CARE

Here we are concerned with the psychological response to the intensive care unit experience that manifests itself after the patient is discharged from such a unit. How will the patient react to routine hospital care after a week or more of constant electronic observation? How will the patient respond to hospital discharge after having had this type of intensive medical observation? Certainly, constant monitoring can emphasize to the person how critically ill he is. For some patients, transfer out of the intensive care unit can, therefore, represent tangible evidence of improvement. However, others report their concern regarding the loss of attention and constant observation.

Klein[9] reported a study in which he found that five out of seven patients transferred from a coronary care unit showed an emotional reaction to transfer and associated cardiovascular complications, such as reinfarction or arrhythmia. Five showed a coincidental increase in urinary catecholamine excretion. Although the transfer was intended to be a sign of getting well, the patient's feeling of rejection by those who had been caring for him was far more frequent. This was more likely to occur when a patient was transferred abruptly because there was an urgent need for the monitored bed. When the patient arrived on the new ward, he was "a transfer patient" whose major medical problem had already been handled by others. He was seen as "just convalescing," with the associated relative diminution of medical or nursing attention. The patient, therefore, was reacting to both a symbolic and a real rejection.

Klein, therefore, suggested the following changes in coronary care routine:

1. All patients are prepared in advance for transfer out of the unit; they should be told that their stay will be terminated when they no longer need intensive care, and that abrupt transfer may indeed occur.

2. Arrangements are made for one physician to follow the patient throughout his course and after hospital discharge. This physician is the patient's "doctor."

3. One nurse follows each patient through the coronary care unit onto the hospital ward. It is her responsibility to contact the nursing staff in the new hospital area and alert them to this patient's special needs and problems.

4. This nurse spends an hour each day with the patient, carrying out nursing procedures, providing information about his illness, and allowing discussion of his feelings.

Following institution of these changes, Klein followed another seven patients and found there were no cardiovascular complications after transfer from the coronary care unit. Certainly, Klein's series is very small; however, good clinical sense would confirm the wisdom of his recommendations. The provision of continuity of care, and easing the transition to the routine hospital setting, would appear to have valuable medical benefits. Shannon[14] has also outlined ways in which the nurse can make the transition out of the CCU easier.

Transfer from a surgical ICU to the ward may be less psychologically stressful than transfer from a CCU, since patients are probably aware of the sudden death potential with myocardial infarction that does not exist in most surgical conditions. On the other hand, some surgical patients are kept in the ICU setting for a very long period of time, and the problem of leaving the ICU and the familiar staff can also present problems. These problems can be diminished by giving the patient adequate notice of the impending transfer; allowing him to talk about his fears of leaving the familiar environment; providing an opportunity for the patient to meet the new staff and see the new unit to which he is going; and, of course, providing for some continuity of care.

One should be aware of the possibility that some patients coming off respirators may suffer from what psychiatrists refer to as a "traumatic neurosis." This is seen in patients who have experienced an unexpected or prolonged severe threat to life. It is more likely to have occurred in patients who had not anticipated the ICU respiratory care experience. These patients suffer from anxiety, insomnia, nightmares, tremors, listlessness, general irritability, and depression. These symptoms usually disappear with time; however, the healing process can be accelerated if the patient is given an opportunity to discuss his reactions to what he has experienced.

One must also consider the possible effects of the ICU experience that manifest themselves after discharge from the hospital. Druss and Kornfeld[4] studied 20 such patients after discharge from a coronary care unit. Ten had experienced cardiac arrest and had been resuscitated. Ten had cardiac problems without arrest. Patients had been treated in a coronary care unit not especially constructed for such use. It incorporated all the stressful features found in such units as previously described.

In evaluating the impact of the room on these patients after discharge, it was impossible to separate the effect of cardiac arrest and cardiac illness from the effect of the room itself. It was clear, however, that most of these 20 patients were suffering from persistent psychological symptoms, such as restlessness or irritability. Insomnia was also quite common. Many had become extremely dependent and had modified their life habits beyond what had appeared to be medically indicated. This, of course, is often seen in patients after cardiac disease. It is possible, however, that the effect of the coronary care unit experience is an additive one; that is, while these patients were reassured at the time by the constant attention in the coronary care unit, they were simultaneously made especially aware of the great danger in which they found themselves.

The constant awareness of danger may produce some chronic apprehension, perhaps similar to the traumatic neurosis described in respirator patients after they come off the machine. Most patients interviewed stated that they would have preferred a larger unit with less congestion. Most of these patients did deny experiencing any anxiety during their stay in the coronary care unit. It may indeed be an important protective mechanism at that time. However, the unexpressed concerns may contribute to later adjustment problems.

Therefore, it is important that physicians spend some time with patients prior to hospital discharge to give them an opportunity to work through some of the anxiety-provoking experiences they may have undergone there. This may reduce the likelihood of a prolonged anxiety reaction after discharge. Medical advice upon discharge, such as "You should take it easy," should be spelled out more specifically, thus reducing the likelihood of misinterpretation. This type of injunction may have a greater effect than one wishes on a patient who is already terrified at having been so close to death. Some patients may need to deny the serious nature of their illness and be overly active, whereas others become excessively terrified and invalided. A detailed discussion between the patient and his doctor can do much to produce a more realistic reaction. The physician, however, must take the initiative. The frightened patient is not likely to talk openly of what he may have viewed as an unspeakable topic—his near demise.

PSYCHOLOGICAL PROBLEMS OF THE INTENSIVE CARE UNIT STAFF

One must not overlook the psychological hazards for the staff in the intensive care unit setting. The unit is a special environment not only for the patient but also for those people who work there.[7] While they may eventually adapt to the multitude of stresses, the baseline of stress persists for both nurses and physicians.

The intensive care unit nurse is beset by a variety of problems. She must deal constantly and exclusively with the seriously ill. Opportunities for relaxation are reduced, since every patient is critically ill. The consequences of an error can be catastrophic, yet the equipment with which she works is most complex and demanding. She must face death more frequently than she would in a general medical setting. This requires her to experience all of the emotional turmoil that one experiences with the death of a patient, only she must experience it more frequently. Her exposure to visitors is much more stressful, since each visitor is concerned about a critically ill patient, and each of the nurse's words are carefully weighed. She may be working with physicians who have much less experience in the handling of the special equipment and problems seen in these units, and yet she must strive to preserve the traditional doctor-nurse relationship.

The charge nurse is in a particularly difficult role. She is in charge of a group of very independent individuals who have chosen to work in the ICU because they wish to have more responsibility and freedom. They expect responsibility to be delegated and often resent having their freedom restricted. However, they retain the need for recognition from a maternal figure. The charge nurse, often a contemporary of her staff, is, therefore, in a very difficult position, since she must deal with their unconscious ambivalence. She must also deal with a nursing administration, often of an older generation and without ICU experience. They often do not appreciate the special needs of the ICU staff. Therefore, the charge nurse can fail to elicit the support she needs to keep her staff content. Her failures can then fuel whatever latent resentment exists for this woman with whom the staff unconsciously competes.

The physicians must be aware of the special problems they face. The ICU expert can become so involved with the gadgetry that he can overlook some of the emotional needs of his patients. The referring practicing physician can feel so overwhelmed by the machinery that he feels useless and, therefore, afraid to participate in the care of his patient. He can thus overlook the patient's very real need for his presence at the bedside. Old and young physicians must also learn to deal with the specialist-nurse who may have greater knowledge in certain technical areas. Mature physicians of all ages have always been able to learn from an experienced nurse.

In the intensive care unit, the areas of responsibility in an emergency must be clearly spelled out. There may not be time to wait for the attending physician to answer his page. The cardiac surgeon may be in the operating room and, therefore, not immediately available. An inexperienced house officer may feel ill-equipped to assume the decision-making responsibility. The intensive care unit nurse may be the only professional person with the training and experience to deal with the problem. She may thus feel the need to make medical decisions; for example, at the Columbia-Presbyterian Medical Center, the coronary care unit nurses are permitted to do electrical conversion of ventricular fibrillation if a physician is not available. The authority is logically delegated to the experienced cardiac nurse, but this policy simultaneously places her in conflict with her previous training to act only on the direct order of a physician. Thus, another emotional burden is added. This is a problem that should be openly discussed with the medical staff.

The availability of effective life-support devices has also created some very special psychological problems for the ICU staff. Their machines can prolong "life"; however, the situation often calls for a new definition of "death." The staff members will ask themselves, when the patient can survive only when on the machines, for how long such devices should be used. To continue their use may only add to the financial and emotional burden of the family. For how long should valuable staff, space, and equipment be utilized in this cause?

Should the medical profession alone be asking such questions, since the issues are not just medical, but legal and philosophical as well? Certainly no obvious answers are available, and in the meantime, the issues represent tremendous potential stress. The best I can offer is the suggestion that staff members share the burden of these responsibilities and concerns with each other. Group discussions led by a psychiatrist, not directly involved in the patient's care, may help to clarify the issues, but he is no more likely than the others to have the answers.

What can be done to ease these problems for the ICU staff? Perhaps an awareness of these emotional stresses could help in selecting the best qualified people. What kind of individuals, then, should be recruited? It is difficult to establish criteria that are not clichés, such as emotional maturity, good clinical judgment, and so on. Since these units are usually staffed by nurses who volunteer, they tend to acquire the youngest graduates, who have been trained in the use of the equipment as students. Perhaps more experienced nurses with proven clinical judgment and skills could be recruited if they were provided with good training in the theory and application of the new technology. For the experienced nurse, possibly already in charge of a ward, it is important that she retain her role as an expert. She may hesitate to volunteer for a new untested experience without considerable assurance that she will be trained well enough to assume a leadership role. It should be noted that some of today's nurses have had considerable theoretical education; therefore, good training must now be more than a quick course on which button to push. Today's nurse needs to know *why*.

Intensive care unit training, of course, emphasizes emergency, lifesaving techniques and thus inadvertently downgrades the satisfactions available to nurses from other nursing skills. It thus makes it more likely that a death will be taken as a total personal failure. Therefore, training programs and intensive care unit leaders must emphasize that complete nursing care is still important. It would also help if a nurse could be given an opportunity to follow her patients after they leave the unit. She would then get the important satisfaction of seeing her patients discharged from the hospital.

What else can be done to reduce emotional pressures on the intensive care unit nursing staff? Above all, the nurses must feel that the physicians with whom they work understand the special stresses of the job. The physician in charge should hold regularly scheduled meetings with the nursing staff to allow them to communicate their questions and problems directly to him. It is important that the head nurse have ready access to him. Regularly scheduled meetings are essential. It is imperative that a clear line of command for all situations be established.

The necessity for close surveillance of patients often will not allow the time required to handle some of the more routine nursing chores. A good intensive care unit should be adequately staffed with a ward secretary and nurse's aides to handle the tasks for which the nurse may not be available. In addition to getting the work done, this relieves the conscientious nurse of the chronic sense of uneasiness that will occur when these tasks remain undone.

Every opportunity should be provided for the relief of unit nurses during the course of the day. There is no reason why they should be forced to work through mealtime or without an opportunity for brief breaks to provide some anxiety-free moments. The coffee break should be a scheduled activity so it can be taken without guilt. This is necessary to maintain a high level of efficiency. Regular meetings should be instituted by the charge nurse with her staff. This is important to maintain the morale of a staff whose members are working under pressure.

SUMMARY

This article is intended to provide the staff of intensive care units with an overview of the psychological hazards that may exist there. Such problems may complicate a patient's course while in the unit or perhaps manifest themselves after discharge. The effectiveness of the staff can also be impaired by a failure to recognize and adequately deal with the special working conditions found in such units. These problems are, for the most part, solved by the application of relatively simple measures. I believe we have reached a level of sophistication that allows us now to look beyond purely technical matters. In doing so, the intensive care unit can be made an even more effective medical instrument.

REFERENCES

1. Bendixen, H. H., Egbert, L. P., Hedley-White, J., et al.: Respiratory Care. St. Louis, C. V. Mosby Company, 1965.
2. Blachly, P. H., and Starr, A.: Post-cardiotomy delirium. Am. J. Psychiatry, *121*:371, 1964.
3. Bruhn, J. G., Thurman, E., Jr., Chandler, B. C., and Bruce, T. A.: Patients' reactions to death in a coronary care unit. J. Psychosom. Res., *14*:65, 1970.
4. Druss, R. G., and Kornfeld, D. S.: The survivors of cardiac arrest. A psychiatric study. J.A.M.A., *201*:291, 1967.
5. Egerton, N., and Kay, J. H.: Psychological disturbances associated with open heart surgery. Br. J. Psychiatry, *110*:444, 1964.
6. Hackett, T. P., Cassem, N. H., and Wishnie, H. A.: The coronary care unit, an appraisal of its psychological hazards. N. Engl. J. Med., *279*:1365, 1968.
7. Hay, D., and Oken, D.: The psychological stress of intensive care unit nursing. Psychosom. Med., *34*:109, 1972.
8. Heller, S., Frank, K. A., Malm, J. P., et al.: Psychiatric complications of open-heart surgery: a re-examination. N. Engl. J. Med., *283*:1015, 1970.
9. Klein, R. F., Kliner, V. S., Zipes, D. P., et al.: Transfer from a coronary care unit. Arch. Intern. Med., *122*:104, 1968.
10. Kornfeld, D. S., Zimberg, S., and Malm, J. R.: Psychiatric complications of open-heart surgery. N. Engl. J. Med., *273*:282, 1965.
11. Lazarus, H. R., and Hagens, J. H.: Prevention of psychosis following open-heart surgery. Am. J. Psychiatry, *124*:1190, 1968.

12. McKegney, F. P.: The intensive care syndrome. Conn. Med., *30*:633, 1966.
13. Parker, D. L., and Hodge, J. R.: Delirium in a coronary care unit. J.A.M.A., *201*:702, 1967.
14. Shannon, V. J.: The transfer process, an area of concern for the CCU nurse. Heart Lung, *2*:264, 1973.
15. Viederman, M.: Adaptive and maladaptive regression in hemodialysis. Psychiatry, *37*:68, 1974.
16. Wilson, W. M.: Intensive care delirium. Arch. Intern. Med., *130*:225, 1972.

CHAPTER 14

ETHICAL AND LEGAL CONSIDERATIONS IN THE INTENSIVE CARE UNIT

SAMUEL R. POWERS, M.D.

Technologic advances in health care delivery have improved the ability of the physician to care for his patient, but have paradoxically raised ethical and legal questions that have resulted in the interposition of society between the physician and the patient he wishes to treat. The techniques of modern medicine have raised the specter that a selected group of individuals may have their lives almost indefinitely prolonged and, when life is lost, may under certain circumstances have it restored. Society, suspicious of the motives and objectivity of the medical profession, has demanded a role in the decision as to who shall have life prolonged or restored and under what circumstances. There are at least four ethical and legal questions that must be considered in the everyday management of the modern intensive care unit. These questions are:

1. Assuming that the number of adequately staffed and equipped intensive care beds will never be sufficient to provide care for all individuals who may require them, how shall the decision be made as to who will be admitted to such a unit?

2. Assuming that individuals admitted into an intensive care unit are suffering from severe illnesses, for which the probability of survival is greatly reduced, what freedom does the physician possess to depart from established medical practice and utilize extraordinary methods of treatment?

3. Assuming that most patients in an intensive care unit are incapable of making decisions concerning their own welfare and particularly of providing informed consent to their physician, what is the extra liability of treatment without the patient's expressed permission?

4. Assuming that modern technology will permit the prolongation of a lifelike state well beyond the time when life has any legal or religious sig-

nificance, at what point should the life be terminated, and who shall participate in this decision?

These ethical and legal questions will pose a direct conflict in the or-
derly course of therapy as traditionally carried out by a physician in the care
of his patient. It is no longer possible for the physician to remain aloof from
the wishes of society and to proceed as if the perceived therapeutic goal was
the sole determinant of a course of action. A decision to withhold or discon-
tinue life-support devices in patients with presumed irreversible brain injury
or terminal metastatic cancer symbolizes the direct conflict between the
miracle of therapeutic technology and the ethical and economical requirements of a society.

WHO SHALL BE ADMITTED TO AN INTENSIVE CARE UNIT?

Intensive care units in a modern hospital represent the greatest concentration of expert personnel and advanced equipment that can be brought to
bear for the management of a patient's illness. It is almost a truism to state
that a patient who is sufficiently ill to be admitted to a hospital would have a
greater chance of recovering from his illness, if placed in the confines of an
intensive care unit rather than in some other part of the hospital. It is not
uncommon for a surgeon at the end of a long and difficult operation to order
that a patient be placed in the intensive care unit "in case something hap-
pens." This is a referral to the intensive care unit not because of an actual
need for intensive care, but because of a concern that such a need might
arise. This attitude is reasonable unless the placement of the patient with a
possible requirement of intensive care management replaces a patient with
an immediate requirement. In addition, it is a convenience for the nursing
service to place patients who require highly specialized nursing care, such as
the maintenance of tracheostomy tubes or of intravenous hyperalimentation
catheters, in the intensive care unit even though the patient's medical condition does not in fact require intensive care nursing. All patients who are
dependent on life-support systems, on the other hand, require the intensive
care unit for the maintenance of these systems. If the patient's disease is
thought to be reversible, then this situation represents intensive care utilization at its best. When such devices are used to support a patient who has no
expectation of survival, the utilization of the facility cannot be justified. If
one patient on a general ward succumbs who might have survived in an
intensive care unit, and if this occurred at a time when there were patients in
the intensive care unit who had no hope of surviving, then we have failed to
accept the ethical responsibilities inherent in the intensive care concept. The
most difficult aspect of this problem is that the distinction between these two
groups of patients is frequently impossible to make with medical certainty.
Every intensive care unit has had the experience of telling a patient's family
that there is no hope whatever for survival only to have the patient survive,
flourish, and return to a perfectly normal existence.

Few hospitals have developed a mechanism for managing admissions and discharges to the intensive care unit, but some mechanism must be found. The cost of an intensive care bed is now approaching $1,000 per day in some centers, so that it is no longer possible to leave the decision as to who shall occupy such a bed to a haphazard hierarchical system. Society pays for these facilities and must have a role in deciding who will use them. An intensive care utilization committee should be established in each hospital, with the committee composed of specialists in intensive care medicine as well as hospital administrators, representatives of the nursing service, and nonmedical professionals with interests in the ethical and legal aspects of medicine. Such a committee would serve to assist the patient's physician in making decisions concerning admission and discharge from the intensive care unit and would also serve as a buffer between the physician and the patient's family to explain the reasons for a particular decision, and to remove the sole liability from the physician in circumstances where a decision was counter to the family's wishes. The increasing role of the federal government in the financing of health care has led to the requirement of utilization review committees to determine the appropriateness of hospital admission and the quality of care provided. The intensive care utilization review committee would function in a similar fashion for these specialized facilities. It would have as its sole function the determination of the need for a specific patient to be in the intensive care unit.

WHAT FREEDOM DOES THE PHYSICIAN POSSESS TO DEPART FROM ESTABLISHED MEDICAL PRACTICE AND UTILIZE EXTRAORDINARY METHODS OF TREATMENT?

Intensive care units by their very nature tend to become the arena for explicit or implicit clinical research. New procedures and techniques, such as the balloon tip flow-directed pulmonary artery catheter, will often find their initial applications in the intensive care unit. The additional information that may be made available from these relatively untried techniques is felt to provide an increased chance for survival of the patient. Whenever a new technique is introduced into clinical practice, there will be an implied scientific question as to the validity and usefulness of the information obtained as well as of the hazard of the device. Drugs of unproved value and with possible unknown side-effects are frequently administered under situations of medical desperation. Pharmacologic doses of corticosteroids in patients suffering severe hemorrhagic hypotension and the administration of loop diuretics in patients with suspect acute tubular necrosis are current examples. Each of these drugs is widely used in the intensive care setting, although convincing scientific evidence as to their therapeutic efficacy is currently lacking. It is only a short step from this type of unproved therapy to the performance of a cardiac transplantation on a patient dying of myocardial disease, and from there only a very short jump to the use of animal donors for the required diseased human organ. If one could be certain that the patient who is considered for such extraordinary therapy has no chance for survival without it, or, if there is a chance for survival, that the proposed therapy cannot under any circumstances diminish this possibility of survival, then the course of action might be countenanced. Unfortunately, neither requirement can generally be met in clinical practice.

A further problem that has received recent attention concerns the use of patients in an intensive care unit who are thought to be dying as subjects for clinical research. In a recent case in the state of California, it has been ruled that a patient who has been judged brain dead as evidenced by absence of electrical activity in the brain may not be made the subject of a muscle biopsy even though it could clearly have no deleterious effect upon the patient. Paul Ramsey has argued on ethical grounds that a subject can be "wronged without being harmed."[6] This occurs whenever the subject is used as an object or as a means only rather than as an end in itself.

One possible solution to this dilemma is to adopt rigid criteria for the use of new or experimental methods of treatment and to apply the same criteria in the intensive care unit as in other parts of the hospital. This will usually require the approval of the Human Experimentation Committee. The committee should be composed not only of physicians who are knowledgeable in this particular area of human disease, but also of members of other professional but nonmedical disciplines such as the ministry and law. The clinical expectation of impending death should not be sufficient ground to abrogate established ethical and scientific procedures. A physician should not carry out extraordinary procedures on patients in the intensive care unit if they are unacceptable in other clinical areas.

WHAT IS THE ETHICAL AND LEGAL LIABILITY OF PROCEEDING WITH THE COURSE OF TREATMENT WITHOUT THE PATIENT'S EXPRESSED PERMISSION?

Consent for a physician to proceed with a course of treatment can occur in a variety of ways. Thomas J. O'Donnell has noted that these may be at least four in number.[4] The first of these is true informed consent where the patient is fully aware of the possible consequences and benefits of such treatment and of his own will makes the decision to proceed. This form of consent will rarely be obtainable in the intensive care unit. A second form is presumed consent. Lifesaving measures that are clearly in the interest of patient survival belong in this category. In addition to the ethical requirement for the physician to proceed, there is ample legal justification under the good samaritan laws, which specifically exempt a physician from charges of assault under these circumstances. Third, there is implied consent. When a patient voluntarily goes to his physician for a complete examination, the mere fact of his appearing in the physician's office is considered an implied consent to the tests that are necessary for the medical evaluations. Finally, and of most concern in the intensive care unit, is vicarious or substituted consent. This occurs when a member of the family provides consent for someone who is either medically or legally incapable of providing his own informed consent. There would appear to be little question that if the vicarious consent is provided under the same circumstances that presumed consent would be operative, then the physician may proceed with appropriate treatment. Specifically exempted from this form of consent is the permission to carry out experimental procedures, if such procedures have no reasonable likelihood of improving the health of the incompetent subject. A special case in clinical research is the use of incompetent patients for control studies. The withholding of a possible beneficial drug in order to obtain an evaluation of its efficacy in other patients cannot be permitted. A recent federal decision concerning the withholding of a method of therapy that might have been beneficial in the treatment of syphilis was deemed illegal. The application of the concept of vicarious consent for removing an organ from a healthy incompetent donor to be given to a diseased recipient is under careful scrutiny at the present time. Richard McCormick has stated, "I would conclude that parental consent for a kidney transplant from one noncompetent 3-year-old to another is without moral justification."[3] The removal of a small amount of bone marrow from a infant for transplantation to an incompetent sibling is ethically identical but might be justified on the grounds that although some risk to the donor may exist, the potential benefit to the recipient is significant and far outweighs that risk. It is in this area of vicarious consent that much further study will be required before a final answer is available. There are at least four legal strategies that are receiving varying degrees of acceptance as possible solutions to this problem. The first is the use of judicial decisions. The Farrelli Case involving bone transplantation from one legally incompetent sibling to another has received detailed legal consideration. The hospital administration ruled that the parents could not give permission for a minor to provide the required donation of bone marrow, since there was no possibility that this donation could be of any therapeutic value to the donor. The court appointed an advocate for the incompetent proposed donor to argue in his behalf against his providing the desired bone marrow, whereas the parents provided an advocate to argue that the risk to the donor was insignificant in terms of the probable benefit to his sibling recipient. After hearing the arguments, the court ruled for the parents and provided a judicial order permitting the transplantation to take place. There is precedent for the courts to intervene in the health care of an incompetent, as for example in the case of the Jehovah's Witness patients, who refuse to permit the administration of blood to a minor. The courts have ruled that such transfusion may be permitted if the attending physician can provide substantial evidence to indicate that the risk of transfusion is insignificant, whereas failure to administer the required blood might result in the death of the infant. A serious limitation of this method is that each case must be presented for judicial opinion on an individual basis.

A second method in widespread use consists in the appointment of watchdog committees at both the local and national levels whenever federal funds are involved in order to pass on the possible risks of a procedure and to be certain that the probable benefit exceeds such risk. It now appears doubtful that the approval of such committees could be considered as a valid permission to carry out procedures involving an incompetent individual, even with parental permission, where no clear-cut benefit to that individual could be ascertained.

A third possibility is a legislative act permitting the parents or some other duly authorized individual to act for the incompetent and give permission for such studies. This solution could conceivably lead to widespread use of prisoners or other undesirable groups for experimentation, and therefore is ethically unacceptable.

A final possibility that appears most reasonable at the present time could be to combine the watchdog committee and a system of no-fault insurance, which would guarantee compensation to any individual who suffered harm resulting from a clinical investigation whether there was evidence of negligence on the part of the investigator or not. Such legislation could take the same form as current compensation law and would protect the rights of an incompetent should any harm occur.

At variance with these positive suggestions is a significant body of legal opinion which states that under no circumstances should an incompetent individual be involved in a procedure which cannot be clearly demonstrated to be directly in the interests of that individual. The implication of this procedure is that vicarious or substituted consent can never be provided.

AT WHAT POINT SHOULD THE LIFE BE TERMINATED, AND WHO SHALL PARTICIPATE IN THIS DECISION?

Active or passive termination of a human life poses the most complex ethical and legal problem in the intensive care unit. It would be stated at the outset that statements such as "death with dignity" and "the right to death" are catch phrases that attempt to reduce a complex issue to the level of an advertising slogan. I am highly suspicious of the validity of conclusions based on this approach. Public concern about the prolongation of life frequently places the burden of implicit or explicit manslaughter at the door of the physician. It may be worth examining some of the reasons for this concern. The issue is not a recent one. In 1624, John Donne wrote an essay on euthanasia and asked "whether it was logical to conscript a young man and subject him to risk of torture and mutilation in war and probable death and refuse an old man escape from an agonizing end."[1] The role of the physician in providing such an escape was stated by Francis Bacon, who wrote, "I esteem it the office of a physician, not only to restore health but to mitigate pain and dolours; and not only when such mitigation may conduce to recovery but when it may serve to make a fair and easy passage."

Careful review of much of the current writing indicates that the despair associated with the dying patient is more often in the eyes of the observer than in the sufferer. This point has been beautifully expressed in a book entitled *Last Rights—A Case for the Good Death,* by Marya Mannes.[2] All too frequently, the argument for active or passive euthanasia is stated in terms of the anguish of the members of the family in having to observe the presumed suffering of a loved one. It is unfortunate that not only the family, but frequently the patient's physician, is uncomfortable in the presence of suffering or impending death. A simple though usually subconsciously appreciated solution to the family's dilemma is to either induce or permit death to occur, thereby absolving everyone of the responsibility of further visits which they, not the patient, find emotionally intolerable. It seems ethically unacceptable to permit the family to make a decision as to when the patient should have life-support devices removed, since directly or indirectly this decision must certainly be at least to some extent self-serving. If the decision to terminate life cannot be made by the family, should the patient himself be assigned this irrevocable role? Studies of the literature on psychosomatic illness suggest that severe depression and even a death wish may be a part of reversible disease, and if observed would often lead to the unnecessary death of patients with reversible illness. Should this decision then be made by the patient's physician? I submit that the traditional role of the physician at the bedside of a terminally ill patient is not so much concerned with the taking or the saving of life as with the relief of suffering. The decision to carry out a particular therapeutic maneuver or to withhold it should not be based upon its effects on the continuance or cessation of life. The test is whether this therapeutic maneuver has a reasonable likelihood of alleviating suffering. A patient dying of intestinal cancer and unable to ingest oral fluids may suffer the extreme anguish of thirst. To provide such a patient with intravenous fluids is not an act to prolong life, but rather a therapeutic effort to alleviate the suffering of a symptom. A terminal cancer patient with intestinal obstruction and severe abdominal cramps should be subjected to a surgical procedure to relieve the obstruction if there is a reasonable likelihood that this procedure will relieve the excruciating pain of intestinal obstruction. Conversely, there is no possible indication for providing intravenous fluids, blood transfusion, or other life-support maneuvers to a patient when the anticipated maneuver offers no opportunity of either treating the underlying illness or relieving the suffering.

When a physician makes the decision to provide or withhold treatment based on a conviction that the patient be allowed to die, he is in the same moral position as if he had given a lethal injection. As stated by James Rachels, "If the physician's decision is wrong, if for example, the patient's illness was, in fact, curable, the decision to withhold therapy would be equally regrettable no matter what method was used to carry it out."[5] The legal implications for withholding therapy that might prolong life have recently received widespread public concern in the case of Dr. Edelin following the death of an abortus. Although the reasons for the jury's decision in finding Dr. Edelin guilty of manslaughter will never be known, one possible interpretation is that he failed to introduce lifesaving measures at a time when such measures might have resulted in the survival of the infant. The implications of this principle are that if a physician withholds therapy in the belief that the patient is dying of an incurable disease or is nonviable, and subsequent autopsy demonstrates that a treatable disease was present, then the physician would be subject not only to a civil action in malpractice but to a criminal action for manslaughter as well. This principle of law, if upheld, would be in direct violation of a principle of common law which states that an individual is under no obligation to take affirmative action to preserve another individual's life. A citizen, for example, is not required to rescue a drowning person from a swimming pool even though it is clear that such intervention might have resulted in the saving of the person's life. On the contrary, it has been stated that an officious volunteer who behaves in a negligent manner in an attempt to save the life would be subject to an action for failure to successfully complete the unrequested interference.

The solution of these problems is certainly not simple or explainable by slogan, nor is it likely that a single answer will be acceptable in all cases. There are, however, at least two areas where solutions may be found. The first is in the definition of death. It is clear that the physician is under no obligation to continue a "life-support system" on a patient who has been legally deemed to be dead. The American Bar Association has suggested that each state modify its laws governing the definition of death to include the cessation of cerebral activity as indicated by absence of brain waves and other neurologic findings. Dr. Earl Walker, a noted neurosurgeon, has recently studied cerebral death in over 500 patients and has suggested specific criteria for declaring that death has taken place.[7] If these were to become law, then a large number of patients being kept "alive" in our intensive care units would automatically be legally dead. All life-support systems would immediately be discontinued. The second area where much can be done is the education of patients' families and physicians concerning the process of dying and death. The commentator Stuart Alsop, writing about his own fatal bone marrow disease, stated, "when you feel sick enough, you don't much fear death."[2]

Doctors, patients, and their families must face the question of dying honestly, preferably in conversation together. The Reverend Cassem, staff psychiatrist at Youville, has stated, "the greatest fear the dying have is the fear of dying alone and this is a fear we can treat."[2] It is the responsibility of the physician in an intensive care unit to bring the family into the room with the patient and to explain in the presence of all concerned what the true situation is and what the expectations are. Marya Mannes quotes from a network program on ABC in which an elderly terminal patient complained to her doctor that her nurse kept offering her fruit juice when what she desperately wanted was attention. There is a crucial need for talk and for the acknowledgment of all concerned that only by facing death squarely and fearlessly can the dread of death dissipate or be transformed into acceptance and peace. Once the initial shock has been faced, the patient and his family may enter into a final experience together that will leave the family enriched and aid the patient in achieving what Francis Bacon called "a fair and easy passage." When suffering is apparent, the physician should direct his therapy at those measures that will relieve the suffering, with the realization that such treatment may result in some instances in the prolongation of life, and in other instances in the hastening of death. The decision of who shall die and when is not properly within the physician's province. The relief of mental and physical suffering is the essence and the extent of a physician's role at the approach of death.

REFERENCES

1. Donne, J.: Deaths Duell, 1624.
2. Mannes, M.: Last Rights—A Case for the Good Death. New York, William Morrow and Company, 1973.
3. McCormick, R. A.: Proxy consent in the experimentation situation. Reprinted from Perspectives in Biology and Medicine, Vol. 18, Autumn 1974.
4. O'Donnell, T. J.: Editorial: Informed consent. J.A.M.A., 227:73, 1974.
5. Rachels, J.: N. Engl. J. Med., 292:78, 1975.
6. Ramsey, P.: The Patient as a Person. New Haven, Yale University Press, 1970.
7. Study suggests new, less rigid criteria for declaring death. Medical World News, January 27, 1975, pp. 26–27.

Part III

MANAGEMENT OF SPECIFIC CONDITIONS

CHAPTER 15

THE CONTROL OF INFECTION

HARVEY R. BERNARD, M.D.

Infectious disease in the intensive care unit, although basically no different from that found elsewhere, poses additional problems. Several factors serve to intensify the difficulties: the patient is seriously ill, more than one organ system is usually involved, decisions and therapy must be hastily accomplished, more than one discipline may be involved, multiple breaks in the normal host resistance mechanism for treatment or monitoring are frequent, and some degree of crowding is usual.

Although infectious disease may constitute the most serious aspect of an illness, it is usually not the primary reason for admission to an intensive care unit and may not be accorded the attention it requires. If relegated to a lower level of priority, its cure, though essential, may be considered only a minor episode necessarily tolerated during the therapy of more interesting problems. The urgency surrounding treatment and monitoring utilized in an intensive care unit encourages the staff to abrogate the rigid techniques that are necessary to prevent infections.

RECOGNITION OF INFECTION

The first step in the management of the infected patient begins with recognition that a consequential infection exists; while this seems an easy matter superficially, those of experience are aware that this decison is frequently most difficult. The discovery of bacteria on a smear or culture is not always sufficient evidence of infection. Similarly, a change in the organism cultivated during a patient's hospital care does not necessarily indicate a change in therapy. The therapist is faced with a dilemma. In general, he would like to treat patients suffering from infection at the earliest possible moment, or perhaps even attempt to prevent the bacterial infection. On the other hand, he is aware that unnecessary treatment is expensive, exposes

203

the patient to the risk of drug reactions, or may increase the difficulty in treating infections in the future.

Commensal bacteria of little or no significance to healthy human beings may become significant in the intensive care patient who has become, by virtue of his illness, a compromised host in the host-pathogen relationship. The normally sterile tracheobronchial tree rapidly becomes colonized after tracheostomy; and despite the most careful precautions, urinary tract infections eventually follow indwelling catheterization of the bladder. There is good evidence that colonization of the pharynx by gram-negative bacteria, rare in health, is associated with hospitalization and that the frequency correlates directly with the seriousness of the illness.[5]

Although a hard and fast definition of infection is difficult to derive, the presence of pus in a wound, in the urinary tract, or in the tracheobronchial tree is almost certainly diagnostic, especially if accompanied by fever, leukocytosis, and the isolation of appropriate bacteria. Infection is of more consequence if systemic effects are pronounced, and if there is remarkable fever, positive blood culture, and the like. The definition of infection around indwelling tubes or catheters is somewhat more difficult, since skin bacteria are always present at their egress from the skin. However, the combination of induration and otherwise unexplained fever or systemic response with or without inflammation around the catheter constitutes sufficient reason for the removal and study of such a device for the presence of bacteria.

All too often recognition of wound infection is delayed because of a reluctance to admit the possibility. The attentive surgeon will, upon evidence of infection, immediately assume that the wound is infected until he can demonstrate to his satisfaction that it is not. Frequently, unnecessarily bulky or extensive dressings are employed and direct visualization of the wound is delayed because of a reluctance to disturb an artistic bandage or dressing. Although occlusive dressings and dressings that immobilize may be of importance under specific circumstances, e.g., fractures, burns, or infections of the extremities, the usual clean wound requires only a small dressing or none at all. Wounds occluded with plastic films or large amounts of tape produce a soggy environment with a reduced oxygen tension, the more so if some drainage is present. A change of dressing when saturated with drainage is preferable to the addition of more and more gauze.

Unusual wound pain indicates the possibility of infection with *Clostridium perfringens*. Examination with the gloved hand may disclose crepitus, suggesting the presence of gas. Such gas may also be detected through the use of the stethoscope or soft tissue x-ray techniques. The presence of gas is not necessarily synonymous with the presence of clostridial infection, since bacteria other than clostridia produce gas. It is, however, a serious sign that must not be ignored. Occasionally, crepitus will be found around drain sites, ileostomies, or colostomies when infection is not present, simply from the escape of air left within the peritoneal cavity at the time of closure.

Erythema associated with infections of wounds closed with sutures may be minimized if the skin has been closed with plastic tapes. It is difficult to determine whether the use of these tapes has resulted in a lower incidence of infection in subcutaneous wounds, but the appearance of these wounds has changed, perhaps since the foreign body effect of the sutures themselves is minimized. Subcutaneous wound infection is most certainly defined by exploration of the wound, using a clamp or probe to penetrate to the fascial depth in the most suspicious area, or in multiple areas should this be advisable. The risk is minimal if such explorations are performed under suitable conditions, i.e., with good light, adequate preparation of the skin with antiseptic solution, sterile instruments, gloved hands, and adequate help. The reward is the drainage of infected blood or frank pus when the only symptom of early infection is tenderness localized to a specific area in the subcutaneous wound.

Careful examination of the temperature course expressed on a graph is of continuing importance. Examination of the leukocyte count with a differential examination of the cells is equally important and may be overlooked in favor of more esoteric studies in the modern intensive care unit. However, such studies give considerable information about the presence or absence of an infection and the patient's ability to respond to it. The gallium scan has been described recently for detection of abscesses but has not been of great help in our experience. Examination of the chest and liver by radioisotope scanning is occasionally helpful when searching for abscesses within the liver or beneath the diaphragm, and should be added to simple x-ray examination of the chest and abdomen in search of abnormal accumulations of fluid or the presence of gas in large bubbles or small flecks. Observation of the classic findings of infection may be obscured if the infection is contained beneath investing fascia. Here the surgeon must be persistent, examining and reexamining the patient until the source of the infection is found.

Examination of exudates, almost a lost art, provides a remarkable opportunity for study of bacteria during the early stages of infection by use of the Gram stain. Information thus achieved provides knowledge of the actual numbers of bacteria involved, and their ratio to polymorphonuclear leukocytes provides information about the host's reaction to them. Accurate definition of the bacteria and their speciation through cultivation and biochemical manipulation requires a relatively long period of time with resulting delay, ineffectual therapy, and the possibility that the organisms cultivated represent the ones easily cultivated rather than the ones causing the infection. In general, samples of wound exudates should immediately be transferred to the appropriate culture medium. The samples for culture should be taken from the walls of abscesses or the edges of advancing infection, and samples of tissue or actual pus are preferable to a wound swab. The most effective culture techniques involve direct plating on the culture medium with a minimum of handling and exposure to the environment; when investigating anaerobic bacteria, this is best accomplished by taking the anaerobic media, a gas pack, and an anaerobic jar to the bedside. Failing this, transfer media suitably deprived of oxygen by boiling, or media commercially prepared to supplant oxygen with inert gases, may be utilized.

THE BACTERIA

The types of bacteria encountered in infections that develop in hospitals, especially in intensive care units, vary from time to time and from hospital to hospital. This may result from changes in the bacteria, the type of patient, and the types of operations that are prevalent.

The microorganisms that are cultivated from hospitalized patients, except for unusual circumstances, are characteristic of the bacterial flora of the area of the body which has been compromised, or of the bacteria of the environment which gained access to the patient through a break in his host defenses. The latter usually means an injury to the integument or a mucosally lined surface as a result of either trauma or the introduction of a device for therapeutic or monitoring purposes.

In the relatively healthy and normally resistant patient, unencumbered by necrotic debris, infection is usually caused by *Staphylococcus aureus,* the hemolytic streptococcus, or a combination of the bacteria found within his gastrointestinal tract except when contamination of his tissues by external trauma introduces a greater risk of clostridial infection.

If the patient is severely ill, his illness has been prolonged, his wound is large and associated with much debris, or his treatment has been associated with prolonged therapy utilizing a multiplicity of antibiotic drugs, the wound flora will more likely include gram-negative bacteria, which usually do not cause primary infections, or fungi, which rarely infect patients with normal host resistence, e.g., *Pseudomonas aeruginosa, Serratia marcescens,* and *Candida albicans.*

Much that has been written in the last two decades would indicate that bacteria have undergone remarkable changes, perhaps as a result of antimicrobial intervention. The only changes that can be denoted with certainty relate to *Staphylococcus aureus* where at least one generally recognized worldwide epidemic with a specific bacteriophage type occurred (type 80–81). The reason for the waxing and waning of this bacteriophage type is conjectural. The alterations in antibiotic resistance that have been noted are probably a consequence of effective therapy, a risk which must be borne if antimicrobials are to be used at all. There is, of course, the possibility of change in antimicrobial resistance, through one of several mechanisms, caused by unnecessary use of antimicrobials, but the definition of this is difficult. Some of the changes in the names of bacteria reported reflect alterations in the interest of bacteriologists, who have from time to time become interested in the more specific identification of organisms and as a result of such interest have given the impression of an altered incidence of bacteria. The most recent example is the "rediscovery" of the anaerobic bacteria and an awakening interest in their cultivation. While there is no evidence at the present to indicate that anaerobic bacteria are more prevalent in the intestines or wounds contaminated by soil and intestinal material in the modern patient than was found three to four decades ago, improved methods of bacterial cultivation, especially of fastidious anaerobic bacteria, have made physicians and surgeons aware of the presence of a variety of bacteria previously rarely discussed. Careful, energetic utilization of modern methods of bacterial cultivation will decrease the incidence of what was formerly called "sterile abscess" and will increase the complexity of the bacteria found in the flora of a mixed bacterial infection. Decisions concerning treatment will depend upon observation of the important clinical effects of these bacteria in addition to the simple knowledge of their presence. Anaerobic bacteria and appropriate surgical and antimicrobial therapy for them should be considered whenever contamination by the gastrointestinal or genitourinary tracts has taken place, especially if the infections are malodorous.

There has been, on the other hand, an obvious change in the host, particularly in the intensive care unit. Patients are no longer denied operative treatment at either end of the age scale. Size does not represent any contraindication, since the surgical experience encompasses the tiny premature and the excessively obese. Since modern surgical therapy and antimicrobial drugs are capable of eliminating most organisms that cause infections, the ones that remain are of low pathogenicity but have significant antimicrobial resistance and are capable of invasion in the severely compromised host. The new flora, then, is that of the antibiotic-treated, immunologically paralyzed, seriously ill patient whose host defenses have been penetrated by many tubes and catheters.

The introduction of the indwelling plastic venous catheter and the prolonged use of the endotracheal tube have caused a major alteration in the infective pattern. The effects of these devices may be minimized through the use of Silastic materials.

SURGICAL TREATMENT OF THE INFECTIOUS PROCESS

The primary objectives of surgical therapy are a decrease in the size of the bacterial inoculum and an increase in the resistance of the host. The former objective is obtained, preferentially, through excision of the infective process along with necrotic debris and foreign material. As a corollary, surgical wounds are less likely to develop infection if the amount of foreign material used is minimized, is composed of material that causes the least tissue reaction, and has a smooth surface avoiding braiding, twisting, and the like. Since complete excision of the infected locus is frequently impossible, incision and drainage with removal of foreign material and necrotic tissue is the next goal. This has the additional advantage of relieving pressure within the infected area, which otherwise tends to promote the drainage of infected material and its by-products into the lymphatics and the venous circulation.

When the decision has been made to treat an infected wound, the surgeon is well advised to choose his time and place carefully. The usual surgeon is an optimist and frequently underestimates the difficulties that may be encountered. For this reason, good preparation including lighting, sufficient help, and adequate anesthesia is advisable before wounds are explored.

Drainage should be effected via the most direct route consistent with preservation of the important anatomic structures in the area. The opening should be of sufficient size to allow the free egress of pus, and the skin edges should be kept from reapproximation through the insertion of adequate drains or sterile fine-meshed gauze. The use of tight packing should be avoided, for it will serve as a plug to impede the passage of pus. The surgeon should be alert to the probability of remarkable bleeding from surface vessels just beneath the skin. Ligation of these at the time of the incision and drainage will prevent loss of blood in the early postoperative period and the need for painful and obstructive packing to control hemorrhage. The use of stiff rubber or plastic drains and tubes should be avoided when such instruments may impinge upon vessels or other viscera.

Vigorous and thorough irrigation of wounds has become a surgical ritual that may have some value in removing gross debris and purulent material. It is, however, unlikely to remove significant numbers of bacteria in viable tissue or to aid in the removal of necrotic material that has not as yet undergone lysis. The injudicious use of irrigation may actually spread infection. Irrigation through small openings under pressure may open tissue planes that have previously been closed. Solutions used for irrigation should be physiologic in content, tonicity, and temperature to avoid additional tissue destruction. The addition of antibiotics to such irrigations is probably inadvisable because of the variable dose of the antibiotic that may be absorbed, the unnecessary environmental spillage of the antibiotics, and the comparative inefficiency of this dosage route as compared with the intravenous one. The cytotoxic effects of various halogen-containing solutions, such as the iodophors and Dakin's solution, make their value questionable except in chronic, neglected infections. Hydrogen peroxide has the same effect on the red blood cells as does water, and the bubbling effect of oxygen may produce additional tissue damage. Accurate anatomic debridement with sterile sharp instruments is preferable.

Host resistance may be improved locally by improvement in the blood flow through a part by reconstruction of vessels and by the addition of an improved supply of oxygen through improved respiratory function, the addition of blood transfusions to elevate the percentage of oxygen-carrying hemoglobin, and the relief of either hypovolemia or extracellular fluid volume deficit as a cause of hypoperfusion.

TREATMENT OF THE OPEN WOUND

Open wounds should be treated as described above during their early stages. Careful, sharp debridement followed by frequent changing of fine-meshed gauze kept moistened with physiologic saline solution remains the basic standard. If employed diligently, this will result in a clean, healthy surface that will permit direct closure or closure through the application of autogenous skin covering. Krizek's estimate of 10^5 organisms per gram of tissue[8] gives a rough approximation of the maximum bacterial contamination that will permit healing. Additional information may be obtained by observation of the wound edges for evidence of epithelialization, which indicates the likelihood of clean healing.

The time for closure depends upon the mobility of the tissues and the degree of undermining. If there is sufficient mobility and no undermining, closure with sterile plastic or paper tapes provides a simple, painless, and secure closure that permits ready inspection of the wound at all depths. We have avoided the insertion of sutures, which result in tissue tunnels containing foreign bodies, and do not employ skin adhesives because of the blisters that frequently attend their use if overzealous approximation is attempted or if distention beneath the wound occurs. Large fixed defects may be favorably influenced through the use of thin split-thickness grafts that have been separated into small stamps or whose surface area has been increased through the use of a meshing device. Wound contracture is evident within 24 to 48 hours when skin grafting has been effective.

We have utilized delayed primary closure of the skin and subcutaneous tissue of wounds considered likely to develop infection and have generally closed these with sterile tapes within 48 to 72 hours, relying on a normal appearance of the wound as the indication for closure. While such early closure does not guarantee clean healing, systemic or spreading infection is rare.

INFECTION ASSOCIATED WITH INTRAVENOUS LINES, URINARY CATHETERS, ENDOTRACHEAL TUBES, AND OTHER DRAINAGE DEVICES

Infections associated with the insertion of foreign devices for monitoring and care of physiologic functions constitute the next most important group after infections of the wound or primary illness itself. In the intensive care unit, the frequency of such infections probably exceeds that of wound infection. The treatment of infection associated with such devices is usually comparatively simple, i.e., most are cured by the removal of the offending catheter or drain with or without the addition of an antimicrobial effective against the organism involved. The complete prevention of these infections is probably impossible and the reduction of their incidence is difficult because, first, the devices are unphysiologic and can never be made physiologic. Each breaches the normal host resistance (skin or mucosal barrier) and provides a foreign body bridge for external contamination. Second, the devices are used so frequently that personnel within areas like intensive care units come to regard them carelessly. Although intravenous catheters, urinary catheters, and other monitoring devices are frequently inserted into the most vital areas, they are usually packaged in a single wrapper, are placed carelessly in carts and bins by untrained personnel, and are inserted and manipulated with comparative disregard for the risks that might be involved. Fortunately the risks with modern, minimally reactive devices are comparatively minor for each individual device; however, since many patients in intensive care units are treated with several such devices, and since such treatment may be prolonged for days, weeks, and even months, the risk mounts steadily as the use increases.

The endotracheal tube is an even greater problem, since its use eventually guarantees colonization of the lower respiratory tract, as does the use of the tracheostomy. The endotracheal tube must of necessity pass through an unsterile area before its insertion into the previously uncontaminated lower respiratory tract, and this realization plus the difficulty in caring for such an airway leads to many lapses in technique. Infections associated with endotracheal tubes may be minimized through the use of minimally reactive plastic materials, the use of occlusive cuffs which avoid pressure on the mucosa and tracheal rings, and careful technique for suctioning of secretions to avoid the implantation of extraneous bacteria or the damage of the mucosal surface from the catheter tip itself. A careful program of sterilization and maintenance of the respiratory therapy equipment must be mounted to preclude the possibility of inoculation of bacteria through humidification and other devices.[9] Perhaps most important of all, infection is avoided by the initial skillful and careful insertion of the endotracheal tube and its removal at the earliest possible moment.

Intravenous solutions are used so frequently in modern hospitals that they have become commonplace and have lost much of the respect originally accorded them. Particularly in areas where frequent changes of drugs and rapid administration are performed, the intravenous lines are contaminated with a frequency inversely proportional to the care that is utilized.

The use and introduction of the indwelling plastic catheter in the last several decades has altered the pattern of infection in the hospitals remarkably and with a frequency that is undeterminable. It is fortunate that the human can absorb and control a remarkable number of bacteria given intravenously, for such contamination is probably frequent.

Individual punctures with small, sharp, sterile, stainless steel needles connected to a single intravenous tubing and a single use intravenous bottle constitute the technique least likely to result in infection following the administration of intravenous solutions. However, most intravenous solutions will be administred in intensive care units through an indwelling plastic catheter. These catheters and their tubing and bottles are usually changed infrequently because of inconvenience to both the personnel and the patient himself.

A decreased risk of bacterial contamination of intravenous therapy should follow the use of the system detailed on Figure 1, which provides for the administration of intravenous fluids, the administration of intravenous medications, and the change of the various containers with a minimum of contamination. All reconstitution or adaptation of fluids to be given intravenously should be carried out by specially trained and equipped pharmacists under the most careful conditions, thus avoiding risk, inefficiency,

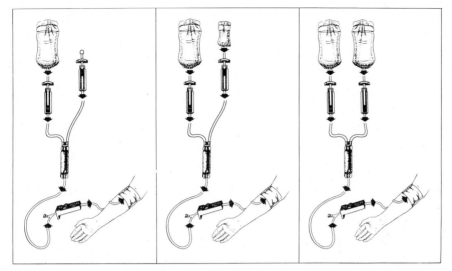

Figure 1.   A "Y" shaped, plastic intravenous delivery device, which permits regulation of rate of fluid delivery at each of its limbs, intermittent delivery of medications (here shown in plastic "mini bottles"), or administration of additional intravenous fluid with minimal risk of contamination. The side arm post remains for emergency injections but should rarely be used.

expense, and untidiness of reconstitution of solutions at the bedside. The fluids given in this manner should be connected to a Silastic catheter implanted in an appropriate vessel through a wound made in skin prepared as carefully as it would be for a standard surgical operation, and maintained securely to avoid movement to and fro through the skin. Although the need for the urgent injection of an unexpected drug will arise, this should be infrequent. Reperforation of rubber seals to gain access to intravenous lines should be avoided, since the technique for resterilizing these seals is totally inadequate, is never employed properly, and is probably impossible after the seal has been perforated previously.

Prevention of infection following the insertion of urinary catheters is difficult and probably impossible in the long term, but infection may be minimized by utilizing the principles enunciated by Kunin: the skillful insertion of a catheter under near sterile precautions and its connection to a closed drainage system, the integrity of which is never disturbed except for the periodic removal of urine through a system which avoids ascending contamination of the urine.[6] Several devices are available that make this at least theoretically if not practically possible. The major difficulty is insurance of the proper employment of these devices, particularly under urgent or hurried conditions.

Skillful, gentle, aseptic insertion of catheters and tubes followed by skillful dressing changes with intermittent reprep with an iodophor is probably preferable to local use of antibiotic ointments.

ANTIMICROBIAL USAGE

There are several principles that are basic to effective antimicrobial therapy, especially in surgical patients: (1) antimicrobial therapy is most effective when employed early in the illness when the inoculum is small; (2) necrotic debris, impaired blood flow, and retained foreign bodies minimize or negate the effectiveness of antimicrobials; and (3) laboratory descriptions of antimicrobial sensitivity of bacteria cultivated from surgical infections do not always coincide with clinical evidence of antimicrobial effectiveness; when this discrepancy occurs, the clinical observations are probably the most valid.

There are few instances in the intensive care setting that demand the use of antimicrobials as prophylaxis, although antimicrobial administration of an effective drug should be utilized to protect patients about to undergo drainage of an established infection through previously uncontaminated tissue planes. Otherwise, almost all antibiotic usage in the intensive care unit is therapeutic.

Antimicrobials will not be effective against localized infections accompanied by necrotic debris, retained foreign bodies, or inadequate blood flow unless a concomitant surgical attack upon these problems is made. Reliance upon antimicrobial therapy alone to treat surgical infections is usually a vain hope, and although a few patients may recover after prolonged therapy, expeditious surgical treatment of the infection will usually result in a safer and more rapid recovery. Antimicrobial drugs are more useful in the prevention of lymphatic spread from established infection, in the treatment of spreading cellulitis, and for the minimization of the systemic effects of blood-borne bacteria. Certain seeming contradictions include antimicrobial treatment of urinary tract and respiratory tract infections, although even in these instances cure is usually asssociated with eventual intraluminal drainage and removal of obstruction.

Unfortunately, the popular usage of antimicrobial drugs is remarkably influenced by commercial considerations. Careful day-to-day observations of the effects of the antimicrobials on specific medical problems must be heeded. Since differences are reported concerning the effectiveness of various antimicrobials, depending upon geographic and temporal relationships, it is far better for a hospital to decide upon a few drugs with well known side-effects which, based on experience, are effective in that setting and which are changed when a need is perceived, not when a new drug needs to be sold. Intensive care units are busy places and poor areas for the careful observation and documentation of side-effects that are common to all drugs; it is therefore advisable to utilize drugs with known side-effects whenever feasible.

Table 1 lists information about six antimicrobials with established utility. The author uses others under urgent conditions only after appropriate reflection and consultation. For a more encyclopedic dissertation, see Weinstein's chapter on antimicrobials in Goodman and Gilman.[11]

There is a recent trend toward multiple drug usage, which has resulted from a realization of the polymicrobial nature of many infections plus the physician's natural desire to control all possibilities. However, this trend toward the use of a separate antibiotic for every germ cultivated should cease. The infections requiring a combination of antibiotics are rare,[2] and the use of combinations of antibiotics usually indicates ignorance of the etiology of the infection or insecurity about the therapist's ability to assess the likely offender. An educated estimate based upon observation of the bacteria usually observed and the chemotherapy usually most effective, aided by a smear and Gram stain of available specimens, must always constitute the basis of informed therapy in all but the most trivial infections.

A change of the organism in the culture during treatment does not dictate a need for change of antimicrobial. However, a change in the clinical course always requires reassessment of therapy; the surgeon under these circumstances should look again for evidence of the presence or increase in size of a specific bacterial inoculum with accompanying necrotic debris or foreign body, and seize the opportunity for extirpating it. Failing this, alteration of the antimicrobial in search of an effective one is appropriate. However, addition of more than one antimicrobial to the original selection always adds risk, always adds cost, but rarely results in clinical benefit. If the original selection is effective, it should not be changed; if it is not effective, there is little benefit in retaining an ineffective antimicrobial, and a change to a more effective one is in order.

Significant renal failure is encountered frequently in the intensive care unit. Drugs that are excreted by the kidneys require modification of the amount administered when renal excretion is impaired to avoid undesirable accumulation of these drugs. The extent of renal impairment is most practically and accurately assessed through determination of the creatinine clearance and by monitoring the serum level of the drug. Modifications of the dose of these drugs and the timing of administration may be approximated by comparison of their elimination constants with creatinine clearance nomograms or special tables and formulas.[1] The package inserts for relevant drugs provide specific information about modification of dosage. These should be consulted and their directions followed explicitly when renal failure complicates antimicrobial therapy. Since the extent of renal failure may change rapidly, the creatinine clearance must be studied repeatedly. For example, the information dealing with the dosage of gentamicin in the face of renal impairment as listed on the package inset is given in Table 3.

ISOLATION PRECAUTIONS

An intensive care unit is a place where patients who are exceedingly ill are cared for; it is also a medical philosophy and a window on medical happenings for the public as a whole. Much of the public's image of the medical profession results from its perception of our activities in the inten-

Table 1.   ANTIMICROBIALS RECOMMENDED FOR GENERAL USE UNDER URGENT CONDITIONS IN INTENSIVE CARE UNITS

DRUG	INDICATIONS	ROUTE	DOSE	DILUENT	INCOMPATI-BILITIES	EXCRETION OR INACTIVATION	COMPLICATIONS
Penicillin G	Penicillin-sensitive gram-positive and gram-negative bacteria	IV	1.2–12 million units/day	Normal saline solution; 5% glucose in water	—	Renal 60–90% (hepatic)	Hypersensitivity
Nafcillin	Gram-positive bacteria; penicillin-resistant *S. aureus*	IV	500 mg–1 gm every 4 hours	Normal saline solution; sterile distilled water	—	Hepatic 90% (renal)	Hypersensitivity
Cephalothin	Sensitive gram-positive and gram-negative bacteria; penicillin-resistant *S. aureus*; chemoprophylaxis of general and gynecologic surgery	IV	4–12 gm/day	Normal saline solution; 5% glucose in water	Aminoglycosides furosemide	Renal 60–80%	Hypersensitivity; thrombophlebitis locally

Gentamicin	Sensitive gram-negative bacteria in seriously ill; *P. aeruginosa*	IV	3 mg/kg/day in 3 divided doses in adults with normal renal function; otherwise *see package insert*	Normal saline solution; 5% glucose in water, 1 mg/ml; should not be mixed with other drugs	Cephalosporins furosemide	Renal	Ototoxicity; nephrotoxicity
Chloramphenicol*	Serious infections with anaerobic bacteria or mixed aerobic and anaerobic flora	IV	50 mg/kg/day in 4 doses	5% glucose in water	—	Hepatic (renal)	Blood dyscrasia
Clindamycin†	Bacteriologically proven serious infections caused by *Bacteroides fragilis* or other sensitive anaerobic bacteria	IV	600–1200 mg/day in 2–4 doses in adults; otherwise *see package insert*	All IV solutions in usual clinical concentrations	Vitamin B complex erythromycin	Hepatic	Ileocolitis

*The risk of aplastic anemia may have been overstated when chloramphenicol is limited to intravenous therapy of serious surgical infection.[4]
†The author prefers to limit administration of clindamycin to infections of established etiology until the relationship of clindamycin to ileocolitis is established.[10]

Table 2.   Dosage Schedule Guide for Garamycin Injectable[7] in
Adults with Normal Renal Function

Patient's Weight kg	Usual Dose for Serious Infections 1 mg/kg every 8 hours		Dose for Life-threatening Infections (Reduce as Soon as Clinically Indicated) 1.7 mg/kg every 8 hours	
	mg/dose	ml/dose	mg/dose	ml/dose
40	40	1.0	66	1.6
45	45	1.1	75	1.9
50	50	1.25	83	2.1
55	55	1.4	91	2.25
60	60	1.5	100	2.5
65	65	1.6	108	2.7
70	70	1.75	116	2.9
75	75	1.9	125	3.1
80	80	2.0	133	3.3
85	85	2.1	141	3.5
90	90	2.25	150	3.75
95	95	2.4	158	4.0
100	100	2.5	166	4.2
105	105	2.6	175	4.4
110	110	2.75	183	4.5
115	115	2.9	191	4.75
120	120	3.0	200	5.0

Table 3.   Dosage Adjustment Guide for Garamycin Injectable[7] in
Patients with Renal Impairment

Serum Creatinine mg/dl	Approximate Creatinine Clearance Rate ml/min/1.73 m^2	Percent of Usual Dose Shown in Table 2 every 8 hours
≤ 1.0	> 100	100
1.1 to 1.3	70 to 100	80
1.4 to 1.6	55 to 70	65
1.7 to 1.9	45 to 55	55
2.0 to 2.2	40 to 45	50
2.3 to 2.5	35 to 40	40
2.6 to 3.0	30 to 35	35
3.1 to 3.5	25 to 30	30
3.6 to 4.0	20 to 25	25
4.1 to 5.1	15 to 20	20
5.2 to 6.6	10 to 15	15
6.7 to 8.0	< 10	10

sive care area both in real life and in the public media. Since intensive care usually includes a rather large number of personnel involved with each patient, and since the concept also frequently includes multiple occupancy of a given patient area, there is an obvious need for planning, discipline, and general tidiness. Control of the traffic is an obvious necessity that many times is not carried out.

There are no data that would indicate the requisite level of bacteria in the atmosphere about intensive care patients. It is unlikely that this is of great significance except in the nursing of patients who are immunologically paralyzed. Although numerical guidelines are lacking, a reasonable level of hygienic housekeeping and satisfactory air filtration and control is advisable, not only for the maintenance of a satisfactory level of environmental bacteria, but also as a method of increasing public confidence. The housekeeping must be especially controlled, since those involved in this effort are usually not medically educated.

Isolation is usually a crude, ineffective device and must be reckoned with in that light. The rules that hospitals make must fit the circumstances and will not replace intelligent understanding of individual problems. Many hospitals attempt to invoke one form of isolation to cover all possibilities, and this absurdity is usually followed by a lack of cooperation on the part of the staff.

In the active intensive care unit, a sensible balance must be struck between isolation of patients who require it and the avoidance of interference with necessary intensive care. The U.S. Public Health Service manual on Isolation Techniques should serve as a standard for hospitals in the United States.[3]

Fortunately, most of the infections seen in the intensive care unit are not highly contagious. The prevalent organisms may change, but since the outbreak of the epidemic *Staphylococcus aureus* infections of the 1950s and 1960s, there has been little evidence of virulent bacterial epidemics. Patients are usually infected with bacteria of endogenous origin, bacteria normally present within the gastrointestinal tract or on the skin surfaces of normal patients. The risk of transfer of the usual mixed bacterial wound exudate is no greater than that associated with the care of colostomies or the products of the normal gastrointestinal tract.

Infections associated with intravenous tubing, respiratory tubing, drains, catheters, and the like require proper handling by the disposal team, which of course requires constant supervision; but the risk of cross-contamination is nil, provided the initial technique of insertion is satisfactory.

In conclusion, the control of infection in intensive care units relies less upon complicated devices and antimicrobial drugs and more upon intelligent understanding of the cause of infection and careful application of sound principles of aseptic technique, especially when working under urgent or desperate circumstances.

REFERENCES

1. Bennett, W. M., Singer, I., and Coggins, C. J.: A guide to drug therapy in renal failure. J.A.M.A., *230*:1544, 1974.
2. Brumfit, W., and Percival, A.: Antibiotic combinations. Lancet, *1*:387, 1971.
3. Department of Health, Education, and Welfare: Isolation techniques for use in hospitals. Publication No. (HSM) 71–8043. Washington, D.C. Reprinted 1973.
4. Gleckman, R. A.: Warning—chloramphenicol may be good for your health. Arch. Intern. Med., *135*:1125, 1975.
5. Johanson, W. G., Pierce, A. K., and Sanford, J. P.: Changing pharyngeal bacterial flora of hospitalized patients—emergence of gram-negative bacilli. N. Engl. J. Med., *281*:1137, 1969.
6. Kunin, C.: Detection, Prevention, and Management of Urinary Tract Infections. 2nd Ed. Philadelphia, Lea and Febiger, 1974.
7. Product Information, Garamycin Injectable. Schering Pharmaceutical Corporation, Kenilworth, New Jersey.
8. Robson, M. C., Krizek, T. J., and Heggers, J. P.: Biology of surgical infection. Curr. Probl. Surg., 1, March 1973.
9. Sanford, J. P.: Infection control in critical care units, Crit. Care Med., *2*:211, 1974.
10. Tedesco, F. J., Barton, R. W., and Alpers, D. H.: Clindamycin-associated colitis: a prospective study. Ann. Intern. Med., *81*:429, 1974.
11. Weinstein, L.: Antimicrobial Agents. *In* Goodman, L. S., and Gilman, A. (Eds.): The Pharmacological Basis of Therapeutics. 5th Ed. New York, Macmillan Publishing Company, 1975, pp. 113–1247.

CHAPTER 16

VENTILATORY COMPLICATIONS: PREVENTION AND TREATMENT

Michael A. Rie, M.D.

Henning Pontoppidan, M.D.

The last 25 years have witnessed an ever expanding body of knowledge relating to the normal and abnormal physiology of respiration in man. The advent of modern respiratory care and its successful therapeutic and prophylactic application to ventilatory derangements has paralleled this information explosion.[2,14,15] Paradoxically, the number of patients requiring such care has continued to increase. This trend reflects two fundamental changes in contemporary surgery: (1) large numbers of poor-risk patients are undergoing surgical procedures that require intra- and postoperative multiorgan system interventions and mechanical respiratory assistance; (2) modern intensive care units are able to support gas exchange in the lungs for prolonged periods of time in patients who continue to manifest failure or instability of other vital systems that precludes the withdrawal of respiratory support. While patients in prior years might have died (and still do) with prolonged wound sepsis, starvation and cardiorenal failure, the advent of total parenteral nutrition, improved circulatory monitoring, newer cardiotonic drugs, and coronary revascularization with mechanical circulatory assist devices has created an expanding population of patients who continue to require mechanical respiratory assistance for nonpulmonary causes.

This chapter attempts to present a physiologic approach to the diagnosis and therapy of respiratory derangements in the surgical patient. The interrelationship of respiration with the ongoing care of other vital organ systems is stressed.

Supported by Grant GM–15904–08 from the National Institute of General Medical Sciences.

219

ETIOLOGY OF RESPIRATORY DECOMPENSATION IN SURGICAL PATIENTS

Acute respiratory failure (ARF) in this chapter denotes an acute insult to the respiratory apparatus in patients with near normal lung function prior to operative intervention or trauma. While surgery may lead to acute decompensation of gas exchange in patients with previous chronic obstructive lung disease (COPD), pathophysiologic and therapeutic considerations in the care of chronic respiratory failure are different from those of ARF and will be alluded to only briefly in this chapter.

Hypoxemia as measured by the arterial blood oxygen tension is the hallmark of ARF, being present when Pao_2 is below the predicted normal range (supine position) for the patient's age at the prevalent barometric pressure (in the absence of intracardiac right-to-left shunting). Hypoxemia commonly manifests as *tachycardia, tachypnea, disorientation,* and *hypertension.* Severe acute hypoxemia ($Pao_2 < 40$ mm Hg) may present with cyanosis, hypotension, and bradycardia.

Hypercapnia ($Paco_2 > 50$ mm Hg) is *not* a feature of ARF except as a preterminal event. Mild ARF is usually associated with normocapnia. As hypoxemia worsens, hypocapnia ($Paco_2 < 40$ mm Hg) develops and there is a progressive fall in arterial $Paco_2$ (in the absence of CNS depression or injury) with advancing hypoxemia culminating in an abrupt return of $Paco_2$ to normal or elevated levels at or near the time of total cardiopulmonary collapse.

While a multitude of situations may contribute to the development of ARF (pneumonia, aspiration, congestive heart failure, contusion emboli, and so on), little is known of the specific effects of each on lung structure and cellular function. Until more is known, the physician must assess and treat the two physiologic disorders present in all patients with ARF: alveolar collapse and pulmonary edema.

ALVEOLAR COLLAPSE

Functional residual capacity (FRC).   Functional residual capacity of the lung is that volume of gas residing in the lungs at the end of expiration. It is elevated in emphysema and acute asthmatic attacks but decreased in other acute lung diseases. As FRC falls, the number of open alveoli that may participate in gas exchange decreases. Acute loss of alveoli will lead to the appearance of perfused but nonventilated areas (shunt), which results in hypoxemia.

Airway closure.   In normal man, the small airways (less than 1.0 mm diameter) show a progressive tendency to close as lung volume falls during expiration. With closure of the small airways there is nonventilation of distal alveoli until reopening of the airways occurs. The longer the closure period continues, the greater the "damage." The critical lung volume at which closure of the airways is first detected is referred to as the closing volume (CV). The FRC usually exceeds CV in the upright position; with the supine position or an acute decrease in FRC from disease and pulmonary restriction, FRC will fall below CV and further alveolar collapse with aggravation of hypoxemia will occur. Common restrictive factors are the supine position, abdominal distention, pain-induced splinting, abdominal binders, and body casts. Depressive factors such as narcotics, residual neuromuscular relaxant drug effects, and central and peripheral neurologic depression also contribute to diminished lung volume. With alveolar collapse, the stage is set for further deterioration as outlined in Figure 1.

Pulmonary Edema

Pulmonary edema is defined as a greater than normal pulmonary extravascular water (PEVW) content and is a universal finding in ARF. The accumulation of PEVW is a complex process dependent on the multiple factors that enter into the Starling equation.[20] Two basic mechanisms for the genesis of pulmonary edema have been advanced.

Hydrostatic Pulmonary Edema.   Left atrial hypertension leads to passive increase in the pulmonary vascular pressures with transudation of fluid into

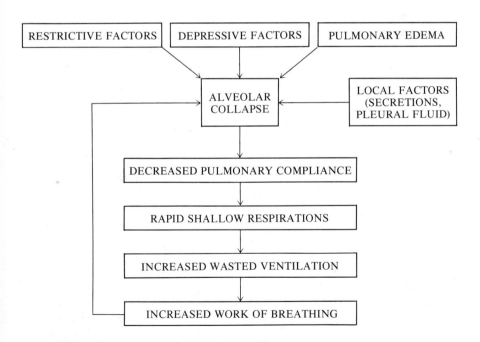

Figure 1.   Pathophysiology of acute respiratory failure.

the pulmonary interstitium (congestive heart failure). When the rate of transudation exceeds the resorptive capacity of the pulmonary lymphatics, alveolar flooding occurs.

Pulmonary Capillary Leak Syndrome. Disruption of the alveolar-capillary membrane leads to exudation of protein-rich plasma into the pulmonary interstitium in the presence of a normal or decreased left atrial pressure. This is a nonspecific response of the lung to a wide range of insults. Some of the commonly encountered causes in surgical practice of this capillary injury include prolonged shock of any cause, endotoxemia, bacterial and viral infections, disseminated intravascular coagulopathy, allergic reactions with release of vasoactive substances, fat embolism, massive transfusions (particularly when fine-pore filters are not used), and inhalation of noxious substances and smoke. In dealing with patients who suffer from any degree of pulmonary capillary leakage, it is important to realize that small increases in left atrial pressure and fluid balance, which would normally be well tolerated, may result in a major increase in edema with aggravation of hypoxemia.[20] Fluid management is discussed in further detail in the section on Fluid and Electrolyte Balance in Respiratory Failure.

DIAGNOSTIC–THERAPEUTIC PRIORITIES ALGORITHM FOR RESPIRATORY INSUFFICIENCY

In everyday practice the surgeon is surrounded by patients who manifest "respiratory distress" of difficulty in breathing. Every patient should be rapidly screened in a systematic manner to arrive at a correct diagnosis and treatment. The scheme outlined in Figure 2 is offered as one such approach for patients not previously intubated or receiving positive pressure ventilation.

For patients already intubated and receiving mechanical respiratory assistance, "respiratory distress" will usually manifest as: (1) being "out of phase" or fighting the ventilator; (2) hypertension, tachycardia, and/or arrythmias; (3) sweating; (4) agitation. When such a situation arises, the first priority is to assume that the F_{IO_2}, ventilation, and ventilatory pattern are inadequate until proven otherwise. Sedatives are always of secondary concern (see section on Sedatives and Neuromuscular Relaxants).

AIRWAY MANAGEMENT

AIRWAY OBSTRUCTION

When called to see a patient with "respiratory distress," one should remember that (1) noisy breathing indicates obstructed airways. (2) Inspiratory stridor and wheezing usually indicate upper airway obstruction, while expiratory wheezing is more typically associated with lower (small airways)

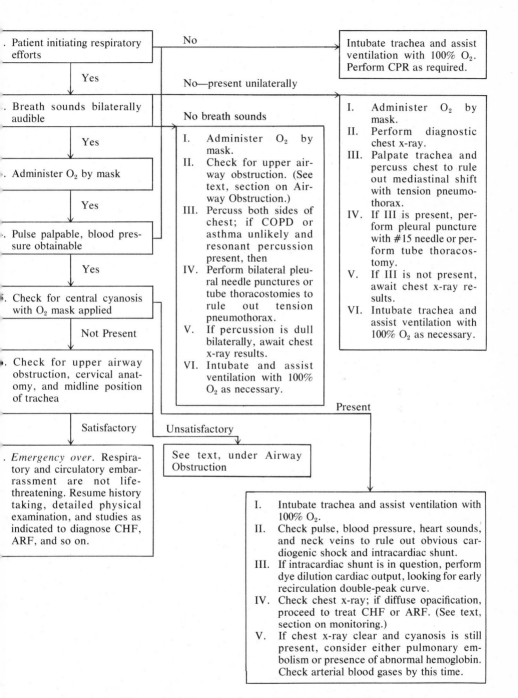

Figure 2. Diagnostic-therapeutic priorities for respiratory insufficiency.

obstruction. (3) Never use sedatives or neuromuscular relaxants when an abnormal airway is in question.

The most common form of upper airway obstruction occurs in sleeping or somnolent people in whom the base of the tongue falls back in the pharynx, obstructing the glottic opening. Frequently seen in elderly individuals during normal sleep (snoring), it may rarely become pathologic with total airway obstruction, chronic nocturnal hypoxemia, and insomnia requiring chronic tracheostomy for its cure. The treatment of choice for individuals recovering from anesthesia and surgery is to position the patient on the side; if necessary, insert an oral or nasal artificial airway. Always rule out the presence of excessive pharyngeal secretions by gently suctioning the mouth and pharynx. If these simple maneuvers fail to ameliorate the situation, other possible causes must be immediately sought. These are:

Postextubation Edema of the Vocal Cords. This problem, uncommon in adults, is not infrequently encountered in children.[9] It is more often seen following multiple or traumatic intubations in the adult and can present immediately or within one to two days following extubation. If detected early, a trial of conservative therapy is indicated and includes the following procedures:

1. Sit the patient upright in bed.

2. Administer cool humidified mist inhalation.

3. Administer racemic epinephrine, 0.25 to 0.50 ml of a 1:200 solution in 3 ml of saline via a nebulizer face mask (e.g., Updraft Neb-U-Mask, Hudson Oxygen Therapy Sales, Temecula, California) or via intermittent positive pressure breathing every 3 hours.

4. Administer pharmacologic doses of systemic corticosteroids for 72 hours (e.g., dexamethasone 4 mg intravenously every 4 hours).

5. Fluid restriction and use of diuretics may be helpful if time permits but is usually of little immediate benefit.

External Compression of the Cervical Trachea. This complication is occasionally seen after head and neck surgery and is usually detected by inspection and palpation of the neck. Hematoma accumulation following thyroidectomy or anterior cervical fusion may develop rapidly with little warning. In such situations, reestablishment of the natural airway may be achieved by opening the surgical wound and attempting to evacuate the hematoma; attempted intubation, if possible, should be tried first.

Tracheal Stenosis Secondary to Prolonged Intubation and Tracheostomy. This problem has risen in its incidence since the advent of modern respiratory intensive care.[14] This lesion should be suspected in any individual who has a history of prolonged placement of an artificial tracheal airway in the past. While most individuals manifest symptoms of obstruction within days to weeks after decannulation, some patients may present several years later often having been erroneously diagnosed as having asthma or chronic lung disease. Differentiation of large airway obstruction from lower airways obstruction in this case is made by: the history; inspection of the tracheal air column on routine radiographs of the chest; lateral and oblique views of the neck will give further definition of the lesion; auscultation of "wheezing" over the mouth and neck with clear lung fields; and the flow volume loop at pulmonary function testing will show "amputation and flattening" of the peak flow, while small airways disease will show diminished flow at 25 per cent of vital capacity.

It is important in dealing with these patients to recall that superimposed upper respiratory infections may exacerbate the obstruction with edema and accumulation of secretions at the site of obstruction. A program as outlined for vocal cord edema will often improve the situation. If an artificial airway is needed, a small bore rigid endotracheal tube should be placed cautiously by an expert anesthesiologist after spontaneous ventilation preoxygenation by face mask. If the situation suggests imminent cardiorespiratory collapse, a pediatric bronchoscope may be advanced under direct vision with aspiration of secretions and passage through the lesion. This procedure carries the potential hazard of perforation into the mediastinum and great vessels. Once an airway is established from above, a new tracheostomy may be created through the previous incision and lesion. This will spare further loss of viable tracheal rings, which will simplify the ultimate resection and reconstruction that will be required. Definitive reconstruction may be considered only if it is clear that mechanical respiratory assistance and high inspired oxygen tensions will not be required postoperatively.

In summary, patients with upper airway obstruction require prompt reestablishment of the airway as the first therapeutic priority. The majority of these problems are solved by intubation of the larynx and trachea. For patients with *direct laryngotracheal trauma* and *external compression* who cannot be intubated, *tracheostomy* will be *required*. If this is necessary, remember that valuable time is wasted in setting up and performing a tracheostomy. During these moments, cricothyrotomy or placement of a transtracheal polyethylene catheter by tracheal puncture will allow insufflation of oxygen and aspiration of secretions until the stoma may be properly created. This may be lifesaving.

ARTIFICIAL AIRWAYS

The indications for endotracheal intubation are:

1. The establishment of a secure airway in patients who cannot be treated adequately with an oropharyngeal airway.

2. Institution of positive pressure ventilation.

3. Prevention of aspiration.

4. Removal of tracheobronchial secretions by catheters or fiberoptic bronchoscopy.

The safety of prolonged (greater than 72 hours) intubation by either the nasal or oral route is well established. The choice between oral or nasal intubation is largely dependent on the technical considerations summarized in Table 1. The introduction of large residual volume, highly compliant cuffs

Table 1. CLINICAL REQUIREMENTS AND TECHNICAL CONSIDERATIONS IN
CHOICE OF NASAL AND ORAL INTUBATION

NASAL INTUBATION	ORAL INTUBATION
Advantages	
Easily held in place	Large bore and shorter length make
Better tolerated by patients	suctioning easier
May be inserted blindly without	More easily inserted by
laryngoscopy when neck motion or	inexperienced intubationist
visualization is limited	
Allows surgical and nursing access	
to oral cavity if required	
Disadvantages	
Choanal size limits the diameter of	Easily dislodged and may be occluded
tube that can be inserted	if precautions are not taken to
Occasional difficulty in passing	prevent patient from biting the tube
suction catheter	May be poorly tolerated by some
Relative contraindications:	patients
Risk of epistaxis in anti-	
coagulated patient or	
patients with bleeding	
tendency	
Inability to drain sinuses if	
active infection is present	
Maxillary and facial fractures	

and improvements in the biocompatibility of material from which endotracheal tubes are fabricated have increased the margin of safety even when
tubes remain in place for one or more weeks. Thus, it is now common
practice to maintain endotracheal tubes in situ for a minimum of seven days,
provided that certain simple precautions are taken. After one week, the
future needs for an artificial airway should be assessed. If extubation seems
imminent (within a few days), tracheostomy is usually delayed. In our experience, laryngeal injury following prolonged intubation has not occurred
with greater frequency than that following short-term (less than 72 hours)
intubation.

COMPLICATIONS OF ARTIFICIAL AIRWAYS

Red rubber tubes used in some anesthesia departments have non-
compliant cuffs. They are rigid and easy to insert during emergencies, but
because of high pressures in the cuff they will readily cause necrosis of the
tracheal mucosa. They should be electively changed postoperatively or following emergencies if prolonged use is foreseen.

When using nasal tubes, it is wise to employ a small nasogastric tube (especially in comatose patients). If air leak occurs around the cuff and cannot escape via the mouth, gastric distention and potential rupture may occur. If there is difficulty passing a gastric tube in the intubated patient, laryngoscopy of the esophagus and McGill forceps may help.

The cuff should be periodically deflated (after pharyngeal suction) and reinflated to the volume where air leakage audibly disappears. The volume required to reach this point should be recorded daily. Large increases in the required volume may signal the development of tracheomalacia. A sudden increase in cuff air requirement may indicate that the cuff is in the larynx.

After intubation and fixation of the endotracheal tube, an x-ray of the chest should be taken to confirm the position of the tip relative to the carina; oral tubes migrate easily into the right mainstem bronchus, and sudden changes in blood gases or compliance should suggest auscultation and/or x-ray of the chest to rule out this common occurrence.

If airway pressures rise suddenly, always suspect obstruction of the tube. A suction catheter should pass freely, and secretions removed if found. If this does not work, deflate the cuff, removing all previously instilled air to rule out the possibility of cuff herniation around the tip. If this fails, change the tube position and auscult for breath sounds. One may have a well functioning tube sitting on the carina or sudden development of tension pneumothorax.

If the cuff of a tracheostomy ruptures, requiring change within the first two days after creating the stoma, thread a thin red rubber suction catheter through the original tube and remove it over the catheter; the catheter may then be used as a guide for the new tube. If the stoma collapses, laryngoscope it with a straight blade infant laryngoscope. In some obese patients with short necks, the standard tracheostomy tubes may be too short. In such emergencies an armored flexible endotracheal tube (Tovell tube) may be temporarily inserted until an appropriately long tracheostomy tube may be obtained.

INDICATIONS FOR MECHANICAL RESPIRATORY ASSISTANCE

Respiratory insufficiency frequently develops in a slow insidious fashion.[14] Morbidity and mortality can be most effectively reduced if physiologic derangements are detected and reversed early by simple prophylactic measures. The development of intensive care units has allowed the physician to safely employ mechanical ventilation in the care of his patients; as survival rates for respiratory failure have risen, a fundamental change in the indications for mechanical ventilation has occurred in the past decade. While in a prior era intubation and mechanical ventilation were reserved for patients at or near cardiorespiratory arrest, it is now accepted that ventilatory support is essential and preventive in the support of certain patients as a natural continuation from intra- to postoperative periods.

BEDSIDE ASSESSMENT OF RESPIRATORY FUNCTION

Isolated measurements cannot adequately assess the respiratory reserve or likelihood of acute failure in any given patient. It is, therefore, necessary to use sequential measurements to evaluate patient performance trends; some test of ventilation, mechanics and oxygenation should be done in each patient. Those parameters which have been found to be of value are depicted in Table 2.

Numerical guidelines should not be followed to the exclusion of clinical judgment. For example, a vital capacity below 15 ml/kg body weight may be sufficient if the patient is cooperative and can cough effectively, provided that hypoxemia is not progressive.

Marginal numerical performance may be entirely insufficient to avoid respiratory assistance if other vital organs are severely failing or gross sepsis and increased metabolic rate are present.

Insufficient monitoring, nursing, and chest physiotherapy, when they are present, suggest that an aggressive program of conservative respiratory care cannot be carried out. It is often poorly appreciated that vastly greater time and effort need to be expended in the effective care of the nonintubated patient; in similar fashion, it may often be too simple to intubate, mechanically ventilate, and then diminish the intensity of overall effort directed at respiratory care.

Inspiratory force is a measurement well suited to the comatose, anesthetized, or uncooperative patient.

Table 2.   SEQUENTIAL MEASUREMENTS TO EVALUATE THE EFFICIENCY OF PULMONARY MECHANICS, OXYGENATION, AND VENTILATION

DATUM	NORMAL RANGE	TRACHEAL INTUBATION AND VENTILATION INDICATED
Mechanics		
Respiratory rate	12 to 20	>35
Vital capacity (ml/kg of body weight*)	65 to 75	<15
FEV_1 (ml/kg of body weight*)	50 to 60	<10
Inspiratory force (cm H_2O)	75 to 100	<25
Oxygenation		
P_aO_2 (mm Hg)	100 to 75 (air)	<70 (on mask O_2)
P (A—aDo$_2$) $^{1.0}$ (mm Hg†)	25 to 65	>450
Ventilation		
P_aCo_2 (mm Hg)	35 to 45	>55‡
V_D/V_T	0.25 to 0.40	>0.60

*"Ideal" weight is used if weight appears grossly abnormal.
†After 10 minutes of 100 per cent oxygen.
‡Except in patients with chronic hypercapnia.

Table 3. THERAPEUTIC INDICATIONS FOR MECHANICAL VENTILATION

Resuscitation from total or impending cardiopulmonary collapse

Hypoventilation and apnea (Definition: $Paco_2 > 50$ torr during spontaneous ventilation except in the case of COPD)
1. Anesthesia
2. Drug overdose
3. Need for muscle paralysis (status epilepticus, tetanus)
4. CNS dysfunction
5. Peripheral neuromuscular failure (polyneuritis, myasthenia gravis, and so on)

Hypoxemia ($P_aO_2 < 70$ torr on oxygen mask except in the case of COPD)
1. Adult respiratory distress syndromes (viral pneumonia, postcardiopulmonary bypass, fat embolism, and so on)
2. Hydrostatic pulmonary edema inadequately responsive to conservative therapy
3. Acute major ventilation perfusion imbalance (pulmonary embolism, lobar atelectasis, pneumonia)

Loss of mechanical integrity of the respiratory apparatus (crushed chest with flail, lacerated diaphragm, sternal instability poststernotomy, and so on)

Discoordination syndrome

Nonspecific weakness—inability to meet demands of increased respiratory work

PROPHYLACTIC VENTILATION

In addition to the conditions requiring therapeutic ventilatory support (see Table 3), there is a constellation of situations in which mechanical ventilation is initiated prophylactically (see Table 4). In such circumstances the rationale for intervention dictates that a period of stability exist and that

Table 4. PROPHYLACTIC INDICATIONS FOR MECHANICAL VENTILATION

Prolonged shock of any cause

Postoperatively
1. With extreme obesity (especially in abdominal procedures)
2. Where likelihood of massive sepsis is high (e.g., bowel content soilage of the peritoneal cavity)
3. In the patient with chronic obstructive lung disease undergoing major abdominal surgery
4. Debilitation and marked electrolyte imbalance
5. With left lung contusion following thoracic aneurysm repair

Situations in which reduced oxygen consumption and work of breathing will remove additional stress on the cardiovascular system
1. Following open heart surgery—especially in the case of mitral stenosis with severe pulmonary hypertension
2. Shivering during postoperative rewarming in the patient with coronary artery disease (sedate, ventilate, and curarize if necessary)

Acid aspiration syndrome

Cachexia–debilitation with major superimposed physiologic insult

the patient "prove his respiratory apparatus is not going to fail" prior to the elective discontinuation of ventilatory assistance. For example, a patient coming to surgery with gross fecal contamination of the peritoneum is at risk of developing severe sepsis with diffuse pulmonary injury in the immediate postoperative period despite appropriate surgical cleansing and antibiotics. In such cases (even young, previously healthy individuals), it is prudent to keep the patient intubated for a period of time postoperatively until progressive hypoxemia is ruled out. A clear chest x-ray in such cases in the recovery room is no guarantee of healthy lungs and will change more slowly than changes in gas exchange and pulmonary compliance.

CONSERVATIVE RESPIRATORY CARE

BASIC CONCEPTS

For the patient convalescing from surgery and anesthesia, a general program of care (with modifications for each individual) will avert the more obvious though easily reversible respiratory complications that develop within the first postoperative days. In formulating a program of care, basic facts need to be kept clearly in mind.

There is no substitute for both physical and psychological preoperative preparation of the patient.

The supine position will diminish FRC approximately 20 per cent below that found with erect posture in normal individuals. Accordingly, catheters, drains, and dressings in themselves do not contraindicate the sitting position postoperatively.

Intermittent positive pressure breathing (IPPB), "blow bottles," and other such devices are adjunctive therapy that are secondary in importance to effective cough, deep breathing, and clearing of secretions by the patient's own efforts. In this regard chest physiotherapy techniques, breathing exercises, relaxation, and patient encouragement are irreplaceable.

PATIENTS WITH PREVIOUSLY NORMAL LUNGS

For patients with normal lungs undergoing elective abdominal surgery (e.g., cholecystectomy), the following might be appropriate:

Preoperatively advise the patient of what he may expect in the way of pain, drains, ileus, and the like. Egbert and coworkers[5] have objectively demonstrated in a controlled study that preoperative instruction and encouragement will alter the patient's perceptions and response to pain, leading to decreased requirements for analgesics postoperatively.

On the day of surgery the patient should be frequently aroused out of his sedated state and made to change his position. Deep breathing and coughing (with the aid of hand or pillow splinting of the incision) every 2 hours should be sufficient to prevent atelectasis and retention of secretions.

The patient should be sat up in a chair on the first postoperative day. For obese patients or those with marked abdominal distention, this should be considered on the evening of the surgical day.

Humidified oxygen should be administered by face mask in the recovery room until the patient has recovered from the effects of anesthesia; the ability to raise the head and neck off the pillow usually indicates adequate reversal from the effect of neuromuscular relaxants.

PATIENTS WITH UNDERLYING CHRONIC LUNG DISEASE

For patients with underlying lung disease:

Begin preoperative preparation as soon as the possibility of operation is raised.

Smokers (one package of cigarettes per day or greater) all have some degree of chronic bronchitis. Cessation of smoking for even one or two weeks preoperatively will diminish their cough and sputum production.

For patients with chronic bronchitis, evacuation of retained secretions preoperatively will often alleviate the need for prolonged postoperative respiratory assistance. Such a program will require at least three to five days if secretions are copious and purulent. This should include:

1. Use of continuous high humidity aerosols by mask or face tent.

2. Administration of bronchodilators and/or mucolytics via IPPB four times a day. This should be ordered to immediately precede chest physiotherapy and postural drainage; remember that this is most effectively done prior to meals on an empty stomach as these modalities frequently induce regurgitation. Typical bronchodilator and mucolytic therapy via IPPB might be: isoetharine (Bronkosol) 0.5 to 0.75 ml in 3 ml of saline; N-acetylcysteine (Mucomyst), 2 to 3 ml of 20 per cent solution in 2 ml of saline (this drug induces bronchospasm in some patients and the first treatment should consist of only 1 ml of 20 per cent solution with 4 ml of saline).

3. Chest physiotherapy and postural drainage. It is helpful for the therapist to see the patient preoperatively (even if surgery is urgent), as instruction in breathing exercises and coughing for only a brief visit will be much easier to recall in the face of postoperative pain than to learn anew.

4. Schedule operation for elective surgery at such time that chest physiotherapy and clearing of secretions may be accomplished in the hour preceding surgery.

5. For patients who have significant reversible airways obstruction and wheezing, terbutaline (Astra Pharmaceuticals), half to one tablet (2.5–5.0 mg) per os four times a day, is helpful. Alternately, 0.25 to 0.5 ml (1 mg/ml) solution may be administered subcutaneously every 6 hours and in conjunction with preanesthetic medications at the discretion of the anesthetist.

6. Sputum culture and sensitivity and appropriate antibiotics may be helpful in specific cases, but in no way substitute for physical evacuation of secretions.

Postoperatively, the chronic bronchitic should continue to receive chest physiotherapy and aerosol as soon as he is awake in the recovery room. If surgery is long and many secretions are still present with suctioning of the trachea, one may consider transiently keeping the patient intubated until he is brought to the recovery room. He may then receive bilateral deep breathing with a self-inflating bag in conjunction with chest physiotherapy and IPPB aerosol therapy if necessary. N-acetylcysteine should not be nebulized via red rubber endotracheal tubes, since it reacts with the rubber to liquefy it. Once awake the patient should be promptly extubated, since the tube will only irritate the airway and further inhibit effective cough once it is present. For patients who refuse to cough, gentle pressure with a finger over the first few tracheal rings will often elicit a cough.

For patients who manifest minimal secretions and no cough preoperatively in the face of significant chronic lung disease (emphysema or restrictive disease), one may anticipate little benefit from a program as outlined for chronic bronchitis. In this case one should proceed to surgery and anticipate the need for prophylactic postoperative mechanical respiratory assistance, which should be discussed in advance with the patient, the anesthetist, and the postoperative intensive care unit (ICU).

Poor preoperative performance with studies of the mechanical pulmonary function should not in itself exclude surgery upon the abdomen if the indications for surgery are clear. This does not apply to pulmonary and noncardiac thoracic surgery, for which the reader is referred to other references.

MANAGEMENT OF VENTILATORY ASSISTANCE

VENTILATORY MODES

Mechanical respiratory assistance may be given by a variety of methods and devices and is beyond the scope of this chapter. Important features of the commonly used systems are as follows.

Pressure Preset Ventilators.   These devices (such as the Bird Mark VII and Bennett PR–I) deliver inspired gas to the lungs until a prescribed pressure level is reached. They are relatively inexpensive. The inspired oxygen concentration is variable and requires frequent measurement at the airway unless a reliable oxygen-air blender is added to the system. These ventilators will deliver a variable tidal volume to the patient, depending on changes in compliance of the lungs and chest wall, and frequent checks of the tidal volume are essential. The peak pressure attainable rarely exceeds 45 cm of H_2O, and positive end-expiratory pressure (PEEP) is generally not available. They are best suited for either IPPB aerosol treatment or for ventilation of patients with normal lungs and mechanical ventilatory failure (coma, anesthesia, paralysis) or for patients with emphysema.

Volume Preset Ventilators.   These are designed to deliver a constant predetermined tidal volume to the patient at whatever pressure level is required (pressure limit may be set by an inspiratory relief valve which then reduces the volume delivered).

These machines may be of the "assistor-controller" variety (like the pressure cycled ventilator) in which the ventilator breathes for the patient, or the patient may trigger the ventilator himself with negative pressure (the level being determined by a sensitivity adjustment). Examples of this type of ventilator are the Bennett MA–I and Searle VVA. These ventilators are dependent on electric power; they have built in PEEP devices, inspired O_2 control, variably controllable inspiratory flow rates, and reasonably accurate respiratory rate controls. They are useful in ventilating patients with decreased respiratory compliance, such as patients with ARF or crushed chest, and are, therefore, more versatile than pressure cycled units.

Ventilators such as the Emerson Postoperative Ventilator are strictly "controllers" and do not allow respiratory effort on the part of the patient (unless the IMV mode is used). These ventilators are less costly than the assistor-controllers and are electrically and mechanically simpler in design. Use of the controller mode requires the use of sedatives or neuromuscular relaxants on rare occasions to keep the patient "in phase" with the ventilator; when used in the IMV mode this problem is eliminated.

Continuous Positive Airway Pressure (CPAP). In this system, the patient breathes spontaneously from a gas reservoir and exhales against a water column of the desired pressure resistance to be used. This system requires gas flow rates of two to three times the patient's minute ventilation in order to avoid rebreathing from the long tubings required. Desired inspired fractions of oxygen (FIO_2) are obtained by blending oxygen and compressed air. Any leakage from nebulizers, tubing, or reservoirs may be extremely hazardous, as the circuit may then permit rebreathing in "an infinite deadspace." We have seen a patient develop hypercarbia to $PaCO_2$ values of 215 mm Hg in such a situation. The CPAP system may be easily achieved by using an Intermittent Mandatory Ventilator (IMV) in which the ventilator pump has been turned off. CPAP is useful for patients who are weaning from prolonged mechanical ventilation with marginal mechanical function and who have a tendency to airways closure and progressive hypoxemia during weaning. CPAP is very useful in the acute postoperative setting where pulmonary mechanics may be appropriate for extubation, but the patient continues to require positive airway pressure for increased intrapulmonary right to left shunting (Qs/QT).

Intermittent Mandatory Ventilation. In this system the patient may breathe spontaneously from a fresh gas source with low resistance (with or without PEEP) while receiving active inflations from the mechanical respiratory at preset intervals.[4] This is achieved by the use of special valves within the ventilator that close off the fresh gas reservoir source at the time a mechanically ventilated breath is delivered. In clinical use for four years at the time of this writing, it has already achieved widespread popularity. It is discussed in further detail in the section on Weaning from Mechanical Ventilation.

The ventilatory pattern is defined by (1) the inspiratory and expiratory flow rates and pressures, (2) the tidal volume, (3) the duration of inspiration and expiration, and (4) the frequency and magnitude of passive hyperinflations.

The optimal ventilatory pattern varies from individual to individual and is not easily predictable. A basic pattern of large tidal volume (12–15 ml/kg) and a slow rate (10–12 breaths/minute) without periodic hyperinflations (sigh) remains the best choice for most patients without serious derangements of lung function. Ventilation with small tidal volumes (less than 10 ml/kg) without periodic sighing generally leads to progressive airways closure and increasing shunt. Patients ventilated at low tidal volumes often complain of dyspnea and the sensation of inadequate chest wall expansion. With the advent of PEEP it has been possible to ventilate patients at such low tidal volumes without further deterioration in gas exchange. This fact is of some importance when ventilating patients with ARF with markedly decreased compliance, and is discussed in further detail in the section on Therapeutic Approach and Priorities for Noncardiogenic Pulmonary Edema and Multiorgan Dysfunction. If the wasted ventilation is great (anatomical plus physiologic deadspace) and minute ventilatory requirements exceed 12 to 15 liters/minute, the respiratory rate should be raised to achieve a $Paco_2$ value in the normal range. For rates in excess of 20 breaths/minute, it is important to adjust the inspiratory flow rate upward as necessary to maintain a pattern in which total inspiratory time does not exceed expiratory time (I:E ratio = 1:1). If this should happen, one can anticipate significant increases in mean airway pressure, potentially incomplete expiration of inspired gas volumes, and significant depression of cardiac output. Always remember that arterial $Paco_2$ level depends on both metabolic rate and ventilation. In many surgical patients the former may be grossly elevated; if this is a problem, hyperpyrexia should not be permitted, and active surface cooling at least to normothermia may significantly decrease the minute ventilatory requirement.

VENTILATION ORDERS

When a patient is to receive respiratory assistance of any variety, it is important that all concerned in the patient's care (physician, nurse, physiotherapist, and respiratory therapist) have a clear idea of what is desired. This should be clearly written in the patient's order, as orders for antibiotics or vasoactive agents would be. These orders are best divided into three categories.

Ventilator Orders

1.   Desired Fio_2.
2.   Desired tidal volume.

3.   Desired level of PEEP.

4.   Permissible peak airway pressure (what level of pressure relief should be set to signal alarm).

Weaning Orders (if not to wean, write "no weaning")

1.   Desired F_{IO_2}

2.   Desired PEEP (if it is to be used)

3.   If conventional "T-piece" weaning, specify how often, how long (see section on Weaning from Mechanical Ventilation), and in the upright posture if feasible. Orders like "wean today" are inadequate and fail to appropriately direct the nurse, who must carry out this difficult process with the patient.

4.   Measurements desired and permissible limits (Should the nurse terminate weaning if blood pressure rises above 200 mm Hg or respiratory rate exceeds 40 to 50 per minute?).

Adjunctive Orders

1.   Chest physiotherapy—how often? If it is known that the patient has an abscess in a particular location, alert the therapist to it.

2.   Aerosol medications—dose, frequency, diluent, ultrasound nebulizer, and so on.

3.   Deep tracheal suction and any specimens desired for laboratory analysis.

4.   Miscellaneous (e.g., "may have sips of clear liquids if methylene blue test negative").

SEDATIVES AND NEUROMUSCULAR RELAXANTS

Before narcotics or sedatives are given to depress respiratory efforts of the patient, check that the ventilatory pattern being provided is adequate. Disconnect the ventilator and try to override the patient's urge to inspire by using manual ventilation with self-inflating bag and delivering frequent deep breaths; if this fails to bring the patient "in phase," then blood gases should be obtained and examination of the chest performed to rule out hypoxemia or other unforeseen problems. In similar fashion, blood pressure and hemodynamic performance should be thoroughly scrutinized, as agitation and dyspnea are typical of the hypovolemic or shock patient. When these maneuvers are performed and Pa_{CO_2} is slightly depressed (35–40 mm Hg), most patients will be content and often fall asleep on the ventilator. Circumstances where this is not the case include: (1) severe pain from surgery or discomfort that the patient is unable to communicate (e.g., distended urinary bladder); (2) severe ARF, particularly where FRC has been reduced 50 per cent or more below predicted normal; (3) florid systemic sepsis with or without shock; (4) in certain individuals (especially the young) who are bothered by orotracheal tubes; (5) shivering and increased metabolic rate in hypothermic patients who are rewarming in the recovery room; (6) central neurologic dysfunction or injury; (7) patients in metabolic acidosis of whatever cause.

In the first five situations narcotics and sedatives are indicated. Small frequent doses of morphine intravenously to titrate against the patient's needs are useful. Young, previously healthy individuals may require large doses of narcotics (morphine, 20–30 mg intravenously every 1 to 3 hours), and these drugs should be dispensed as needed in each case. When this is necessary, frequent blood gas analysis should be done to prove that ventilation and oxygenation are adequate.

An occasional patient in one of the first five situations mentioned above may require neuromuscular relaxants as well. In the case of neurologic dysfunction, sedatives and narcotics should be avoided and neuromuscular relaxants used to control ventilation. The effects of these drugs may be electively reversed with cholinesterase-inhibiting drugs, permitting periodic assessment of neurologic function. A few practical pharmacologic facts about the nondepolarizing (long-acting) neuromuscular relaxants may be helpful to those physicians infrequently employing these drugs:

D-Tubocurarine (curare or DTC) is the oldest natural compound of this drug class in clinical use. It blocks acetylcholine receptors at postsynaptic neuromuscular junctional membranes to inhibit impulse transmission. *It has no sedative or depressant effect on the central nervous system.* This drug has a mild ganglionic blocking and histamine-releasing effect, and if given rapidly may induce transient hypotension. It has no effect on impulse formation and transmission in the heart and is ideal for patients with heart disease and tachyarrythmias. It should be given slowly in 3 mg (1 ml = 3 mg) increments to an initial dose of approximately 0.3 to 0.5 mg/kg (60 kg adults usually require 25–30 mg). Thereafter, 6 to 9 mg every 30 to 60 minutes are usually required to maintain the desired neuromuscular relaxation. An alternate method for long-term use in the ICU is to mix an infusion (e.g., 200 mg DTC in a total volume of 100 ml with 5 per cent dextrose in water and initially infuse 15 to 20 ml over 20 minutes, thereafter controlling the drip rate at 5 to 15 ml/hour as necessary via a controlled infusion pump. This method obviates undesirable hypotensive effects from sudden bolus administration of drug and is more easily employed by nursing personnel in a well staffed ICU. Dosages should be periodically reassessed by terminating the drip to assure that large stores of the drug are not accumulating in the patient. This drug is partly metabolized in the liver and excreted in the urine and bile. It may be used in patients with acute renal failure in reduced dosage.

Pancuronium bromide (Pavulon) is a synthetic drug of the same class as DTC with approximately the same duration of action as DTC. It has no clinically significant ganglionic blocking effect, and therefore hypotension is not a side-effect. It generally increases intrinsic sinue rate of the heart and may produce supraventricular and nodal tachycardias in susceptible patients. It may aggravate or precipitate fatal ventricular arrythmias in patients with unstable ischemic heart disease and should be used with extreme caution in these patients. Usual initial dosage for neuromuscular blockade approximates 0.06 to 0.10 mg/kg given in slow increments intravenously (4–6 mg in a 60 kg adult). This may then be supplemented with 0.01 to 0.02 mg/kg (1–2 mg) every 40 to 60 minutes as necessary. The route of excretion is via the kidneys; it cannot be recommended for use in acute renal failure at this time.

Positive End-Expiratory Pressure (PEEP)

PEEP during assisted ventilation, IMV, or spontaneous breathing is widely employed to reduce Qs/Qt and to improve arterial oxygenation. This most likely results from increasing FRC and keeping small airways open throughout the respiratory cycle, thus permitting gas exchange in previously nonventilated or partially ventilated alveoli.[6] The magnitude of increase in Pao_2 with PEEP coincides with the resulting increase in FRC. In some patients (particularly those with unilateral or assymetric parenchymal lung disease), PEEP may worsen Pao_2. This may be explained by overdistention of normal compliant lung regions with redistribution of pulmonary blood flow to less ventilated regions, thus increasing net intrapulmonary shunting of venous blood.

Criteria for use of PEEP during mechanical ventilation are difficult to establish; while most experienced physicians would use PEEP if Pao_2 could not be maintained above 60 mm Hg with $Fio_2 = 0.5$, many would use PEEP in a prophylactic manner whenever Pao_2 was less than 100 mm Hg with 40 per cent oxygen or greater.

In general it may be said that:

1.   PEEP of 5 cm or less will be tolerated by all patients with ARF.

2.   No patient is "too sick to tolerate PEEP"; hypotension and decreased cardiac output are discussed in the section on Cardiovascular Effects of Positive Pressure Ventilation and PEEP.

3.   The optimal PEEP for a given patient must be determined by clinical trial. The customary approach is to raise PEEP in 3 to 5 cm of water increments while monitoring Pao_2, cardiac output, and Qs/Qt. That this level of "best PEEP" may coincide with maximal total respiratory compliance and least dead space as suggested by Suter and coworkers[21] should not be considered a substitute for detailed assessment of hemodynamic performance, particularly when compliance is severely reduced and high levels of PEEP (greater than 20 cm of water) are employed.[11]

4.   There is little or no evidence at this time to suggest that barotrauma (pneumothorax, subcutaneous emphysema, and pneumomediastinum) occurs with greater frequency in patients receiving PEEP. Barotrauma in general reflects the severity of underlying parenchymal injury.

MONITORING

LABORATORY AND BEDSIDE STUDIES

Clinical Laboratory

BACTERIOLOGY.   While frequent cultures of sputum are helpful in defining resident organisms and their antibiotic sensitivities, there is no substitute for daily Gram stains of the sputum to decide whether or not the cultured growths represent active infection in need or antibiotic treatment. Gram stains also allow early recognition of changes in the respiratory flora.

HEMATOLOGY.   Screening for intravascular coagulopathy should be done in all patients with ARF. In these patients, slow progressive decrease in thrombocyte count usually precedes the appearance of fibrin split products (FSP) in the plasma and usually suggests severe ARF (in the absence of other causes).

CHEMISTRY.   Sodium, potassium, chloride, and osmolality measurements in serum and urine should be performed daily.

Respiratory Function in the Patient

OXYGENATION.   For patients with ARF, frequent measurements of FIO_2 (at least every 6 hours) and arterial oxygen tension are essential. The potentially harmful effects of continued exposure to high concentrations of oxygen (> 60 per cent) have been demonstrated to alter pulmonary function and structure in experimental animals.[26] Pulmonary defense mechanisms (e.g., macrophage function) in animals have been shown to be impaired in a dose-related manner for the entire spectrum of FIO_2 in excess of room air concentrations. The measurement of Pao_2 while breathing 100 per cent oxygen with calculation of $D(A-a)o_2$ and Qs/QT has been popular for assessing lung function. This is based on the assumption that hypoxemia during ARF is due to nonventilated perfused areas or "true physiologic shunt." It has recently been demonstrated that in ARF a large number of alveolar units are present with very low but finite ventilation/perfusion ratios (VA/QT).[13,24] One hundred per cent oxygen breathing promotes absorption atelectasis in these alveoli and converts them from units of low VA/QT to true shunt units.[22] It has been confirmed from several investigators that short-term breathing of 100 per cent oxygen produces increases in Qs/QT and decreases in FRC not found at lower FIO_2s. Thus, it is probably safer and clinically relevant to calculate $D(A-a)o_2$ and Qs/QT at an FIO_2 of less than 1.0.

VENTILATION AND MECHANICS.   Tidal volume, respiratory rate, peak inspiratory pressure, and PEEP should be checked hourly to avoid subtle or gross changes in ventilatory pattern. Measurements during weaning are discussed in the section on Weaning from Mechanical Ventilation.

Compliance of the lungs and chest wall is a valuable measure and is invariably reduced in ARF. Effective dynamic compliance is

$$C_{Dyn} = \frac{tidal\ volume}{inflation\ pressure}$$

when an inspiratory plateau of 1 second or greater is employed. For patients receiving PEEP, the inflation pressure is the plateau inspiratory airway pressure minus PEEP. The tidal volume, if measured at the expiratory port of the ventilator, contains the expired tidal volume of the patient plus the compressible volume in the ventilator when inspiration ended. To calculate the C_{Dyn}, the compressible volume should be subtracted from the measured exhaled gas volume. To calculate the compressible volume of the ventilator, the inflation pressure should be multiplied by the compression factor for the individual ventilator. Progressive loss of compliance over a period of several days in the face of PEEP dependence and acceptable oxygenation may be indicative of progressive pulmonary fibrosis (in the absence of fluid overload).

CARDIOVASCULAR MONITORING IN RESPIRATORY FAILURE

Mechanical and Technical Problems in Line Placements and Management

ARTERIAL CANNULATION. With severe ARF, prolonged placement of an indwelling arterial cannula may be necessary. With appropriate materials and care, a percutaneous radial arterial cannula should be able to function for at least 7 to 10 days. We have seen numerous lines remain functional for 2 to 4 weeks, and these catheters are rarely if ever a source of systemic bacteremia. In our experience a useful system has consisted of:

1.   Percutaneous or cutdown placement of a Teflon 2-inch 18-gauge Longdwel catheter (Becton Dickinson Company, Rutherford, New Jersey).

2.   Luer locking 1-foot male-female Cobe tubing (Cobe Laboratories, Lakewood, Colorado). Once the catheter and tubing are luer-locked, this connection is dressed firmly to the wrist, and blood samples are then removed distally. This minimizes direct arterial trauma at the wrist, which occurs if a three-way stopcock is applied to the catheter directly. There is no risk of "line disconnects" at the wrist.

3.   At the distal end of the tubing a luer-locked three-way stopcock is connected to the Cobe tubing.

4.   The stopcock is then luer-locked to a Continuous Flush System Intraflow (Sorenson Research Company, Salt Lake City, Utah).

5.   The distal end of the CFS Intraflow has a luer lock port for tubing attachment to pressure transducers or aneroid systems if desired.

CENTRAL VENOUS CANNULATION FOR SWAN-GANZ CATHETER. The customary approach to placement of large cannulae such as a 7 French Swan-Ganz catheter has been to perform a cutdown on the brachial vein. While this will solve the problem in general, we have found that catheters positioned away from the central axis of the body tend to move particularly with frequent turning, proning, and chest physiotherapy that is required for patients with respiratory failure. It has been found that percutaneous placement via the internal jugular vein using a Seldinger technique (Cordice 8F Catheter Sheath Introducer System, Cordice Corp., Miami) is relatively easy, quick, and successful in the majority of cases.[27]

For patients being turned and receiving chest physiotherapy, the application of 1-foot Cobe tubing to subclavian catheters allows greater flexibility and avoids the problem of air embolism when stopcocks disconnect at the catheter.

When Should A Swan-Ganz Flow-Directed Pulmonary Artery Catheter Be Employed in Patients With Respiratory Failure?   There is no absolute answer to this question, and each patient must be evaluated individually. The use of this catheter should be considered if (1) the contribution of left atrial hypertension to pulmonary edema is in question; (2) large volume requirements and fluid shifts exist in a patient with ARF; (3) a previous history of cor pulmonale or right ventricular failure exists in a patient with a new pulmonary injury; (4) severe ARF is present and one is concerned about pulmonary hypertension and increased right ventricular afterload with its deleterious effects on hemodynamic performance (see sections on Cardiovascular Effects of Positive Pressure Ventilation and PEEP, and Therapeutic Approach and Priorities for Noncardiogenic Pulmonary Edema and Multiorgan Dysfunction for further information).

When the Swan-Ganz catheter is employed, measurement of mean pulmonary artery and capillary wedge pressures should be made at the same point in the respiratory cycle (usually end-expiration) when taken during mechanical ventilation. Whatever method is chosen, measurements should be recorded consistently from hour to hour and from one observer to another if serial measurements are to serve as guides to the trend of hemodynamic performance.

Several commercial models of these catheters allow measurement of cardiac output by the thermodilution method; this is accomplished by injecting the indicator into a right atrial lumen while recording a change in temperature at the catheter tip in the pulmonary artery. These measurements are essential for optimal hemodynamic monitoring and therapy of patients with severe ARF. These methods are not adequate for assessing the presence of an intracardiac right to left shunt that may be an issue in selected instances. If an intracardiac shunt is suspected, the diagnosis is confirmed by use of a dye dilution indicator technique in which the indicator is injected in the superior vena cava, with sensor sampling from the systemic arterial blood yielding the characteristic double-peaked curve.

CARDIOVASCULAR EFFECTS OF POSITIVE PRESSURE VENTILATION AND PEEP

For almost 30 years since the classic experiments of Cournand and coworkers[3] it has been known that positive pressure breathing (and specifically mean airway pressure elevation) will produce decreases in the cardiac output in man and animals. The circulatory effects of positive airway pressure depend on the extent to which airway pressures are transmitted to the pleural space and intrathoracic great vessels. Maximal transmission will occur with a stiff chest wall and a highly compliant lung (COPD), while less positive pleural pressure change will occur in ARF where the pulmonary compliance is reduced. In a spontaneously breathing man (see Fig. 3)[23] the CVP and left atrial (LA) pressures as measured by vascular transducers are accurate approximations of transmural filling pressures of right and left ventricles at end-expiration because the pleural pressure approximates zero mm Hg. When pleural pressure rises above zero, the measured CVP and LAP may rise, but the transmural filling pressures of the ventricles will fall (Fig. 4). This phenomenon has been well studied by Qvist and coworkers[16] in close chested dogs in which the pleural pressures were directly measured by an implanted pleural sensor. In this study, Qvist demonstrated that decreases in cardiac output with use of 12 cm PEEP in healthy

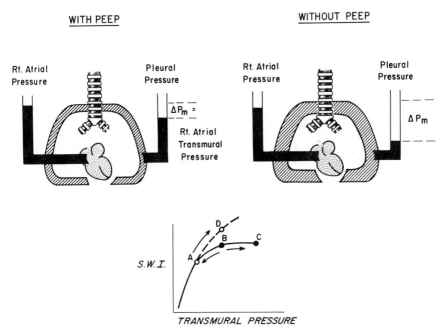

Figure 3.   Effect of change in airway pressure (i.e., mechanical ventilation with or without PEEP) on blood flow. Right and left ventricular preload are determined by transmural atrial pressures, in turn the algebraic sum of atrial and pleural pressures measured relative to atmospheric pressure. If addition of PEEP to the ventilatory pattern increases functional residual capacity, then pleural pressure will rise more than left or right atrial pressure and the transmural pressure (preload) will decrease. The magnitude of the associated decrease in cardiac output will depend on ventricular function as defined by the Frank-Starling curve shown below. If the patient is in failure (point C), a decrease in transmural pressure (from C to B) will result in virtually no change in stroke work index (SWI). If ventricular function is normal (point D), addition of PEEP will decrease transmural pressure and SWI (from D to A). Decreases of FRC and pleural pressure removal of PEEP, as shown by an increase in the width of the crosshatched area. In the hypervolemic patient, the fall in right atrial pressure (relative to atmospheric) will be offset by redistribution of blood volume into the thorax and will result in a rise in transmural pressure (ΔP_m). *Reproduced with permission.*[23]

dogs were directly related to decreases in the transmural filling pressures of the ventricles and that this effect could be reversed with the administration of blood volume expanders to increase transmural filling pressures. This effect of PEEP on measured vascular filling pressures complicates the interpretation of CVP (or RVEDP) and pulmonary capillary wedge (PCW) pressure as depicted in Figure 4.[16] The absolute values of CVP and PCWP will be higher for a given level of cardiac performance for patients receiving positive airway pressure. We favor measurements of vascular pressures "on the ventilator," as this is the steady physiologic state. Acute disconnections of the airway may yield lower measured pressures but are not relevant to hemodynamic performance as it exists during positive airway pressure administration. Thus, arbitrary allowable limits to PCWP in the clinical setting are probably unwarranted and in some cases will lead to suboptimal hemodynamic performance from inadequate ventricular filling.

In addition to the effect of PEEP on ventricular preload, increases in mean airway pressure are also known to elevate pulmonary vascular resistance (PVR), which is derived by the formula: $PVR = \dfrac{PA - LA}{CO}$. In a spontaneously breathing human, LAP is closely approximated by the PCWP. During positive pressure breathing with PEEP, PCWP may accurately reflect LAP at low levels of PEEP, while higher levels of PEEP may lead to spuriously high PCWP recordings.[12,30] This is an artifact caused by the catheter tip's presence in a region of the lung where alveolar pressure

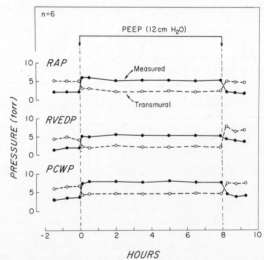

Figure 4.   Hemodynamic effects of airway pressure on ventricular filling pressures. Measured (relative to atmosphere) and transmural (calculated) right and left heart filling pressures: right atrial pressure (RAP); right ventricular end-diastolic pressure (RVEDP); pulmonary capillary wedge pressure (PCWP). Note that while pressure measured relative to atmosphere rose, transmural pressure fell when PEEP was applied; trend was reversed when PEEP was removed. See text for additional discussion. *Reproduced with permission.*[16]

exceed perfusion pressure;[29] in this instance the catheter reflects alveolar pressure instead of downstream vascular pressure. In addition to elevating alveolar pressure, PEEP may raise the right ventricular afterload via its effect on raising the PVR as previously described. This will result in right ventricular dilatation and displacement of the interventricular septum toward the left ventricular free wall. The result of this phenomenon is to alter the compliance and pressure-volume relationship of the left ventricle.[30] The net result is to generate higher recorded PCWP or LVEDP for a given left ventricular stroke volume. Thus elevation of PCWP in the setting of ARF may not necessarily represent acute left ventricular failure for a variety of reasons. Careful correlation of PCWP with cardiac and urinary output is essential in arriving at rational therapeutic decisions.

FLUID AND ELECTROLYTE BALANCE IN RESPIRATORY FAILURE

Patients receiving mechanical ventilation with humidified gases manifest little need for replacement of insensible fluid losses if sweating is minimal. Both Sladen[19] and Gett[7] have documented the fact that patients receiving mechanical ventilation have an abnormal tendency to accumulate excess water in the lungs. We have found it necessary to measure total intake and output of fluids accurately daily; strict neutrality is sought and early use of diuretics is considered. Even for patients with mechanical respiratory failure (e.g., polyneuritis or spinal cord injury), positive fluid balance over several days is directly related to weight gain, increasing Qs/QT, and decreasing pulmonary compliance; this is reversible with diuresis and is frequently seen in the absence of cardiorenal failure or sepsis and ARF. If ultrasound nebulization of the airway is employed, it also must be considered in the daily fluid intake, as considerable quantities of water may be absorbed via the lungs.

For patients with postsurgical ARF, fluid balance is a primary aspect of care. In these patients, daily (and sometimes more frequent) measurements of Na^+, K^+, Cl^-, HCO_3^-, blood urea nitrogen (BUN), creatinine, and serum and urine osmolality are essential. When Qs/QT is elevated and ARF with capillary leakage is present, we attempt to maintain serum $Na^+ > 142$ mEq/liter and osmolality at 300 to 310 milliosmoles in the absence of an elevated blood sugar or BUN. If several vascular catheters are present and multiple infusions of drugs are ordered, it should be anticipated that maintenance intravenous fluids will not be required, as this situation rarely allows fluid volumes of less than 750 ml per 24 hours. Drainage losses (gastric, fistulae, and so on) should be replaced. If intravascular volume therapy is needed, then some form of therapy other than free water should be given. Whether concentrated albumin fraction will increase serum oncotic pressure and aid in the removal of interstitial lung water as suggested by Skillman[18] remains controversial. It has been documented in humans that large molecules (400,000 molecular weight) may cross into the interstitial space, and that electrophoresis of pulmonary edema fluid proteins[10,25] may mirror that of the plasma. Given this information, it remains possible that albumin may cross the injured alveolar capillary membrane and lead to increases in interstitial fluid oncotic pressure as well. Nonetheless, the physician must treat hypovolemia as he finds it clinically. We generally use blood or packed red cells for a hematocrit of less than 30 per cent. Fresh frozen plasma, 5 per cent albumin in saline solution, and 25 per cent salt-poor albumin are used when serum albumin is less than 3.5 gm/100 ml or total proteins are less than 5.5 gm/100 ml (in the absence of acute hemodilution). We attempt to maintain urine flow at 0.75 to 1.0 ml/kg/hour.

In treating surgical patients with ARF, it should be noted that:

1. Mechanically ventilated patients are unable to excrete a free water load.

2. Mechanical ventilation and PEEP are potent stimulators of antidiuretic hormone.

3. PEEP may cause decreased urine flow by redistribution of the renal blood flow from cortical to medullary nephrons.[8]

4. Hyponatremia will regularly be seen if water balance becomes positive.

5. Excessive dehydration with diuretics and hyperosmolarity (serum osmolality >320 milliosmoles) increase the risk of acute renal failure. The combination of ARF with renal failure markedly increases mortality; survival in these patients is rarely seen in our experience.

6. Total parenteral nutrition is a major source of excess water and acid-base and metabolic abnormalities in prolonged ARF. We are currently using 47 per cent dextrose solution with amino acids and vitamin supplements as our basic parenteral cardiorespiratory diet, which permits 1300 calories intake with less than 900 ml of fluid volume. The introduction of concentrated intravenous lipids into American parenteral diets should eventually decrease the fluid volume requirements for parenteral nutrition.

7. Parenteral nutrition should be considered early if prolonged use of sedatives, narcotics, and neuromuscular relaxants will be needed. These drugs and systemic sepsis cause adynamic ileus that is frequently incompatible with gastrointestinal alimentation.

THERAPEUTIC APPROACH AND PRIORITIES FOR NONCARDIOGENIC PULMONARY EDEMA AND MULTIORGAN DYSFUNCTION

Treatment of ARF will require a balanced approach to monitoring and support of all vital organ systems, whose functions are invariably deranged in the course of severe respiratory failure. However, circulatory monitoring may not be permitted to continuously interfere with chest physiotherapy and turning even in the most unstable patients. Dehydration therapy cannot be carried out successfully if overwhelming systemic sepsis, capillary leakage, and large volume requirements (greater than 2 liters/day of plasma and blood) are present. The severity of ARF and its response to therapy will be dependent on the reversibility of the underlying cause. It must be understood that optimal respiratory care is at best a supportive modality that buys time for the natural healing of the pulmonary injury. Suboptimal care may, on the other hand, aggravate existing injury. Understanding the physiologic derangement permits the physician to better stablilize the internal environment during the healing process; respiratory care does not directly treat the alveolar-capillary injury.

Assessment of the severity of ARF will dictate the necessary level of therapy; in this respect, a spectrum of illness and therapy can be distinguished.

Stage I

Acute hypoxemia requiring intubation and mechanical ventilation with or without PEEP.

Stage III

Patients with ARF who either (1) manifest life-threatening hypoxemia with $Pao_2 < 50$ mm Hg with 100 per cent O_2 and maximum tolerable PEEP, or (2) who after 48 hours of maximal conventional therapy manifest (a) $Qs/Qt > 30$ per cent of the cardiac output or (b) $Pao_2 < 50$ mm Hg with Fio_2 0.6 and PEEP ≥ 5 cm H_2O.

Stage II

Patients who have not improved in Stage I after 24 hours of intensive care and who are not classified in Stage III. Patients in Stage I form the vast majority of patients in ARF, and prognosis will be favorable given reversible underlying disease. Stage III defines a very small fraction of all patients with ARF; these patients qualify for entry into the National Heart and Lung Institute's randomized study for Extracorporeal Membrane Oxygenator (ECMO) therapy. To date, 45 patients from nine centers have entered this study over a one-year period with an overall mortality of 90 per cent. These criteria for Stage III, therefore, define a near lethal clinical condition.

Stage I Monitoring

Blood pressure, CVP, temperature, heart rate, urine output, arterial blood gases, Fio_2, effective dynamic compliance, chest x-ray, sputum, and blood coagulation tests.

Stage I Treatment

1. Mechanical ventilation or IMV as necessary to maintain adequate $Paco_2$[11].

2. Fio_2 and PEEP as necessary to keep $Pao_2 > 60$ mm Hg (if circulation is stable). PEEP should be used cautiously if emphysema and supernormal FRC are present.

3. Volume expansion if PEEP depresses blood pressure and urine output.

4. Chest physiotherapy every 4 hours with suction and nebulization as indicated.

5. Appropriate antibiotics if bronchopulmonary or other bacterial infections are present.

6. Appropriate fluid balance (see section on Fluid and Electrolyte Balance in Respiratory Failure).

Stage II and III Monitoring

This should include all monitoring done for Stage I. In addition, a Swan-Ganz flow-directed pulmonary artery catheter should be placed to record (by transducer) the pulmonary artery systolic, diastolic, mean PA, and PCW pressures. In normal individuals and in patients with fluid overload or acute left heart failure, the PA diastolic and PCW pressures will vary little from each other (< 5 mm Hg). With increasing pulmonary capillary injury and ARF, functional and anatomical obliteration of the pulmonary vasculature will occur; with this injury the resistance to blood flow across the lungs increases, and pulmonary hypertension will develop.[28] In such circumstances the PA diastolic pressure will be significantly greater than the PCWP, and a (PA diastolic-PCW) gradient of greater than 10 mm Hg should suggest significant increase in the pulmonary vascular resistance and right ventricular afterload.

If available, serial measurements of the cardiac output should be performed and circulatory status assessed with respect to filling pressures, PVR, sepsis, and therapeutic interventions. Zapol and coworkers[28] have noted an inverse relationship between cardiac output and PVR in patients with severe ARF. These authors noted that at cardiac indices below 4.0 liters/min/m², mean PVR values were 400 per cent greater than predicted normal (in the absence of abnormal venous desaturation), whereas at cardiac indices in excess of 5 liters/min/m², mean PVR values were significantly lower than those during low cardiac output. This phenomenon complicates the interpretation of PVR calculation in ARF. Serious consideration needs to be given to inotropic support for right ventricular function when these abnormalities are demonstrated. In our experience, CVP elevation is a near terminal event.

Stage II Treatment

1. All Stage I therapy plus:

2. Curarization to decrease skeletal muscle oxygen consumption, prevent shivering, and allow perfect control of mechanical ventilation and decreases in chest wall compliance. In our experience these patients require very large minute ventilation, and many of the sickest become hypercarbic and acidotic if normothermia and IMV therapy with PEEP is attempted.

3. Consideration of inotropic support for right ventricular performance and augmentation of cardiac output. Vasodilator therapy may be at-

tempted to decrease pulmonary hypertension, but is usually of little measurable benefit.

4. Chest physiotherapy every 2 hours.

5. Fluid therapy as discussed in the section on Fluid and Electrolyte Balance in Respiratory Failure.

Stage III Treatment

As previously stated, these patients have an overall mortality of 90 per cent given all types of care at this time. Some of these patients will occasionally survive with or without ECMO, but the factors that allow survival of some and not others are unknown. In these patients, continued care requires large-scale commitments of medical, nursing, paramedical, and laboratory resources in well equipped facilities. Patients with life-threatening hypoxemia and hemodynamic instability may be safely transported to regional referral centers given a well organized mobile ICU and transport team.[17]

With the passage of time the incidence of pulmonary infections, bleeding, and fibrosis increases, and patients who fail to improve ultimately succumb to one of these complications. It is clear, however, that some patients with these complications do survive; recovery to the point of spontaneous ventilation may take weeks to months of continued intensive monitoring and care. Whether extraordinary therapies such as ECMO, lung transplantation, and therapy to inhibit pulmonary fibrosis are efficacious is uncertain; at present, these are areas of active research in specialized centers.

WEANING FROM MECHANICAL VENTILATION

Weaning from mechanical ventilation is a poorly understood and often frustrating phase in the management of ARF. With the exception of certain diseases that are known to require prolonged uninterrupted mechanical ventilation (e.g., crushed chest or tetanus), consideration to begin weaning should be given when a few simple criteria have been met.

MINIMAL CRITERIA FOR INITIATING WEANING

1. Major systemic sepsis is controlled without shock.
2. Vital capacity 4 to 5 ml/kg.
3. Inspiratory force at least − 10 cm H_2O.
4. PEEP requirement 10 cm H_2O or less.
5. $D(A-a)o_2{}^{1.0} < 350$ mm Hg.
6. Stable cardiovascular system.
7. Chest wall flailing not severe.

General Principles of Weaning

1.   Correct hypocapnia if present. If the patient has been ventilated to a low $Paco_2$, this should be corrected by reducing the minute ventilation, using mechanical dead space, or employing the IMV technique.

2.   Correct significant metabolic alkalosis (base excess $> + 5$ mEq/liter) prior to weaning with KCl or HCl infusions as indicated.

3.   Regardless of the technique employed, the daily program for the patient should be planned with weaning as the first priority.

4.   Before commencing weaning, the procedure and weaning plan should be explained in detail to the patient, whose confidence in those caring for him is essential. He should be told that dyspnea can be expected, but will not be harmful. Assurance and encouragement are important in overcoming psychological dependence on the ventilator. Each weaning episode should end with a sense of accomplishment, not on a note of failure. Consequently, weaning by the clock according to tolerance is preferred rather than pushing the patient to the point of exhaustion.

Conventional Weaning

1.   Use T-piece high flow and high humidity gas.

2.   For initial weaning and until oxygen requirements have been established, adjust inspired oxygen concentration to 10 to 20 per cent above ventilator maintenance levels.

3.   Most patients benefit from the use of 3 to 10 cm H_2O CPAP to overcome the tendency to small airways closure.

4.   Elevate the body trunk at 20 to 40 degrees in bed or have the patient sit in a chair as tolerated.

5.   Delay nightly weaning until daytime weaning is essentially complete. When nightly weaning is initiated, many patients fear they will "stop breathing" and may initially remain awake when disconnected from the ventilator. Patience and a thorough explanation of the physiological considerations will usually overcome this problem rapidly.

Physiologic Effects of Weaning

Changes in Lung Mechanics.   These are secondary to changes in breathing pattern and lung volumes and include small airways closure, increase in small airways resistance, gas trapping, and progressive diffuse atelectasis. This, in turn, increases ventilation-perfusion inequality, causing a fall in lung compliance and an increase in the work of breathing. The most effective prevention is careful monitoring and use of CPAP and/or IMV technique.

Hemodynamic Changes.   These result from abrupt changes in intrathoracic pressure, causing a sudden rise in the cardiac filling pressures (see section on Cardiovascular Effects of Positive Pressure Ventilation and PEEP). As a rule, cardiac output should rise. Beach, Millen and Grenvik[1] recently documented a group of patients in whom discontinuance of mechanical ventilation resulted in a decrease in cardiac output, unsuccessful weaning history, and the development of hydrostatic pulmonary edema. Presumably these patients are unable to tolerate the increase in ventricular preload and are pushed to the flat portion of their Frank-Starling ventricular function curve. CPAP, IMV, and careful hemodynamic monitoring and intervention should reduce this "autotransfusion" effect seen during weaning.

INTERMITTENT MANDATORY VENTILATION

IMV as an alternate approach to weaning is gaining increasing acceptance and is a superior approach in many patients. As the frequency of the ventilator-provided breaths is progressively reduced, the patient gradually assumes a greater fraction of the alveolar ventilation. The advantages of IMV weaning are:

1. IMV permits an earlier start of weaning and earlier normalization of $Paco_2$ than is the case with conventional weaning.

2. IMV requires less nursing and physician time. (It should not become a reason to devote less attention to the patient.)

3. IMV facilitates gradual circulatory adaption to changes in intrathoracic pressure and may be the technique of choice for patients with chronic heart failure or compromised cardiac performance.

4. IMV, by providing ultrafrequent sighing with large tidal volumes, prevents airways closure and atelectasis.

5. IMV may cause an improvement in the ventilation-perfusion ratio distribution in the lungs by favoring ventilation to dependent lung regions during spontaneous ventilation.

6. IMV may reduce the tendency to systemic and pulmonary water retention to the extent that spontaneous ventilation favors lymphatic drainage from the lungs and thoracic duct.

REFERENCES

1. Beach, T., Millen, E., and Grenvik, A.: Hemodynamic response to discontinuance of mechanical ventilation. Crit. Care Med., *1*:85, 1973.
2. Bendixen, H. H., Egbert, L. D., Hedley Whyte, J., et al.: Respiratory Care. St. Louis, C. V. Mosby Company, 1965.
3. Cournand, A., Motley, H. L., Werko, L., et al.: Physiological studies on the effects of intermittent positive pressure breathing on cardiac output in man. Am. J. Physiol., *152*:162, 1948.
4. Downs, J. B., Klein, E. F., Desautels, D. A., et al.: Intermittent mandatory ventilation: A new approach to weaning patients from mechanical ventilation. Chest, *64*:331, 1973.
5. Egbert, L. D., Battit, G. E., Welch, C. E., and Bartlett, M. K.: Reduction of postoperative pain by encouragement and instruction of patients. N. Engl. J. Med., *270*:825, 1964.

6. Falke, K. J., Pontoppidan, H., Kumar, A., et al.: Ventilation with end-expiratory pressure in acute lung disease. J. Clin. Invest., *51*:2315, 1972.

7. Gett, P. M., Jones, S., and Sheperd, G. F.: Pulmonary edema associated with sodium retention during ventilator therapy. Br. J. Anaesth., *43*:460, 1971.

8. Hall, S. V., Johnson, E. E., and Hedley Whyte, J.: Renal hemodynamics and continuous positive-pressure ventilation in dogs. Anesthesiology, *41*:452, 1974.

9. Jordan, W. S.: New therapy for post intubation laryngeal edema and tracheitis in children. J.A.M.A., *212*:585, 1970.

10. Katz, S., Aberman, A., Frand, U., et al.: Heroin pulmonary edema: Evidence for increased pulmonary capillary permeability. Am. Rev. Resp. Dis., *106*:472, 1972.

11. Kirby, R. R., Downs, J. B., Civetta, J. M., et al.: High level positive end-expiratory pressure (PEEP) in acute respiratory insufficiency. Chest, *67*:156, 1975.

12. Lozman, J., Powers, S., Older, T., et al.: Correlation of pulmonary wedge and left atrial pressures: A study of patients receiving PEEP. Arch. Surg., *109*:270, 1974.

13. Markello, R., Winter, P. M., Olszowka, A., et al.: Assessment of ventilation inequalities by arterial-alveolar nitrogen differences in intensive care patients. Anesthesiology, *37*:4, 1972.

14. Pontoppidan, H., Geffin, B., and Lowenstein, E.: Acute Respiratory Failure in the Adult. Boston, Little, Brown and Company, 1973.

15. Pontoppidan, H., Laver, M. B., and Geffin, B.: Acute respiratory failure in the surgical patient. Adv. Surg., *4*:163, 1970.

16. Qvist, J., Pontoppidan, H., Wilson, R. S., et al.: Hemodynamic response to mechanical ventilation with PEEP: The effect of hypervolemia. Anesthesiology, *42*:45, 1975.

17. Rie, M. A., White, A., Skirm, L., et al.: Interhospital transportation for the severely hypoxemic and hemodynamically unstable patient. Abstracts of Scientific Papers, Scandinavian Society of Anesthesiologists, Oulu, Finland, July 1975.

18. Skillman, J. J., Parikh, B. M., and Tanenbaum, B. J.: Pulmonary arteriovenous admixture: Improvement with albumin and diuresis. Am. J. Surg., *119*:440, 1970.

19. Sladen, A., Laver, M. B., and Pontoppidan, H.: Pulmonary complications of water retention in prolonged mechanical ventilation. N. Engl. J. Med., *279*:448, 1968.

20. Staub, N. C.: "State of the Art" review. Pathogenesis of pulmonary edema. Am. Rev. Resp. Dis., *109*:358, 1974.

21. Suter, P. M., Fairley, H. B., and Isenberg, M.: Optimum end-expiratory airway pressure in patients with acute pulmonary failure. N. Engl. J. Med., *292*:284, 1975.

22. Suter, P. M., Fairley, H. B., and Schlobohm, R. M.: The Response of lung volume and pulmonary perfusion to short periods of 100 per cent oxygen ventilation in acute respiratory failure. Crit. Care Med., *2*:43, 1974.

23. Trichet, B., Falke, K., Togut, M., et al.: The effect of preexisting pulmonary vascular disease on the response to mechanical ventilation with PEEP following open-heart surgery. Anesthesiology, *42*:56, 1975.

24. Wagner, P. D., Laravuso, R. B., Uhl, R. R., et al.: Distribution of ventilation-perfusion ratios in acute respiratory failure. Chest, *65*:325, 1974.

25. Warshaw, A. L., Lesser, P. B., Rie, M. A., et al.: The Pathogenesis of pulmonary edema in acute pancreatitis. Ann. Surg., *182*:505, 1975.

26. Winter, P. M., and Smith, G.: The toxicity of oxygen. Anesthesiology, *37*:210, 1972.

27. Zaidan, J., Lowenstein, E., Hallowell, P., and Lappas, D.: Routine use of Swan-Ganz flow-directed pulmonary artery catheters in adult cardiac surgical patients: Time for insertion, success rate and incidence of complications in 76 consecutive attempts. Abstracts of Scientific Papers, American Society of Anesthesiologists, Chicago, Illinois, October 1975.

28. Zapol, W. M., Snider, M., Rie, M., et al.: Pulmonary hypertension in severe acute respiratory failure. *In* Zapol, W. M., and Qvist, J. (Eds.): Washington, D.C., Hemisphere Publishing Corporation, 1975, p. 435.

29. Powers, S. R., and Dutton, R. E.: Correlation of positive end-expiratory pressure with cardiovascular performance. Critical Care Medicine, *3*:64–68, 1975.

30. Pontoppidan, H., Wilson, R. S., and Rie, M. A.: Respiratory intensive care. Anesthesiology, *47*:96–116, 1977.

CHAPTER 17

PERIPHERAL CIRCULATORY FAILURE

J. R. Border, M.D.

L. Bone, M.D.

THE CLINICAL PROBLEM

Peripheral circulatory failure may be defined as any disorder of the peripheral circulation that reduces cardiac output or alternatively increases cardiac output to a value inappropriate to metabolic needs. This may be subdivided into three categories. The first category includes those conditions that limit cardiac filling. The second category includes conditions that limit systolic ejection of the heart owing to ventricular outflow obstruction. The third category consists of disorders of the peripheral circulation that produce an increase in cardiac output as a response to a fall in peripheral resistance.[16,20,22] The last category includes such hyperdynamic states as cirrhosis and sepsis. In addition, increased cardiac output may result from an increased metabolic need. Peripheral circulatory failure must also be considered in relation to pulmonary function, since the critical parameter is the delivery of oxygen to peripheral tissues.[1]

Shock constitutes a portion of the act of dying. It must be diagnosed rapidly and treated vigorously. The most important ingredient of successful therapy is a trained physician standing at the bedside, rapidly evaluating the patient's condition and response to therapy over and over again until success is obtained.

THE PATHOPHYSIOLOGY

The three types of peripheral circulatory disorders commonly coexist in patients who have been critically ill with sepsis, pulmonary failure, cirrhosis,

Supported in part by National Institutes of General Medical Sciences Grant, GM 15768.

multiple trauma, and so on. Their coexistence leads to difficult problems in judgment. Thus, the patient who has a dilated peripheral vascular bed requires a cardiac output higher than normal, but the optimum level can be determined only from the physiologic response to therapeutic increases of the cardiac output. Values of two to four times normal have been reported.

Ventricular outflow obstruction can induce ventricular failure. With a normal ventricle, this may require arterial pressures of two or more times normal. Conversely, a previously failing ventricle may have a relative ventricular outflow obstruction at normal pressures.[14] This type of ventricular failure constitutes the major indication for use of the intraaortic balloon pump or systemic vasodilators. It may be seen with severe systemic arterial hypertension secondary to acute head trauma, with exogenous vasoconstrictors infused at too great a rate, or with cross-clamping of the aorta in the chest. Left ventricular outflow obstruction as a cause of left ventricular failure, except in the patient with previous severe heart disease or acute myocardial infarction, is uncommon.

In contrast, right ventricular outflow obstruction is common. It may occur because of pulmonary emboli (either macro and micro), fat emboli, or any condition that results in increased pulmonary vascular resistance. The normal mean pulmonary artery pressure in a man is 12 to 15 mm Hg.[9] Doubling this pressure puts it in the commonly observed range of 24 to 30 mm Hg, while quadrupling it would place it in the range of 48 to 60. These increases in pulmonary artery pressure are great enough so that some degree of right ventricle failure may be expected. The requirement for increased central venous pressures in order to achieve adequate cardiac output in the presence of increased pulmonary vascular resistance is not unexpected.

The presence of increased central venous pressure in response to right ventricle outflow obstruction is normal and must be distinguished from left ventricle failure. The more severe the right ventricle outflow obstruction, the higher will be the central venous pressure required to maintain the output of the right ventricle and therefore an adequate cardiac output. In contrast, the occurrence of left ventricle failure with a high central venous pressure plus an elevated left atrial pressure will lead to pulmonary edema. Therefore, there is no single range of central venous pressures that can be used for all patients. One differential diagnosis between right ventricular outflow obstruction and left ventricular failure may be made with the use of the Swan-Ganz catheter to measure the wedge pulmonary artery pressure. This measurement usually approximates the left atrial pressure and provides an index of left ventricular function. Artificial ventilation with positive endexpiratory pressure above 10 cm H_2O may produce pulmonary artery wedge pressures higher than the simultaneously measured left atrial pressure.[18] Pressures of 14 to 18 mm Hg can be used to drive the left heart without danger of pulmonary edema.[17]

The problems at this stage may be summarized, therfore, as to how high a cardiac output is high enough and how high a central venous pressure is high enough to achieve that cardiac output without pulmonary edema. The maximum central venous pressure that can be generated depends upon the venous vasomotor tone, the blood volume, and the colloid osmotic pressure. Within certain limits, the central venous pressure and cardiac output may be maintained in the face of blood loss by venous vasoconstriction, while central venous pressure and cardiac output may also be maintained in the face of increased blood volumes by venous vasodilation.[14] These attributes of the veins allow the clinical patient to do fairly well so long as the blood volume is maintained within plus or minus one liter of normal. Arterial pressure does not in general fall below the range of normal until cardiac output is reduced to one half of normal.[19] This attribute of the peripheral circulation plus the venous vasoconstrictor response commonly allows young healthy persons a blood loss of about two liters (40 per cent) before arterial hypotension occurs. The young healthy patient in shock generally requires an increase in blood volume of one to two liters. The patient with injuries such as femoral shaft fracture or an enlarging pelvic hematoma with known closed space blood loss should therefore receive blood before he becomes hypotensive. The objective of management of a patient with known blood loss is to prevent shock, not to treat it.

All of the normal responses of the circulation to right ventricle cardiac filling may go awry. The patient with spinal cord transection with its associated sympathetic nervous system destruction loses the ability for both venous and arteriolar vasoconstriction.[14] He will therefore require a blood volume above normal and pharmacologic arteriolar vasoconstrictors. The patient with preexisting cardiac failure, on the other hand, has increased sympathetic nervous system activity and thus has both arteriolar and venous vasoconstriction.[8] The arteriolar vasoconstriction allows him to subsist on cardiac outputs below normal, but the rigid veins that also occur secondary to increased sympathetic nervous system activity are associated with increased central venous pressure and the development of arterial hypotension with much smaller blood losses and pulmonary edema with much smaller increases in blood volume. This type of patient requires a much smaller increase of blood volumes during resuscitation. Some patients with sepsis require such large infusions of plasma and blood to obtain a given central venous pressure that it must be concluded that they have loss of venous vasomotor tune.

Central venous pressure and capillary hydrostatic pressure represent the two ends of a pressure scale. In order for blood to flow from the periphery to the heart, the capillary hydrostatic pressure must always be greater than the central venous pressure.[14] The maximal capillary hydrostatic pressure which can be generated is that of the colloid osmotic pressure. Any greater pressure produces fluid transudation with edema and reduced blood volume until the capillary hydrostatic pressure is at the maximum value allowed by colloid osmotic pressure.[13] Under normal conditions of low central venous pressure, the colloid osmotic pressure has little influence on blood volume even at fairly low levels of plasma albumin. However, the higher the central venous pressure required, the more important is the colloid osmotic pressure.[10,17] Stated differently, high central venous pressures and high left atrial pressures simply cannot be generated in the face of low colloid osmotic pressure, since the fluid given ends up as peripheral edema fluid and does not contribute to increasing blood volume except for a short period of time.

Therefore, the colloid osmotic pressure is of importance only under conditions of high atrial pressure. Ringer's lactate is good resuscitation fluid for the previously healthy, well nourished person in acute blood loss shock because the atrial pressures are low and because the liver will synthesize and release large amounts of albumin,[2] and extravascular albumin can be mobilized.[1] In spite of these facilitating factors, approximately four liters of Ringer's lactate are required for each liter increase in blood volume desired, and therefore three liters of increased extravascular fluid is produced. The three liters are partially utilized in correcting the deficit in extravascular volume produced by the cellular edema that occurs with shock.[6] These considerations may not apply if there is primary pulmonary damage, if there is severe hypoxic hepatic damage limiting albumin synthesis, if the patient is previously malnourished, or if there is a primary cardiac failure. Under these specific conditions, more plasma, albumin, and whole blood are indicated in blood volume resuscitation.

There are a number of chronically critically ill patients who may now be recognized to have a number of attributes of peripheral circulatory failure secondary to malnutrition and hypoalbuminemia. These patients commonly have pulmonary failure, central venous pressures of 12 to 15 cm H_2O, oliguria with edema, hyponatremia and hypochloridemia, and have usually been supported on intravenous glucose for prolonged periods. In addition, they are commonly lethargic comatose, are somewhat jaundiced, and have wounds that do not heal in association with decubital ulcers. This can largely be reversed in the acutely ill patient with exogenous albumin, and in the chronically ill patient by supplying adequate amounts of a complete mixture of amino acids. Total caloric support is best given via the gastrointestinal tract and next best as intravenous hyperalimentation.[2,3]

Systemic arteriovenous shunting is associated with hepatic dysfunction occurring in relationship to cirrhosis, sepsis, or the chronically critically ill state. The magnitude of the blood flow involved is such that it almost necessarily involves the muscle beds. Observation in experimental animals has shown increased muscle blood flow and biochemical changes consistent with this deduction.[15] It appears probable at this time that what appears to be muscle systemic arteriovenous shunting is in reality an increased blood flow through the normal capillaries of muscle with an associated physical or biochemical change that reduces oxygen consumption and increases lactate production.

Systemic arteriovenous shunting requires much more study. At present, it can be said only that patients supported on amino acids appear to have both less hepatic dysfunction and less systemic arteriovenous shunting than those supported on pure glucose. These changes may be correlated with hepatic ketogenesis.[5] The patient on isotonic amino acids who has ketonuria is clearly doing well. This observation is of great practical value since the urine may easily be tested with Keto-Diastix.

PRACTICAL EVALUATION

The practical evaluation of the patient with peripheral circulatory shock depends upon knowledge of a large number of parameters. These include the history leading up to the shock; the urine in the bladder when the patient is first seen, and the subsequent quality and quantity of urine output; the blood pressure and heart rate; the central venous pressure and at times the pulmonary artery and pulmonary artery wedge pressure; the arterial blood gases, mixed venous blood gases, and inspired oxygen; the state of cerebral function and neurologic function; the cutaneous circulation and the presence or absence of visible hand and neck veins; and the electrocardiogram.

HISTORY

The history is of great importance, since it quickly directs one's attention to the most probable mechanisms of shock. Clearly, the most common mechanism of peripheral circulatory failure is hypovolemic shock. In posttrauma and postsurgical patients, this usually means blood loss shock, while in patients with burns, peritonitis, and repeated emesis, it usually means extracellular fluid loss hypovolemic shock. In the trauma patient, one must always be alert to the fact that the accident may have occurred because of a myocardial infarction, a cerebrovascular accident, or the use of drugs, so that the shock following trauma is a much more complicated problem than just blood loss shock.

Initial evaluation of this sort of patient should include not only the degree and mechanism of the circulatory failure but also the degree and mechanism of concurrent pulmonary failure. One cannot resuscitate the circulation if there is inadequate oxygen in the blood to support the function of the heart. This degree of hypoxia may easily be ascertained simply by drawing arterial blood and looking at it. Blood that pulsates into the syringe and is black implies severe pulmonary failure that requires immediate ventilatory support. Any patient who maintains black arterial blood in spite of adequate ventilation requires large chest tubes placed bluntly, blindly, inferiorly, and posteriorly. Black arterial blood in the presence of adequate ventilation implies intrathoracic pathologic changes, such as a pneumohemothorax or a tension pneumothorax, and demands immediate therapy in order to obtain survival.[4]

Some other comments may be made about the history. The patient with chest pain preceding his episode of shock must first be suspected of a myocardial infarction. The patient with a temperature spike, a history of sepsis, prolonged intravenous catheterization, or urethral instrumentation must first be suspected of the shock associated with sepsis. Shock of whatever nature produces an elevation in the leukocyte count, so that in the shock state this parameter is not of great value in discriminating the shock associated with sepsis from hypovolemic shock. Cardiac arrhythmias in the shock state may have multiple causative mechanisms. These include head trauma, cerebrovascular occlusion, arterial hypoxia, preexisting cardiac disease aggravated by hypovolemia, direct chest trauma with a myocardial contusion, or an acute myocardial infarction.

RESPONSE

OLIGURIA—THE WARNING OF IMPENDING SHOCK

The onset of oliguria in the patient who was previously putting out urine should be considered as much a surgical crisis as blood loss. A vigorous approach to diagnosis, evaluation, and treatment of oliguria commonly prevents not only oliguric renal failure but also overt shock. The most common cause of oliguria by far is dehydration, with the second most common cause being hypovolemia. The first maneuver in the treatment of oliguria is the rapid administration of a liter of crystalloid fluid under close observation. If the oliguria does not respond within one half hour or so the second maneuver is to increase the blood volume about one liter rapidly and again under close observation. If there is still no response, a central venous catheter is required and a second liter increase in blood volume is produced with plasma under close observation. Most patients respond to this sequence of maneuvers, and overt shock may be prevented.

OVERT SHOCK

Shock is most commonly secondary to hypovolemia. The history quickly directs one's attention to the mechanism producing hypovolemia as to overt blood loss, hidden blood loss, gastrointestinal blood loss, extrarenal fluid loss, and third space fluid loss. In order for overt shock to occur, hypovolemia of at least one liter, and commonly of two liters, has occurred. Patients with preexisting cardiac failure may have hypovolemic blood loss with smaller blood losses.

The first maneuver is to increase blood volume. The rate at which blood volume is increased by infusion of blood, plasma, and crystalloid fluid depends upon how severe the shock is, and varies from three intravenous lines being pumped as fast as they can be to simply hanging up a bottle and letting it flow at its own rate. While this is going on, pulmonary function is quickly surveyed by obtaining arterial blood, first to evaluate color, and second for analysis. Arterial oxygen tension cannot be evaluated unless the patient has a known inspired oxygen. The best by far is room air.

The third maneuver is to evaluate by history and physical examination the mechanisms producing the hypovolemia so that attention may be turned to its correction. At this time the question must be asked as to whether there is a component of sepsis that requires antibiotics, drainage of abscess, or excision of dead bowel or tissue. The presence of localized sepsis generally implies both bacteria and dead tissue or hematoma to provide nutrient for bacterial growth. Both aspects of the septic process require therapy. This is not true of the bacteremias produced with uretheral instrumentation or prolonged central venous catheterization. It may be true of peripheral intravenous lines that produce thrombosis of the vessel with subsequent suppurative thrombophlebitis. This diagnosis must always be considered, since there are very few clinical signs and the diagnosis is commonly not obvious. The choice of antibiotics must largely be based upon guesswork as to customary flora and preexisting cultures if they are available. It is clear that if a correct choice of antibiotic is initially made, the chances of survival are enhanced. This is particularly true if a massive bacteremia has occurred. The choice in the absence of preexisting cultures largely revolves around the organ involved and the anatomic level of involvement.

Most patients in shock quickly respond to increased blood volume. In the young, previously healthy patient with short-term shock, the equivalent of one liter of blood volume may easily be given as four liters of Ringer's lactate. In patients with preexisting malnutrition, those with severe prolonged shock, or those requiring high central venous pressure, the Ringer's lactate is required, but they may also require much more in the way of blood and plasma.

The fourth maneuver in the patient who does not quickly respond to infusions of blood and Ringer's lactate is the insertion of a central venous catheter while the patient is quickly evaluated for continuing fluid and blood loss. The patient who has a central venous pressure of 5 cm H_2O or less clearly requires further increases in blood volume. The central venous pressure in general may be increased to 10 to 15 cm H_2O without danger of pulmonary edema. This does not mean one value of 10 to 15 cm H_2O, but means infusion of blood plasma and fluids to maintain the central venous pressure stable at 10 to 15 cm H_2O. The rate at which such fluids are required is helpful in determining the rate of fluid and blood loss.

The patient who remains in shock with a central venous pressure maintained at 10 to 15 cm H_2O requires further evaluation as to right ventricle outflow obstruction, left ventricle failure, colloid osmotic pressure, and systemic arteriovenous shunting. If the patient has severe pulmonary failure, he will be on the ventilator, and central venous pressures may be safely increased to 20 to 25 cm H_2O without danger. This may also be done if the patient has a clear-cut pulmonary thromboembolus. In the presence of relatively good pulmonary function, the patient who is not out of shock with a central venous pressure of 10 to 15 cm H_2O requires a Swan-Ganz catheter to evaluate the pulmonary artery pressure and the pulmonary artery wedge pressure. Blood volume may be safely increased to maintain the pulmonary artery wedge pressure in the range of 14 to 18 mm Hg so long as the colloid osmotic pressure is normal.

Both the pulmonary artery catheter, when it is not in the wedge position, and the central venous catheter may be used to obtain blood for analysis of blood gases. Clearly the best and most dependable of these is the pulmonary artery blood. The normal oxygen tension of this sort of blood is in the range of 35 to 40 mm Hg. Since these oxygen tensions are on the curvilinear portion of the oxyhemoglobin dissociation curve, they may be used as a rough approximation of oxygen content and thus as a measure of the relationship of oxygen consumption to cardiac output. Percentage of oxyhemoglobin may be directly measured, and for mixed venous blood should be between 70 and 75 per cent. Under normal conditions, cardiac output is carefully adjusted to oxygen consumption so that the mixed venous oxygen content remains constant. Values of mixed venous oxygen tension below 35 mm Hg (70 per cent oxyhemoglobin) imply inadequate cardiac output for the rate of oxygen consumption and thus the need for more cardiac output. Values of mixed venous oxygen tension above 40 mm Hg (70 per cent oxyhemoglobin) imply cardiac output in excess of oxygen consumption.

The knowledge of pulmonary artery and pulmonary wedge pressures and mixed venous blood oxygen tensions allows much more exact diagnosis and therapy. The patient with a low mixed venous oxygen tension and a high pulmonary artery wedge pressure has primary left ventricle failure, which requires positive inotropic agents such as dopamine. In general, such a patient also has an increased total peripheral resistance. The patient who has a high central venous pressure, a low pulmonary artery wedge pressure, and a low mixed venous oxygen saturation has hypovolemia with right ventricle outflow obstruction and requires increased blood volume—even though he has a high central venous pressure. The patient with very severe pulmonary failure may be expected to require a much higher central venous pressure in order to obtain a given pulmonary artery wedge pressure.

The patient who has fairly good pulmonary function but requires a high central venous pressure to obtain an adequate pulmonary artery wedge pressure must be strongly suspected of having a pulmonary embolus. If the history is compatible, he probably should be treated for a pulmonary embolus.

The patient who has an increased mixed venous oxygen tension and remains hypotensive has a hyperdynamic state with systemic vasodilatation. This patient requires increased blood volumes until his pulmonary artery wedge pressure reaches the range of 14 to 18 mm Hg. The patient with systemic vasodilatation commonly also has increased pulmonary vascular resistance, so that increased fluid administration to achieve a high central venous pressure may be required to obtain a pulmonary artery wedge pressure of 14 to 18 mm Hg. These patients may then require positive inotropic agents even though they have been brought out of shock by this maneuver. The positive inotropic agents are utilized to reduce the atrial pressures required to maintain adequate systemic blood flow. If the patient has not been brought out of shock, these drugs are utilized to further increase cardiac output while simutaneously increasing blood volume to maintain the atrial pressures. The agents commonly utilized under these conditions where there is no apparent limitation to coronary flow are Isuprel, dopamine, glucagon, and digitalis. These agents act by different mechanisms, and therefore have an additive effect. The simplest agent to utilize is Isuprel, since it has an immediate onset of action and immediately stops when discontinued. It has three major defects in that it increases the cardiac rate, produces some muscle vasodilation, and may produce arrhythmias. It may be utilized in a dose that does not produce a cardiac rate above 140 while waiting for the onset of action of digitalis given intravenously as digoxin. We customarily give one third the normal digitalizing doses of digoxin (0.5 mg) intravenously as a bolus, with later doses depending on responses and the electrocardiogram. Obviously, a history must be obtained as to previous use of digitalis. The patient who does not respond adequately to digitalis and Isuprel requires glucagon or dopamine as the only other available positive agents. There is great controversy about the effectiveness of steroids in this situation, but if the patient is clearly not responding to conventional circulatory support, they probably should be used. This is seldom necessary if conventional circulatory support is vigorously employed. No amount of circulatory support will help the patient with sepsis unless his abscesses are drained, dead infected tissue is excised, proper antibiotics are employed, and vigorous nutritional support is given.

SUMMARY

The mechanisms of peripheral circulatory failure have been discussed. The shock associated with sepsis is commonly secondary to multiple mechanisms. These commonly include an element of hypovolemia, right ventricle outflow obstruction secondary to pulmonary failure, biventricular failure, and systemic vasodilatation. The shock due to hypovolemia is initially a single mechanism shock, but with time additional mechanisms related to ventricular failure, severe vasoconstriction, and pulmonary failure may supervene. The longer the shock state lasts, the more complicated it is to treat. The more rapidly it is diagnosed and treated, the simpler it is to treat.

REFERENCES

1. Border, J. R.: Cardiopulmonary failure in basic surgery. *In* McCredie, J. (Ed.): Basic Surgery. New York, Macmillan, 1976.
2. Border, J. R.: Metabolic responses to starvation, sepsis and trauma. *In* McCredie, J. (Ed.): Basic Surgery. New York, Macmillan, 1976.
3. Border, J. R., LaDuca, J., and Seibel, R.: Trauma and delayed sepsis. *In* Burke, J. F. (Ed.): The Infection Prone Hospital Patient. Boston, Little, Brown and Company, 1976.

4. Border, J. R., LaDuca, J., and Seibel, R.: Priorities in the management of the patient with polytrauma. *In* Allgower, M. (Ed.): Progress in Surgery. Vol. 14. Basel, S. Karger, 1975, pp. 87–122.
5. Border, J. R., Chenier, R., McMenamy, R. H., LaDuca, J., Seibel, R., Birkhahn, R., and Yu, L.: Multiple systems organ failure: Muscle fuel deficit with visceral protein malnutrition. Surg. Clin. N. Amer., *56*:1147, 1976.
6. Carrico, C. J., Canizaro, P. C., and Shires, G. T.: Fluid resuscitation following injury: rationale for the use of balanced salt solution. Crit. Care Med., *4*:46, 1976.
7. Clowes, G. H. A., Zuschoreid, W., Turner, M., Blackburn, G, Rubin, T., and Grein, G.: Observations on the pathogenesis of the pneumonitis associated with severe infections. Ann. Surg., *167*:630, 1968.
8. Davis, J. O.: The physiology of congestive heart failure. *In* Hamilton, W. F. (Ed.): Handbook of Physiology. Section 2: Circulation. Vol. 3. Baltimore, Williams and Wilkins Company, 1965, pp. 2071–2127.
9. Fishman, A. P., Dynamics of the pulmonary circulation. *In* Hamilton, W. F., and Dow, P. (Eds.): Handbook of Physiology. Section 2: Circulation. Vol. 2. Baltimore, Williams and Wilkins Company, 1963, pp. 1667–1745.
10. Greene, D. G.: Pulmonary edema. *In* Fenn, W. O., and Rahn, H. (Eds.): Handbook of Physiology. Section 3: Respiration. Vol. 2. Baltimore, Williams and Wilkins Company, 1965, pp. 1585–1601.
11. Guyton, A. C.: Textbook of Medical Physiology. 5th Ed. Philadelphia, W. B. Saunders Company, 1976.
12. Guyton, A. C., Coleman, T. G., and Granger, H. J.: Circulation: overall regulation. Ann. Rev. Physiol., *74*:13, 1972.
13. Guyton, A. C., Granger, H. J., and Taylor, A. E.: Interstitial fluid pressure. Physiol. Rev., *51*:527, 1971.
14. Guyton, A. C., Jones, C. E., and Coleman, T. G.: Circulatory Physiology: Cardiac Output and Its Regulation. Philadelphia, W. B. Saunders Company, 1973.
15. Hermreck, A. S., and Thal, A. P.: Mechanisms for the high circulatory requirement in sepsis and septic shock. Ann. Surg., *170*:677, 1969.
16. MacLean, L. D., Mulligan, W. G., McLean, A. P. H., and Duff, J. H.: Patterns of septic shock in man: a detailed study of 56 patients. Ann. Surg., *166*:543, 1967.
17. Morisette, M., Weil, M. H., and Shubin, H.: Reduction of colloid osmotic pressure associated with fatal progression of cardiopulmonary failure. Crit. Care Med., *3*:115, 1975.
18. Powers, S., and Dutton, R. E.: Correlation of positive end expiratory pressure with cardiovascular performance. Crit. Care Med., *3*:64, 1975.
19. Schenk, W. G., Camp, F. A., Kjartansson, K. H., and Pollack, L.: Hemorrhage without hypotension. Ann. Surg., *160*:7, 1964.
20. Siegel, J. H., Greenspan, M., and DelGuercio, L. R. M.: Abnormal vascular tone, defective oxygen transport and myocardial failure in human septic shock. Ann. Surg., *165*:504, 1967.
21. Skillman, J. J.: The role of albumin and oncotically active fluids in shock. Crit. Care Med., *4*:55, 1976.
22. Wilson, R. F., Thal, A. P., Kindling, P. H., Grifka, T., and Ackerman, E.: Hemodynamic measurements in septic shock. Arch. Surg., *91*:121, 1965.

CHAPTER 18

CARDIAC PROBLEMS IN THE SURGICAL PATIENT

J. Francis Dammann, M.D.

Rajindar Singh, M.D.

The successful management of cardiovascular problems occurring after general surgery involves three key concepts: a high level of suspicion, early recognition, and aggressive monitoring and treatment. By the first, we emphasize the importance of an acute awareness of the risk factors of age, preexisting heart disease, preexisting respiratory insufficiency, family history, smoking, obesity, and the like. By the second, we are advocating that a cardiac problem be diagnosed on minimal signs before the full-blown picture has emerged. By the third, we are advising that aggressive monitoring be instituted with even minimal evidence, and treatment begun where a cardiac problem is confirmed. Only in this way can morbidity and mortality be reduced.

Cardiac problems postoperatively are not uncommon, particularly in the older age groups. Their true incidence is unknown. They may be acute or slow in developing. They may be life-threatening or merely nagging. They may trigger the failure of other key systems, as for example acute tubular necrosis, or be triggered by failure of another system, such as respiratory failure. They may occur as isolated phenomena, but frequently they are associated with established heart disease. Their importance can be minimized only by early recognition, aggressive monitoring, and treatment. Their cardiovascular manifestations divide basically into two types, electrical (arrhythmias) or mechanical (pump failure).

There are many extrinsic factors related to major surgery that may play a key role in the genesis of cardiac problems after surgery, in addition to the obvious intrinsic factor of underlying heart disease. It is important to recognize this fact, for adequate control of or compensation for these factors is the best means of prevention and the major basis for treatment. Almost all anesthetic agents have adverse direct effects on the cardiovascular system.[2,23] Myocardial contractility is reduced, and cardiac output may be diminished more than 25 per cent—a reduction well in excess of the reduction in body oxygen needs. Autonomic control of the cardiovascular system is adversely affected so that the hierarchy of control mechanisms that regulates blood flow and blood distribution to the body functions inappropriately. Certain agents, such as cyclopropane, increase circulating catecholamine. Halothane, on the other hand, decreases circulating catecholamine and impairs cardiac contractility. Venous return to the heart (preload) is altered by a change in venomotor tone and also by shifts in intrathoracic pressure secondary to assisted ventilation. This in turn affects myocardial contractility and cardiac output. The patient who retains anesthetic agents and premedication postoperatively tends to have impaired cardiac function. If that patient's normal cardiovascular function is borderline, a further reduction may precipitate an infarct, significant arrhythmias, or acute congestive heart failure.

Anesthesia also affects the heart via a direct effect on ventilation and/or the cerebral cortex. Premedication suppresses the cough reflex and the depth of ventilation. Under anesthesia the sigh is lost. Pulmonary drainage tends to be inadequate owing to a fixed body position on the operating room table, inadequate suctioning, and decreased bronchial ciliary action. All of these factors lead to hypoventilation, progressive miliary atelectasis, pulmonary arteriovenous shunting, hypoxia, and, very occasionally, hypercapnea. Hypoventilation during the early periods after surgery is very common.[22] Significant levels of hypoxia—unsuspected and unrecognized—can be found in every recovery room if one does a spot check of arterial blood gases. Hypoxia must always be looked for when a patient develops arrhythmia, congestive heart failure, or signs of a myocardial infarction postoperatively. It is the most common and most potent factor in the genesis of cardiac problems after surgery.

Surgery itself is a factor to be considered. There is a correlation between the length of the operation and the number and severity of complications, particularly in the elderly.[16] Cardiovascular and pulmonary complications decrease in number and severity as the site of the operation moves away from the chest.[29] Incidence and severity are highest with thoracic surgery, next highest with high abdominal, then low abdominal, and finally lowest in the periphery. The size of the operative area and the amount of soft tissue trauma have an effect primarily through determining the size of the third space and third space fluid loss. Pain, its effect on ventilation and movement, and the amount of narcotics required play a role in ventilatory insufficiency. There are factors peculiar to the type of surgery being performed. For example, atrial fibrillation is the most common significant arrhythmia after pulmonary resection.

Of obvious importance are hemostasis and blood and fluid volume. Efforts directed at maintaining a patient's blood volume precisely at the preoperative level alone are not adequate; blood volume must be considered in relation to the available vascular bed. The patient who returns to the recovery room severely vasoconstricted with his blood volume at the preoperative level may develop high output congestive failure. More commonly, blood volume is not at the preoperative levels in such patients but is reduced and appropriate for the size of the total vascular space. Later, when peripheral dilatation occurs, the patient suddenly becomes hypovolemic, with the consequent risks of hypotension, coronary insufficiency, low output congestive failure, arrhythmia, and renal shutdown. Metabolic acidosis, which decreases myocardial contractility and may produce arrhythmia, also occurs when the patient changes from a severe vasoconstricted state to a normal vascular bed, because metabolic waste products pooled in the periphery are suddenly poured into the circulating blood volume. The key to good management of blood volume is to monitor central venous pressure as well as arterial blood pressure, for then the physician can keep the level of blood volume appropriate to the size of the vascular bed, altering with either fluid or drugs as indicated.[34]

During the postoperative period, electrolyte abnormalities are not uncommon and when present may cause arrhythmias and/or congestive heart failure. Frequently at fault is the vigorous use of diuretics preoperatively without proper potassium replacement. Patients given diuretics preoperatively should have the diuretics discontinued two to three days prior to surgery and adequate potassium ingestion ensured. Preoperative nutritional status may also cause significant electrolyte deviations postoperatively. Use of suction tubes before, during, and after surgery can be a major factor in producing electrolyte imbalance. Frequent electrolyte determinations and early replacement measures are mandatory in such patients postoperatively if the possibility of cardiac problems is to be minimized.

Any postoperative complication can be a precipitating factor in the occurrence of cardiac problems. Bleeding from any site or third space fluid loss can produce significant hypovolemia, leading to failure or arrhythmias. The opposite extreme of excessive fluid infusion is a common cause of acute pulmonary edema secondary to left ventricular failure postoperatively, particularly in the elderly with subclinical ischemic heart disease. Excessive drugs producing myocardial, pulmonary, or cortical depression can lead to hypoventilation, decreased myocardial contractility, hypoxia, congestive heart failure, or arrhythmia. Pulmonary complications such as atelectasis, pneumonia, pulmonary emboli, or excessive work of breathing can all embarrass the heart. Abdominal complications such as infection, ileus, and even pain can embarrass the cardiopulmonary system, precipitating failure and/or arrhythmias. Renal failure, if not recognized sufficiently early, may find the patient hypervolemic or with an electrolyte imbalance, inviting congestive heart failure or arrhythmias. With any postoperative complication, the physician must be concerned that a cardiovascular problem may be added and he must be ready to act accordingly.

MYOCARDIAL INFARCTION

The significance of postoperative myocardial infarctions cannot be overstressed. The incidence of mortality associated with postoperative myocardial infarctions is in the range of 50 to 55 per cent, which is considerably higher than the mortality rate in the range of 25 to 30 per cent associated with nonsurgical infarctions.[16,29] Mortality is significantly greater still among patients who reinfarct postoperatively as compared with those who develop a myocardial infarction for the first time in the immediate postoperative period.[30]

The reported incidence of myocardial infarction in the postoperative period varies anywhere from 0.1 to 1.2 per cent.[29,30] This incidence has been found to be largely dependent upon age, history of previous myocardial infarction, and the type of surgery performed.[16,29,30] The incidence of postoperative myocardial infarction in studies of a large number of patients undergoing general anesthesia was found to be 10 to 50 times higher when there was a history of prior myocardial infarction.[30] Furthermore, the postoperative incidence of infarction is much higher if the surgical procedure is carried out within three months after a myocardial infarction, somewhat less so if the waiting period is six months, and lowest after two years.[30] The reinfarction rate has been found to be significantly more in operations involving the thorax or upper abdomen than in those involving other sites.[29]

The clinical presentation of myocardial infarction in the postoperative period may differ from the usual medical situation because of the effect of narcotics and pain secondary to the surgical procedure itself. Thus, pain, which is the most important and typical single symptom of an infarct, is made difficult to assess. In fact, pain attributable to the infarct may be absent. The most common first indications of a postsurgical infarct are the sudden appearance of tachypnea, tachycardia, hypotension, arrhythmias or congestive heart failure.

Serial electrocardiograms and serum enzyme determinations remain the most important tools with which to make a definitive diagnosis. Routine electrocardiogram evaluation in the postoperative period, especially in high-risk subjects who are elderly or who give symptoms suggestive of coronary artery disease, will unmask many otherwise unrecognized instances of myocardial infarction.[26] The diagnostic electrocardiographic feature of acute myocardial infarction in the postoperative period is specifically the development of new pathologic Q waves rather than ST-T segment change. Changes in the ST-T segment alone may be due to a number of other factors functioning in the postoperative period rather than to the development of acute coronary insufficiency. These include drugs, pericarditis, and electrolyte disturbances primarily, and autonomic imbalance secondarily.

Enzyme changes in the postoperative period are not as helpful as in myocardial infarctions without surgery because surgical injury to muscle produces similar enzyme rises. There are no data available as to the exact degree and specificity of enzyme rise after surgery, although some work has been done on the diagnostic value of serum enzymes occurring with myocardial infarction after surgery.[12]

The management of postoperative myocardial infarctions can be divided into three component parts, each deserving close attention: (1) precipitating and/or aggravating yet reversible noncardiac factors; (2) routine care; and (3) management of complications.

Noncardiac factors include hypoxia, hypotension secondary to hypovolemia, arrhythmias, septic shock, and factors producing increased cardiac workload such as temperature, infection, pain, anemia, or excessive fluid administration. All of these factors must be looked for and, when found, treated vigorously, for all aggravate the degree of coronary insufficiency by producing a greater imbalance between myocardial oxygen supply and demand. On the other hand, some of the above problems, such as hypotension, arrhythmias and hypoxia, may indeed result from acute myocardial infarction, in which case they need to be recognized and managed appropriately as complications, not as precipitating factors.

Routine care of postoperative myocardial infarction today should be comparable to that given in a medical coronary care unit. It has been clearly shown that in-hospital mortality from myocardial infarctions has been reduced by 10 to 15 per cent with the introduction of the coronary care unit. Mortality improvement has resulted almost solely from lowering the incidence of death secondary to arrhythmias (electrical death) and not the incidence of pump failure. That reduction resulted from an aggressive monitoring of the electrocardiogram and early aggressive treatment for arrhythmias. The same aggressive monitoring and treatment should be applied to the postoperative myocardial infarction patient in the postoperative intensive care unit.

The use of analgesics and narcotics for relief from myocardial or surgical pain has to be adjusted according to the status of the cardiopulmonary system and the patient's response. Morphine sulfate intravenously in small doses of 2 mg aliquots is the best analgesic unless there is a specific contraindication. Oxygen therapy should be routinely administered, since increased myocardial oxygenation with high inhaled concentrations of oxygen will help to relieve pain as well as lessen the incidence and magnitude of cardiac complications resulting from the infarction.

The major complications of a myocardial infarction are arrhythmias, hypotension, shock, and acute congestive failure. Later during the recovery period, thromboembolic phenomena become important. The management of these complications is described in more depth elsewhere in this chapter.

ARRHYTHMIAS

Statistics on the incidence of arrhythmias in the postoperative period vary. Arrhythmias are very infrequent (0.1 to 0.4 per cent) in general surgery patients who have a normal cardiovascular system, but are seen in 9 to 21 per cent of patients following special forms of surgery, such as cardiovascular and thoracic operations.[35] Arrhythmias are much more common in patients who have preexisting myocardial disease.

It should be emphasized that arrhythmias are a sign of underlying altered and abnormal physiology, and that in order to manage them, the underlying condition must be diagnosed and corrected. Ultimately, if the causative factor is overlooked and untreated, symptomatic treatment alone may prove unsuccessful. Usually arrhythmias are short-lasting and not particularly serious. They may occasionally be life-threatening, however, and then emergency action is required. It should also be stressed that it is extremely important to make a precise diagnosis of the type of rhythm disturbance present. This can be done only with the help of an electrocardiogram. Usually, there is ample time to obtain an electrocardiogram before any specific therapy is required.

Postoperative arrhythmias are frequently the result of factors existing before or during surgery which are aggravated and then precipitate because of one or more of many diverse additional stresses in the immediate postoperative period. Preexisting heart disease, under- or overdigitalization, use of diuretics, steroids or other cardiac medications, electrolyte and metabolic disorders, age, and preexisting arrhythmias are all significant preoperative factors conducive to rhythm disturbances in the postoperative period.[3,13,31] During the operative period, hypotension which leads to inadequate myocardial perfusion, hypoxia from whatever cause, and certain specific anesthetic agents are all arrhythmogenic.[3,32] Various stresses during the postoperative period may produce arrhythmias, including pain, fever, electrolyte and acid-base disturbances, hypoxia, hypotension, tracheobronchial suction, myocardial infarction, myocardial failure, and pulmonary embolism. Indeed, arrhythmias may be the initial manifestation of either a myocardial infarction or a pulmonary embolus.[11]

With increasing use of electrical devices in patient care, any discussion of arrhythmias would be incomplete without mentioning the possibility of electrical artifacts seen in the electrocardiogram which may simulate certain arrhythmias.[4] The importance of this awareness is obvious, as otherwise one may institute unnecessary therapeutic measures, each carrying the potential of doing harm.

As mentioned previously, the importance cannot be overemphasized of an exact diagnosis of the type of rhythm disturbance present, as well as the need for a search of underlying factors before any therapy is undertaken. Any type of rhythm disturbance can occur postoperatively, though certain arrhythmias, such as atrial tachyarrhythmias or premature ventricular contractions, are more frequent than others. Arrhythmias may produce no symptoms, in which case they are detected during vital sign check or through rhythm monitoring on the oscilloscope. Serious and especially sustained arrhythmias may produce palpitations, dyspnea, chest pain, and even the very significant hemodynamic disturbance of low output congestive failure.

An electrocardiogram is essential for identifying the exact nature of the rhythm disturbance. A detailed discussion of the various kinds of arrhythmias is not possible here, since any known form of arrhythmia can be seen. This discussion will be confined to the more commonly occurring rhythm disturbances and their mode of treatment. These arrhythmias can be divided into three groups: (1) tachyarrhythmias, (2) bradyarrhythmias, and (3) arrhythmias with a normal rate.

TACHYARRHYTHMIAS

Tachyarrhythmias can be sinus, atrial, junctional, or ventricular, depending upon their focus of origin. Even though atrial and ventricular premature beats are usually associated with a normal pulse rate, they will be discussed in this section, since their significance and treatment are quite similar to those of the tachyarrhythmias.

Sinus Tachycardia.   Sinus tachycardia is by far the most common postoperative arrhythmia. In one large published series of postoperative arrhythmias it was the only type.[10] The pulse rate is usually between 120 and 150 beats per minute. In the immediate postoperative period, a sinus rate of up to 120 beats per minute may be expected because of the stress of surgery itself. But if the rate is faster, additional stress should be looked for, such as excessive pain, hypoxia, infection, fever, hemorrhage, hypovolemia, and shock. There is no specific treatment for sinus tachycardia itself; the specific cause must be identified and treated.

Atrial Tachyarrhythmias.   Generally, premature atrial beats are seen when significant underlying heart disease and left heart failure are present. They may be a premonitory sign of later atrial fibrillation or atrial flutter. If premature atrial beats are present in the preoperative state, they should be treated, since the incidence of postoperative atrial tachyarrhythmias is then high. Any underlying cardiac decompensation should be treated. The treatment for both is digitalis. If there is no evidence of any underlying heart disease and atrial extrasystoles just appear during the postoperative period, they may simply be observed.

Atrial Fibrillation.   This is most commonly seen after chest surgery[37] and is probably due to acute atrial dilatation (Fig. 1). The rate is usually fast, 150 beats or above per minute, and irregularly irregular. If it develops suddenly, its effect on the total hemodynamic status will depend upon the underlying cardiac reserve. Thus, it may produce no symptoms or may initiate cardiogenic shock. Frequently, ventricular rate in the immediate postoperative period may be somewhat faster because of coexisting factors of fever, pain, anemia, and the like. A form of treatment of long standing is rapid digitalization via the intravenous route. If the patient has not been on digitalis previously, 0.75 mg of digoxin should be given intravenously followed by 0.25 mg every eight hours, making a total of 1.5 mg the first 24 hours, when usually a maintenance dose of 0.25 mg every day by any route

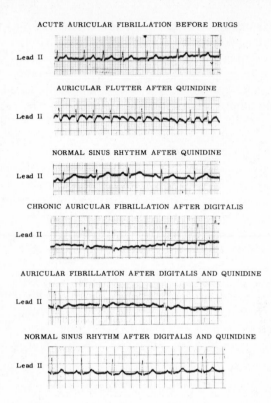

ACUTE AURICULAR FIBRILLATION BEFORE DRUGS

Lead II

AURICULAR FLUTTER AFTER QUINIDINE

Lead II

NORMAL SINUS RHYTHM AFTER QUINIDINE

Lead II

Figure 1. Examples of untreated and treated atrial fibrillation after surgery.

CHRONIC AURICULAR FIBRILLATION AFTER DIGITALIS

Lead II

AURICULAR FIBRILLATION AFTER DIGITALIS AND QUINIDINE

Lead II

NORMAL SINUS RHYTHM AFTER DIGITALIS AND QUINIDINE

Lead II

can be given. If rhythm persists as atrial fibrillation for several days, elective DC cardioversion to a normal sinus rhythm is indicated.

A strong argument can be made for DC cardioversion followed by digitalization, rather than digitalization first. Cardioversion is done at very low risk with a very high success rate, except when atrial fibrillation is chronic. Furthermore, DC cardioversion is immediately effective and brings the immediate benefit of an atrial kick to total cardiovascular function, significantly increasing cardiac output. Finally, patients who are digitalized and then cardioverted tend to develop toxic effects of digitalis with all the potential hazard that this involves. Some advise DC cardioversion first to be followed by slow digitalization, starting with a maintenance dose given orally if possible. If atrial fibrillation recurs, DC cardioversion is again indicated, but digitalization should be pushed a little harder. Elective DC cardioversion is tolerated well. Five to 10 mg of Valium given intravenously immediately before is really all that is necessary. In patients who are not receiving digitalis, 25 to 50 watt seconds is given. If the patient is suspected of being susceptible to the toxic effects of digitalis, a much lower level of 2.5 to 5 watt seconds is tried initially and increased until it is successful.

Atrial Flutter. Like atrial fibrillation, flutter is commonly seen following thoracotomy and suggests the presence of underlying heart disease (Fig. 2). It may sometimes be the presenting manifestation of pulmonary embolism.[11] DC cardioversion is clearly the treatment of choice in atrial flutter, since flutter is successfully converted by a very low level of DC shock and at the same time is known to be a very poor responder to digitalis, in contrast to atrial fibrillation. The poor response to digitalis requires large doses of digitalis in order to increase the atrioventricular block, slow the rate, and eventually convert to atrial fibrillation. This increases the risk of digitalis intoxication after cardioversion. Consequently, the first treatment should be DC cardioversion to be followed by slow digitalization.

Paroxysmal Supraventricular Tachycardia.   Underlying causes for this arrhythmia are the same as for atrial flutter and fibrillation. It may respond to vagal stimulation by physical maneuvers, such as carotid sinus massage. Otherwise, DC cardioversion should be attempted. Cardioversion gives an immediate boost to cardiac output, and therefore is particularly indicated when congestive heart failure is present. If cardioversion is successful, slow digitalization should follow. If it is not successful, rapid digitalization with intravenous digoxin or Tensilon should be tried.

Propranolol, a beta-adrenergic blocking agent, has been used with excellent results to control the ventricular rate in patients with supraventricular tachycardias, such as atrial fibrillation, flutter, and paroxysmal tachycardia. Ventricular slowing results from a prolongation of the atrioventricular nodal refractory period. Propranolol is also effective when the cause of the

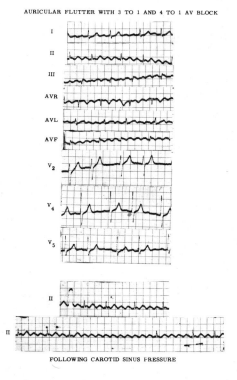

AURICULAR FLUTTER WITH 3 TO 1 AND 4 TO 1 AV BLOCK

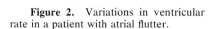

Figure 2. Variations in ventricular rate in a patient with atrial flutter.

FOLLOWING CAROTID SINUS PRESSURE

arrhythmia is digitalis intoxication. Extreme care must be used, for propranolol depresses myocardial contractility. Since incipient congestive failure may have produced the arrhythmia, most investigators now advocate the concurrent use of digitalis. Special care is also necessary in the presence of advanced atrioventricular block. Under such circumstances, propranolol probably should not be used unless emergency pacemaker equipment is available and rhythm monitoring is continuous.

Paroxysmal atrial tachycardia with block and nonparoxysmal junctional tachycardia are usually digitalis intoxication rhythms and are discussed under Digitalis Intoxication later in the chapter.

Ventricular Tachyarrhythmias. Premature ventricular contractions are common after surgery (Fig. 3). In the majority of circumstances, extracardiac factors are responsible for premature ventricular beats. Electrolyte disturbances (especially hypokalemia), tracheobronchial suction or other forms of vagal stimulation, acidosis, hypoxia, hypovolemia, shock, pain, and fever are some of the precipitating factors in the postoperative period. They should be carefully searched for and treated. Arterial blood gases

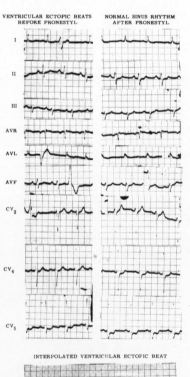

Figure 3. Ventricular extrasystoles before and after treatment in a postoperative patient.

should be determined in all patients with arrhythmias difficult to control, for hypoxia is the most potent and common cause. Digitalis intoxication should be suspected if the patient has been treated previously with one of the digitalis preparations, and cardioversion should be done only with great care under such circumstances for the fear of augmenting digitalis intoxication. If premature ventricular contractions are present in spite of correction of the extracardiac causes, evidence of poor myocardial perfusion and myocardial damage should be looked for and appropriately treated.

Specific antiarrhythmic agents are indicated if premature ventricular contractions are more than six per minute, occur in runs of three or more, or fall on the preceding T waves. Pronestyl, 250 mg, should be given every 4 to 6 hours orally if the patient can take drugs by mouth; otherwise, it is administered intramuscularly. The maximum dosage may be as high as 500 mg every 6 hours in refractory cases. Quinidine at 300 mg every 6 hours may be used if Pronestyl does not work or if digitalis intoxication is suspected. Dilantin at 100 mg four times a day may be given orally. If premature ventricular contractions are very frequent and are present in short runs, Xylocaine should be given intravenously. This should be as a bolus of 1 mg/kg of body weight, which should be followed by a continuous intravenous infusion at a 1 to 3 mg/minute rate. Propranolol has occasionally been used successfully for ventricular ectopic rhythms, but it is not the drug of choice.

Ventricular Tachycardia. Generally, the causative factors for ventricular tachycardias (Fig. 4) are the same as for premature ventricular contractions. Digitalis intoxication should always be suspected and ruled out. A Xylocaine bolus should be given intravenously immediately, and this should be followed by a Xylocaine drip. If significant hemodynamic dysfunction is present, the patient should be cardioverted with DC shock immediately.

Ventricular Fibrillation. Ventricular tachycardia, if prolonged beyond a very short period of time, usually terminates in ventricular fibrillation, which produces zero cardiac output and is rapidly fatal. The patient should be cardioverted immediately by DC shock, unless the patient has been fibrillating for half a minute or more. In the latter event, one ampule of sodium bicarbonate should be pushed intravenously, and the patient should be oxygenated by cardiac massage and bag breathing with 100 per cent oxygen. This should be carried out for one to two minutes before electrical shock is given. If the first shock is not effective, the watt seconds should be increased, and shock should be tried again. If after two or three attempts fibrillation has not been converted to sinus rhythm, or has been converted only transiently so, time should be taken to oxygenate the patient well, treat with more sodium bicarbonate, and depress myocardial irritability with Xylocaine.

Sometimes following electrical shock, asystole appears. The injection of 5 to 10 ml of calcium chloride into the left ventricle and the starting of an Isuprel drip should increase myocardial irritability and establish some sort of

PAROXYSMAL AURICULAR TACHYCARDIA

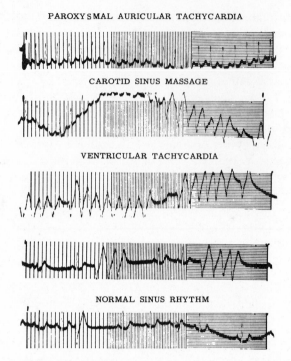

Figure 4. Auricular and then ventricular tachycardia after surgery.

an idioventricular rhythm, which may rapidly progress to a normal sinus rhythm if the heart recovers. Frequently, the heart will not recover because of severe myocardial hypoxia and acidosis. A longer period of vigorous oxygenation and treatment of the acidosis are indicated before the next stimulus is given. External pacemaking can then be tried.

BRADYARRHYTHMIAS

The most common bradyarrhythmia in the immediate postoperative period is a sinus bradycardia, the rate by definition being below 60 per minute. The usual cause is excessive vagal tone. At times, increased intracranial pressure or jaundice may cause sinus bradycardia. Treatment is twofold: correct any factor increasing vagal tone, and decrease the vagal effect by the administration of atropine. If there is marked sinus slowing, an escape rhythm of nodal bradycardia with a rate of 40 to 50 per minute may appear. This usually indicates toxic effects of digitalis. Digitalis should be withheld, atropine should be administered, and a temporary pacemaker should be inserted if response to atropine is not satisfactory. A slow Isuprel infusion may be started after atropine has been tried.

Atrioventricular blocks may be the other cause for bradycardia. Digitalis intoxication or degenerative disease of the conduction system, especially in elderly individuals, may be the underlying mechanism. If the degree of heart block is 2:1 or higher with a slow ventricular response, the patient should be treated with atropine or with a pacemaker.[18]

ARRHYTHMIAS WITH A NORMAL RATE

The principal rhythm or conduction disturbances in this category are first- and second-degree heart block and intraventricular blocks. Their major diagnostic and prognostic implication is that the possibility of digitalis intoxication or advanced conduction system sclerosis, both with the threat of higher degrees of heart block, should be recognized. The diagnosis can be made only with both pre- and postoperative electrocardiograms for comparison in order to be sure that the disturbance is secondary to surgery. If so, electrocardiographic monitoring becomes crucial, for the possibility of an acute cardiac emergency is then real.

DIGITALIS INTOXICATION

Digitalis intoxication deserves a separate discussion and special emphasis because of difficulty in diagnosis, significance, and the presence of certain potentiating factors in the postoperative period. Digitalis intoxication can be overlooked too easily, yet it carries a major mortality risk. Therefore, its diagnosis requires a very high index of suspicion. Appropriate measures, such as withholding digitalis, should be promptly instituted simply on the basis of a strong suspicion, even if the diagnosis is not yet confirmed.

Electrolyte disturbances such as hypokalemia, hypomagnesemia, hypoxia, acidosis, and renal insufficiency can appear as aggravating and precipitating factors in the postoperative period.[36] The common clinical symptoms of nausea and vomiting are hard to evaluate in this setting. The electrocardiogram gives the only clear clue to its presence. Any known form of rhythm disturbance may occur secondary to digitalis intoxication, but paroxysmal auricular tachycardia with block and nonparoxysmal junctional tachycardia are the most specific.[20] Premature ventricular contractions and varying degrees of heart block (Fig. 5) are other common manifestations.

Treatment consists of withholding digitalis and administering potassium. However, potassium should be given only provided that hypokalemia is present, cardiac rate is not slow, and renal function is adequate. Potassium should not be used in cases of bradyarrhythmias that require atropine or temporary pacemaker insertion. In cases of paroxysmal auricular tachycardia with block, or in junctional or ventricular tachycardia, intravenous potassium in a dose of 20 to 40 mEq in 100 to 200 ml of 5 per cent

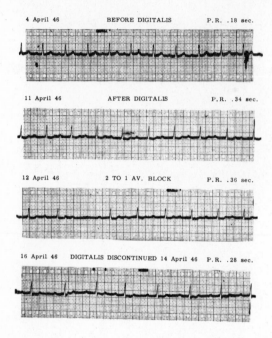

Figure 5. Examples of digitalis toxicity seen in the postoperative patient.

dextrose should be given in a one-half to 1-hour period, provided of course renal function is adequate. Intravenous Dilantin, 100 to 300 mg given slowly over a 10- to 15-minute period, or propranolol 1 to 2 mg, should also be administered if potassium alone is unsuccessful. In cases of refractory tachyarrhythmias with a rapidly deteriorating hemodynamic state, DC cardioversion should be tried. After a bolus of 50 to 100 mg of Xylocaine, a low 2.5 to 5 watt second shock should be given. In the presence of digitalis intoxication, this shock may precipitate ventricular fibrillation, which will require another higher amplitude shock. Thus, cardioversion in this circumstance should be resorted to only when the patient's course goes rapidly downhill.

CONGESTIVE HEART FAILURE

Pump failure is present by definition when the heart cannot deliver an adequate supply of oxygen to the tissues. Very occasionally, this may be seen when total cardiac output is above normal. In cases of severe anemia (decreased oxygen-carrying capacity), thyrotoxicosis or markedly increased body temperature (increased metabolic needs), peripheral resistance may be low and cardiac output high in an effort to increase the net oxygen-carrying power of the cardiovascular system. In the early postoperative period, as the patient comes out of the anesthetic state, severe shivering is not uncommon.

This is to be avoided, since it increases oxygen consumption severalfold, placing an additional load on the heart, and shivering especially should not be permitted in elderly patients. If cardiac function is already marginal, such a load may produce high output failure. The treatment of choice is Thorazine. If the patient's condition is precarious, muscle paralysis may be necessary.

Sepsis or a major infection may also produce high output failure. Elderly patients with sepsis should be watched carefully for signs of congestive failure. Frequent chest roentgenograms are indicated to pick up evidence of pulmonary vascular congestion. Arterial blood gases should be obtained to establish the presence of pulmonary arteriovenous shunting secondary to increased left ventricular end diastolic pressure, increased left atrial pressure, and pulmonary congestion. A low arterial Po_2 along with roentgenographic evidence of congestion may be the only evidence of left ventricular failure. The characteristic rales of left ventricular failure may not be present, especially in the patient on assisted ventilation.

Far more frequent, particularly in elderly patients and in those with ischemic heart disease, is low output failure, at times progressing to the too often lethal low output syndrome. Many factors can cause low output congestive failure during the postoperative period. Congestive heart failure may be the only clinical manifestation of a myocardial infarction and certainly suggests the presence of long-standing heart disease. The most common precipitating factor is acute myocardial depression with a markedly decreased myocardial contractile state secondary to one or more of the many possible myocardial insults. These include hypoxia, routine anesthetic agents, drugs, and metabolic factors such as acidosis, hypokalemia, hypocalcemia, hyponatremia, and significant arrhythmias. Of these, hypoxia is the most common and the most potent. Overtransfusion or the converse, hypovolemia, may also produce low output congestive heart failure. Congestive heart failure can be the first and only manifestation of pulmonary embolism.

The basic mechanism for this form of congestive failure in the postoperative period is decreased myocardial contractility. This may involve the left or right ventricle or both. More commonly, in elderly patients, the left ventricle is involved first, and the right secondarily. Decreased myocardial contractility leads to a lesser stroke volume and decreased cardiac index, while compensatory mechanisms produce a faster pulse rate and generalized vasoconstriction, excepting the brain and the myocardium. This vasoconstriction, mediated by heightened sympathetic nervous activity, leads to greater systemic resistance, maintenance of a normal or only slightly lowered blood pressure, diminished renal blood flow, and decreased urinary output. There is also less heat dissipation. Intense venoconstriction leads to increased right ventricular filling pressure, increasing right ventricular output, and, if the left ventricle is failing, pulmonary vascular congestion with raised pulmonary artery pressure, ventilation perfusion abnormalities, decreased pulmonary compliance, and more labored breathing. The combination of lowered arterial P_{O_2} and intensified vasoconstriction with underperfusion of many areas of the body produces lacticacidemia and metabolic acidosis. The effect of hypoxia and acidosis together is to dilate the precapillary organ sphincters, but without causing dilatation of the postcapillary sphincters, thus leading to an accumulation of blood in the organ, vascular damage, extravasation of blood, and eventually intravascular coagulation and tissue death.

It should be re-emphasized that congestive failure in the postoperative period can run the gamut from marginal increases in venous pressure to cardiogenic shock. Signs and symptoms vary accordingly. Unexplained tachypnea and tachycardia should lead the physician to check an arterial blood gas for evidence of left ventricular failure. Increased restlessness, confusion, excessive cold perspiration, significant peripheral vasoconstriction, and cold, cyanotic hands and feet indicate a far more dangerous level of congestive failure. Urinary output may be decreased below 20 ml per hour. Depending upon the cause and the ventricle involved, either the left atrial pressure or the central venous pressure or both may be elevated. If the left ventricle has failed, the left atrial pressure increases first. An elevated central venous pressure may not be found until late in the course, and then only after significant pulmonary arterial venous shunting with severe pulmonary congestion has occurred. Therefore, particularly in elderly patients with ischemic heart disease in whom the left ventricle is liable to fail first, left atrial pressure is a better determinant than central venous pressure and more critical to proper care. Arterial blood pressure may be normal, borderline, or decreased, depending upon the severity of the failure and the effectiveness of the compensatory mechanisms. When vasoconstriction is maximal, peripheral blood pressure may be unobtainable or markedly lowered, but the central aortic blood pressure will be found to be normal.

Once diagnosed, possible precipitating factors must be looked for and treated vigorously. The presence of hypoxia must be confirmed by the measurement of arterial blood gases. We cannot rely on vision to determine the presence of hypoxia. By the time the patient is clearly cyanotic, hypoxia is already far advanced. Frequent determinations of arterial blood gases constitute one of the major advances in the care of the critically ill patient postoperatively.[22] A central venous catheter should be installed,[34] and we believe that if the failure does not respond rapidly, a Swan-Ganz catheter should be floated into the pulmonary artery. Through this catheter, pulmonary artery pressure can be monitored with the balloon deflated, and pulmonary artery wedge pressure with the balloon inflated.[21,28]

Certain corrective measures are indicated for the heart itself. The primary problem in most low output congestive heart failures is a decrease in myocardial contractility. Therefore, treatment should be aimed at increasing contractility, producing no further arterial constriction but rather moderate vasodilatation.[14,15] If the patient is not on digitalis, he should be digitalized. If he is on digitalis and the low output syndrome is present, one of two drugs should be tried. The choice between the two will depend in good part upon the patient's clinical picture, for the pharmacologic properties of the two are different.[24] Isuprel, a strong inotropic agent, produces significant vasodilatation. The cardiac output response is significantly greater than the decline in systemic vascular resistance. Despite the increase secondary to greater myocardial contraction, net myocardial oxygen consumption may actually be decreased if the patient's heart becomes smaller with improvement of congestive failure. Two additional aspects of Isuprel may be less desirable, depending upon the patient's clinical state. Isuprel exerts a marked beta-adrenergic stimulating effect on the sinoatrial node and increases ventricular automaticity, thus tending to produce marked tachycardia. Too fast a heart rate is also inefficient, and the rate of Isuprel infusion must be varied according to pulse rate as well as systolic pressure, sometimes limiting the total net effect. Isuprel increases renal blood flow only slightly, so that a good diuresis does not occur.[7] Dopamine, on the other hand, produces a marked increase in renal blood flow, promoting good diuresis. It has very little effect on the sinoatrial node, so it does not promote excessive tachycardia.[9,17,25] It does not, however, have as marked a generalized vasodilating effect as Isuprel. Furthermore, the dosage of dopamine must be carefully controlled. Beneficial effects occur at infusion rates greater than 3 micrograms/kg/minute and less than 15 to 20 micrograms/kg/minute. At a dose close to or above 20 micrograms/kg/minute, alpha-adrenergic receptors are increasingly stimulated, and vasoconstriction with an increased peripheral resistance and an elevated diastolic blood pressure occurs. Such a reaction is contraindicated in low output congestive failure. Thus, when using dopamine, the patient's blood pressure and pulse rate, venous pressure, and general evidence of peripheral perfusion must be monitored carefully and the rate of infusion carefully controlled.

Alpha-adrenergic drugs such as norepinephrine and Aramine are contraindicated for they increase peripheral vasoconstriction, thus increasing afterload and augmenting acidosis because of a decrease in the peripheral perfusion. With acute heart failure, a single injection of calcium chloride may improve myocardial tone sufficiently to reverse the state properly. However, the patient must be watched for arrhythmias while the calcium is injected. A massive intravenous dose of synthetic glucocorticosteroids is also effective in treatment of the low output syndrome.[19] Such a dose lowers arteriolar and venular tone, increases blood flow and oxygen consumption, and increases lactic acid and glucose metabolism. There is an additional important benefit, that is, a decrease in myocardial infarct size if an infarct is present.

During the period of treatment, regardless of the specific drug used, the status of the circulation and the ratio of intravascular volume to vascular space must be monitored carefully. Ideally, a pulmonary wedge pressure obtained with a Swan-Ganz catheter should be followed.[28] At a minimum, a central venous pressure should be obtained and followed carefully, with the tip end of the catheter within the chest cage. Central venous pressure should not be permitted to drop below 150 to 200 mm of water, and the mean pulmonary wedge pressure should be kept between 250 and 300 mm of water. The reason for maintaining a high venous pressure is to support a high preload, which increases the ventricular force of contraction, raising cardiac output. If treatment is successful and vasodilatation is produced, circulating blood volume may become inadequate for the increasing vascular space, and venous pressure may tend to drop. Fluids should then be given to maintain the venous pressure and reap the benefits of improved myocardial contraction brought about by an increased preload.

Arrhythmias should be corrected if present. Patients in chronic atrial fibrillation may well be benefited by even a temporary return to a normal sinus rhythm, from which they may obtain some increase in cardiac output from the positive filling effect of an atrial kick. For tachyarrhythmias, electric shock is the treatment of choice. Pushing digitalis too far and too fast may lead to digitalis intoxication and fatal arrhythmias. Other drugs that control tachyarrhythmias tend to be myocardial depressants, and are contraindicated when effective treatment, such as electric shock, is available. Patients with significant bradycardia should have a transvenous pacemaker inserted. If an atrioventricular block is not present, pacing should be done through the atrium. If a block is present, pacing should be done with the electrode at the apex of the right ventricle.

Treatment of the low output syndrome includes those measures taken to decrease oxygen demand. Body temperature should be kept normal. When vasoconstriction is present and severe, there is decreased heat dissipation, and core body temperature may well be elevated. If it is necessary to treat hyperthermia vigorously with methods other than vasodilatation, such as alcohol sponges, ice mattresses, and the like, careful attention should be given to the presence or the absence of shivering. Under no circumstances should the patient be permitted to shiver. Acute vasodilatation can be produced to lower temperature, using drugs such as phenoxybenzamine, nitroprusside, Arfonad, and other alpha blockers. However, it cannot be overemphasized that if such drugs are used the arterial blood pressure must be monitored continuously, using an intra-arterial cannula and pressure transducer. Central venous pressure must be monitored also to make sure that the circulating blood volume is kept adequate and too rapid a drop in the ratio of blood volume to vascular space does not occur.

A major decrease in pulmonary compliance accompanies acute left ventricular failure and pulmonary congestion. Instead of 2 per cent of the body energy being used by the respiratory muscles to ventilate the lungs, energy expended may increase to 15 to 30 per cent or even higher. A material saving in oxygen demand can thus be brought about by taking over respiratory function during the acute low output syndrome, using a volume-controlled respirator with a nasal endotracheal tube. The respirator should be set with a minute volume higher than normal in order to expand atelectactic areas and reduce pulmonary edema. This requires that arterial blood gases be followed carefully, for such hyperventilation may remove an excessive amount of carbon dioxide. Arterial P_{CO_2} should be maintained at close to 35 mm Hg either by lengthening the airway to increase dead space or by adding CO_2 to the mixture of inhaled gases. If the arterial P_{CO_2} is maintained near 35 mm Hg and the arterial P_{O_2} is 80 mm Hg or above, the respirator should take over all respiratory effort, provided that central nervous system problems are not complicating the picture. If significant respiratory effort continues, the patient probably should be curarized.

It should be emphasized again that congestive heart failure can run the gamut between very minimal failure and cardiogenic shock. The treatment must vary according to the magnitude of the failure. To evaluate the effectiveness of treatment and to determine when additional treatment is necessary, aggressive monitoring of arterial, central, venous and left atrial pressures, of arterial blood gases, and of electrolytes is essential.

PULMONARY EMBOLISM

Pulmonary embolism remains a prominent cause of death after major surgery. Pulmonary emboli are reported in roughly 10 per cent of all autopsies, the incidence essentially being equally divided between medical and surgical cases.[5] The frequency of this complication increases with age;[6] thus, its occurrence will probably continue to increase because of the ever-widening application of surgical procedures to the older, and therefore higher-risk, population.

Venous stasis is the main predisposing cause for the formation of intravascular thrombosis, and immobilization after surgery is one of the major factors producing venous stasis. Hypercoagulability, which potentiates thrombus formation, also presents after surgery.[27] Intravascular catheters left in place for a long time can be an additional nidus for thrombus formation. Thrombi initiating in the deep veins of the leg are the most common source of pulmonary emboli, with pelvic veins, particularly in the female, the next most frequent site. Occasionally, pulmonary emboli may originate from thrombi in the right atrium or in the veins of the upper extremities, head, and neck.

Peak occurrence is usually one week after surgery. The diagnosis remains notoriously difficult in spite of improved methods of investigation, and in fact, pulmonary emboli are more often diagnosed at autopsy than considered during life. Thus, a high level of suspicion is essential to diagnosis. The manifestations postoperatively are commonly atypical, subtle, and frequently totally absent. Sudden unexplained dyspnea is the most frequent symptom. A diagnostic but less common symptom, pleuritic chest pain, is present only in cases of the embolic occlusion of a distal pulmonary artery, producing pulmonary infarction with involvement of the overlying pleura. Hemoptysis occurs in one-third of cases. Patients may describe a feeling of apprehension and impending catastrophe. Supraventricular tachyarrhythmias, especially atrial flutter, may be the presenting manifestation, and the patient may experience palpitations and consciousness of an irregular heart beat. Occasionally syncope may occur, spikes of fever are common, and the clinical picture can simulate pneumonia or atelectasis. Circulatory failure may develop from massive pulmonary embolism. Sudden death is not infrequent.

Tachycardia, tachypnea, cyanosis, a pleural friction rub, and signs of pulmonary hypertension, such as left parasternal heave and a loud P2, may be present if embolism is massive. Signs of right heart failure due to acute pulmonary hypertension can also develop. While all signs and symptoms may be transient or recurrent, blood gas determinations remain a very helpful laboratory aid. A low arterial Po_2 is almost always present, the arterial Pco_2 being low secondary to hyperventilation. Unexplained hypoxia should always alert one to the possibility of pulmonary emboli.

A roentgenogram of the chest can be extremely helpful although rather nonspecific, especially in the postoperative period when atelectasis and pneumonia are such common complications. A wedge-shaped opacity in the periphery of the lungs with its apex toward the hilum is a highly suggestive finding. Unfortunately, such an opacity is infrequent and usually late in appearance. Diminution of pulmonary vascularity distal to the occluded pulmonary artery, hyperlucency, platelike atelectasis in the lower lobes, and the appearance of pleural effusions are some of the other helpful roentgenographic signs. The main pulmonary artery segment rarely may become prominent when compared with the preoperative film, and there may be dilatation of the right heart chambers. Such a change is less common and more difficult to recognize than an axis shift to the right and increased amplitude P waves in the electrocardiogram.

Pulmonary scan and angiography are further laboratory aids to establishing the diagnosis. Pulmonary angiography is the more definitive of the two, since the pulmonary scan tends to be nonspecific. The advantage of a pulmonary scan is that it can be easily carried out, whereas pulmonary angiography is a highly specialized procedure and carries a slight but definite risk. The combination of plain chest roentgenogram and scan can be very helpful in making the diagnosis, especially when lung scans show filling defects in an area that appears normal in the standard chest x-ray film. Serially, scans are helpful if new filling defects appear.

The best treatment remains preventive. Early patient mobilization and the use of elastic stockings constitute the two best forms of preventive treatment. Corrective therapy should begin early, when clinical suspicion becomes strong. One should not wait for treatment until the diagnosis is confirmed because of the real likelihood of recurrence, the high mortality rate, and the effectiveness of proper medical treatment in preventing additional emboli. Medical treatment with intravenous heparin and supportive measures such as elastic stockings or bandages remain the treatment of choice. Ten thousand units of heparin should be administered intravenously as the first dose, followed by 5000 to 7500 units every 4 to 6 hours. Heparin administration should be guided by frequent measurements of clotting time, or by partial thromboplastin time estimations, considered recently to be a better guide. Oral anticoagulation can be started after a few days of heparin; the latter may be discontinued when the patient is adequately anticoagulated with oral agents. Oxygen should be administered routinely, and Demerol or morphine sulphate given as required for pain. Digitalization is indicated if heart failure occurs, and vasoactive drugs such as dopamine or Isuprel should be used for shock.

If pulmonary emboli recur in spite of anticoagulation, surgical measures must be considered. These include vein ligation, insertion of caval umbrella, and pulmonary embolectomy. Bilateral common femoral vein ligation entails little or no risk, but pulmonary emboli can recur if clots are present above the site of ligation—a point difficult to establish before ligation.[1] Inferior vena cava ligation below the renal veins is usually highly effective in prevention of further emboli, but carries a 2 to 5 per cent risk in patients without heart failure, and a 20 to 50 per cent risk in patients with heart failure. Recently, the insertion of a vena cava umbrella has been substituted for caval ligation, with a significant decrease in risk. Pulmonary embolectomy is indicated in highly critical situations only because the surgical risk is markedly increased.[33] In cases of massive pulmonary embolism of the main pulmonary artery or of one of the major pulmonary trunks, documented by pulmonary angiography, and with a persistent state of shock that is resistant to treatment, a pulmonary embolectomy should be resorted to.

Fibrinolytic agents have been undergoing trial for several years, but their clinical use has not been well established. The use of a catheter with a small suction cup device at the tip has recently been introduced and has had early success but no systematic trial.[8] The use of such suction catheters to remove pulmonary clots supplemented by circulatory assists may become important in the future for the management of poor-risk patients with major pulmonary emboli.

INTENSIVE CARE ORIENTED TOWARD CARDIAC PROBLEMS

The best treatment for postoperative cardiac problems is intensive preventive care. Elderly patients undergoing major elective surgery should be evaluated carefully before surgery for the presence of marginal function of the key physiologic systems. Such an evaluation with follow-up aggressive monitoring and intensive preventive care avoids a costly progression from marginal function to system failure, thus bringing about a major saving in morbidity, mortality, and the cost of health care.

Before major surgery, the elderly patient should have an electrocardiogram for baseline rhythm abnormalities and evidence of prior infarction or ventricular hypertrophy. Ideally, an exercise electrocardiogram should be done in order to pick up patients with subclinical ischemic heart disease. Roentgenograms of the heart and lung should be obtained for evidence of chronic disease that may endanger the patient after surgery. Pulmonary function studies should be accomplished, including a measurement of blood gases while the patient is breathing room air. This preoperative gauging of blood gases serves two purposes. It establishes the patient's "norm" and it flags the very abnormal patient. In our experience, an MMEFR is a simple, inexpensive test for determining the presence of significant small airway obstruction that potentially can lead to postoperative respiratory insufficiency. It is probably the best screening test available. Chronic smokers should be off cigarettes for at least a week prior to an operation performed under a general anesthetic. Patients with a chronic productive cough should be treated with antibiotics and postural drainage for one to two weeks before surgery. Preoperative training in coughing deeply and in accepting intermittent positive pressure breathing should be given.

Electrolyte studies and a creatinine clearance, or at least a serum creatinine, should be obtained to evaluate renal function. In patients with known heart disease, a careful review of digitalis and diuretic history for evidence of digitalis intoxication and potassium depletion should be carried out. As already mentioned, diuretics should be discontinued for two to three days prior to surgery, and potassium supplemented orally. By so doing, a more normal state of hydration and electrolyte balance will be obtained. In hypertensive patients on treatment, reserpine should be stopped seven days and quanethedine two to three days prior to surgery. Acute or chronic fluid loss should be replaced. By attention to these details, potentially lethal periods of hypotension can be avoided during and after the operation.

Equal in importance to the state of hydration is the nutritional status. Extreme states of nutrition materially decrease a patient's ability to tolerate surgery. If possible, time should be taken to improve the preoperative nutritional state. Muscle training can be helpful. The patient should be in positive nitrogen balance, and obese patients should lose weight. If surgery must be carried out, extreme care must be taken to prevent or minimize respiratory failure and resulting cardiac problems. We have all seen the elderly, obese, or emaciated patient who comes through a major abdominal operation looking well, seems well but tired the night of the operation, and is found dead in the early morning hours. Such a patient has literally worked himself to death. The combination of obesity, age, decreased muscle mass, postoperative thickened secretions, and areas of atelectasis leads to an excessive work of breathing, which in turn leads to excessive fatigue, then respiratory insufficiency, hypoxia, acidosis, and ventricular fibrillation.

Much has been written about the form of anesthesia optimal for the elderly critically ill patient. The probable best answer is that the optimal form is that with which the anesthetist feels most comfortable, provided, of course, that extreme care is taken to prevent any periods of hypotension or hypoxia throughout the operation and afterward. Aggressive action must be taken to prevent hypoventilation, atelectasis, and retained secretions as well as to ensure adequate, but not excessive, fluid intake so that urinary output is kept at acceptable levels.

After surgery, how should the postoperative patient with known heart disease or one who develops a cardiac problem be watched and treated differently from the patient with the same operation and no cardiac problems? Such patients should be monitored aggressively and treated early and vigorously. Monitoring should include a continuous display of the electrocardiogram on an oscilloscope, and rhythm strip recordings should be obtained every four hours to make sure that subtle forms of arrhythmia are not present that can escape detection on a continuously moving oscilloscope.

A central venous cannula should be inserted and connected to a saline water manometer. For insertion, the external jugular, subclavian, and saphenous veins constitute the ideal routes. The tip of the catheter should be in the chest cavity to ensure correct values for venous pressure readings. Using other sites for cannulation is acceptable, although it is more difficult to place the tip of the cannula within the chest.

Ideally, a Swan-Ganz catheter should be passed into a distal pulmonary artery in a position where blowing up the balloon will produce an authentic wedge pressure equal (in most instances) to left atrial pressure. The catheter can also serve as a source for arterial blood (in the wedge position, with the balloon inflated, the blood drawn is pulmonary venous and normally fully saturated) and for mixed venous blood (the blood withdrawn with the balloon deflated is pulmonary artery blood representing mixed venous blood). Arteriovenous oxygen difference gives a good index of the cardiac output at least for serial and trend determinations. An arteriovenous difference of more than 50 ml/liter suggests the presence of low output congestive failure.

Arterial blood pressure must be followed carefully. Ideally, with patients in a critically ill state, intra-arterial pressures are preferable to cuff pressures. The more critically ill the patient, the greater the need for central aortic readings, since peripheral cuff readings become totally unreliable. Usually, the cannula can be left in place for the critical first two to three days. It should then be withdrawn and reliance placed on cuff pressures.

Urinary output should be monitored hourly. This can be accomplished only by inserting a Foley catheter. The measurement of output from all drainage systems should be carried out hourly. Fluid intake must be measured accurately and recorded carefully. Since measurements of fluid input and output are notoriously difficult both to obtain and to trust, daily weight should be obtained using special weight equipment. A special problem arises when the postoperative patient becomes oliguric (less than 20 ml per hour of urine output) and has at the same time a low normal arterial pressure and somewhat elevated central venous pressure. The question is, "Is the patient in low output failure requiring a diuretic, or is he hypovolemic and vasoconstricted, requiring volume?" A safe answer to this question may be obtained by giving the patient 250 ml of 5 per cent glucose in half-strength saline over a 20 minute time period, monitoring central venous pressure, blood pressure, pulse rate, and urinary volume carefully. If congestive heart failure is present, central venous pressure and pulse rate will increase with little or no change in blood pressure and urinary volume. If hypovolemia is present, blood pressure will increase, central venous pressure and pulse rate will stay the same or decrease, and urinary output will increase. If the answer is congestive heart failure, then one should follow with intravenous Lasix and rapid digitalization.

To rule out renal failure as a cause of the oliguria, frequent urinary specific gravity determinations are of value. If the patient concentrates well, renal failure is unlikely. Urine osmolality, daily serum creatinines, and 12-hour electrolytes and hematocrits also assist in assaying renal function and the renal-electrolyte-fluid balance.

It cannot be overemphasized that hypoxia is the most potent and the most common precipitator of cardiac problems. Therefore, the pulmonary status must be watched and treated just as closely as the cardiovascular system. The patient who is permitted to lie quietly in bed hour after hour is destined to develop respiratory insufficiency with consequent hypoxia. A critically ill patient should be returned from the operating room receiving some form of assisted ventilation. This should be continued until the effect of all anesthetic and preanesthetic drugs has worn off, the patient is awake and cooperative, and it has been determined that tidal volume is adequate and can be self-maintained. After the patient is no longer receiving assisted ventilation, care must be taken not to oversedate. Frequent turning, coughing, and suctioning are indicated. Where available, chest physiotherapy and intermittent positive pressure ventilation are very helpful in preventing the development of respiratory insufficiency. Arterial blood gas determinations while the patient is breathing room air and again while breathing 100 per cent oxygen for 10 minutes can be most helpful in assaying the status of the lungs and the magnitude of the intrapulmonary arterial venous shunt. Single determinations are not very useful, since it is the trend that is important and not the momentary status. A knowledge of the trend permits aggressive treatment before the point of danger has been reached—the ideal form of intensive care medicine.

REFERENCES

1. Anlyan, W. G., Campbell, F. H., Shingleton, W. W., and Gardner, C. R., Jr.: Pulmonary embolism following venous ligation. Arch. Surg., 64:200, 1952.
2. Brown, J. M.: Anesthesia and the contractile force of the heart; a review. Anesth. Analg., 39:487, 1960.
3. Buckley, J. J., and Jackson, J. A.: Postoperative cardiac arrhythmias. Anesthesiology, 22:723, 1961.
4. Crampton, R. S., and Hunter, F. P.: False atrial flutter from nasogastric suction pump. J.A.M.A., 223:1160, 1973.
5. Davis, W. C.: Immediate diagnosis of pulmonary embolus. Am. Surg., 30:291, 1964.
6. Freiman, D. G.: Pathologic observations on experimental and human thromboembolism. In, Sasahara, A. A., and Stein, M. (Eds.): Pulmonary Embolic Disease. New York, Grune & Stratton, 1965, pp. 81–85.

7. Goldberg, L. I.: Use of sympathomimetic amines in heart failure. Am. J. Cardiol., *22*:177, 1968.
8. Greenfield, L. J.: Ten-minute vacuum pulls out large pulmonary clots. Med. World News, *10*:15, 1969.
9. Horwitz, D., Fox, S. M., and Goldberg, L. I.: Effects of dopamine in man. Circ. Res., *10*:237, 1962.
10. Howland, W. S., Schweizer, O., and LaDue, J. S.: Evaluation of routine postoperative electrocardiography. N.Y. State J. Med., *62*:1941, 1962.
11. Johnson, J. C., Flowers, N. C., and Horan, L.: Unexplained atrial flutter: a frequent herald of pulmonary embolism. Chest, *60*:29, 1971.
12. Kansal, S., Roitman, D., Kouchoukos, N., and Sheffield, L. T.: Ischemic myocardial injury following aortocoronary bypass surgery. Chest, *67*:20, 1975.
13. Katz, R. L., and Bigger, T. J.: Cardiac arrhythmias during anesthesia and operation. Anesthesiology, *33*:193, 1970.
14. Mason, D. T., and Braunwald, E.: Studies on digitalis. X. Effects of ouabain on forearm vascular resistance and venous tone in normal subjects and in patients in heart failure. J. Clin. Invest., *43*:532, 1964.
15. Mason, D. T., and Braunwald, E.: Digitalis: new facts about an old drug. Am. J. Cardiol., *22*:151, 1968.
16. Mauney, F. M., Jr., Ebert, P. A., and Sabiston, D. C., Jr.: Postoperative myocardial infarction: a study of predisposing factors. Diagnosis and mortality in a high risk group of surgical patients. Ann. Surg., *172*:497, 1970.
17. McDonald, R. J., Jr., Goldberg, L. I., McNay, J. L., and Tuttle, E. P., Jr.: Effects of dopamine in man: augmentation of sodium excretion, glomerular filtration rate, and renal plasma flow. J. Clin. Invest., *43*:1116, 1964.
18. McNally, E. M., and Benchimol, A.: Medical and physiological considerations in the use of artificial cardiac pacing. Parts I and II. Am. Heart J., *75*:380 (March); 679 (May), 1968.
19. Motsay, G. J., Dietzman, R. H., Ersek, R. A., and Lillehei, R. C.: Hemodynamic alterations and results of treatment in patients with gram negative septic shock. Surgery, *67*:577, 1970.
20. Pick, A., and Dominguez, P.: Nonparoxysmal A-V nodal tachycardia. Circulation, *16*:1022, 1957.
21. Porter, C. M., Karp, R. B., Russell, R. O., Jr., and Rackley, C. E.: Pulmonary artery pressure monitoring in cardiogenic shock. Arch. Intern. Med., *127*:304, 1971.
22. Rawitscher, R. E., Lefer, A. M., and Dammann, J. F.: Influence of artificial respiration on cardiovascular performance after open heart surgery. J. Thorac. Cardiovasc. Surg., *53*:685, 1967.
23. Rodman, T.: The effect of anesthesia and surgery on pulmonary and cardiac function. Am. J. Cardiol., *12*:444, 1963.
24. Rosenblum, R.: Physiological basis for the therapeutic uses of catecholamines. Am. Heart J., *87*:527, 1974.
25. Rosenblum, R., Tai, A. R., and Lawson, D.: Cardiac and renal hemodynamic effects of dopamine in man. Clin. Res., *18*:326, 1970.
26. Schweitzer, O., and Howland, W. S.: The value of the electrocardiogram in the immediate postoperative period. Surg. Gynecol. Obstet., *113*:33, 1961.
27. Sharnoff, J. G., Bagg, J. F., Breen, S. R., Rogiano, A. G., Walsh, A. R., and Scardino, V.: The possible indication of postoperative thromboembolism by platelet counts and blood coagulation studies in the patient undergoing extensive surgery. Surg. Gynecol. Obstet., *111*:469, 1960.
28. Swan, H. J. C., Ganz, W., Forrester, T., et al.: Catheterization of the heart in man with the use of a flow directed balloon tipped catheter. N. Engl. J. Med., *283*:447, 1970.
29. Tarhan, S., Moffitt, E. A., Taylor, W. F., and Guiliani, E. R.: Myocardial infarction after general anesthesia. J.A.M.A., *220*:1451, 1972.
30. Topkins, M. J., and Artusio, J. F.: Myocardial infarctions and surgery. Anesth. Analg., *43*:716, 1964.
31. Turville, C. S., and Dipps, R. D.: Anesthetic management of aged. Pa. Med. J., *51*:434, 1948.
32. Vanik, P. E., and Davis, H. S.: Cardiac arrhythmias during halothane anesthesia. Anesth. Analg., *47*:299, 1968.

33. Warren, R.: Current status of pulmonary embolectomy. *In* Sasahara, A. A., and Stein, M. (Eds.): Pulmonary Embolic Disease. New York, Grune & Stratton, 1965, pp. 283–287.
34. Weil, M. H., Shubin, H., and Rosoff, L.: Fluid repletion in circulatory shock: central venous pressure and other practical guides. J.A.M.A., *192*:668, 1965.
35. Wheat, M. W., Jr., and Burford, T. H.: Digitalis in surgery: extension of classical indications. J. Thorac. Cardiovasc. Surg., *41*:162, 1961.
36. Williams, J. F., Jr., Boyd, D. L., and Border, J. F.: Effect of acute hypoxia and hypercapnic acidosis on the development of acetylstrophanthidin-induced arrhythmias. J. Clin. Invest., *47*:1885, 1968.
37. Wylie, R. H., and Bowman, F. O., Jr.: Immediate complications following thoracotomy for pulmonary disease. Surg. Clin. North Am., *44*:325, 1964.

CHAPTER 19

THE PATIENT IN RENAL FAILURE

WILLIAM M. STAHL, JR., M.D.

In spite of improvements in conservative and dialytic management, acute renal failure remains a serious complication when it occurs after surgery or trauma, or in patients suffering from severe sepsis. Over the past 20 years the mortality for such patients has changed very little, and remains at 60 to 65 per cent even in the best of hands. Deaths due primarily to the complications of uremia have declined, but because an increasing number of patients are more severely ill when acute renal failure occurs, the mortality related to the underlying trauma, surgery, or sepsis has increased. The occurrence of renal failure in such seriously ill patients increases the mortality rate, and although therapeutic maneuvers result in the survival of 35 to 40 per cent of the patients, it is clear that prevention of renal failure is much to be preferred.

INCIDENCE

The frequency of occurrence of established acute renal failure (ARF) in the general population is somewhat difficult to determine, since studies have not usually been done from this point of view. However, Eliahou and co-workers studied the annual incidence among the Jewish population in Israel, and found the frequency to be 4.8 to 5.7 per 100,000 in 1965 and 1966, with a male to female ratio of 1 to 6.[14] A decrease in the incidence of occurrence of this serious complication with improved early care of the injured has been demonstrated in military personnel. Whelton compared statistics from Korea and Vietnam and showed that in Korea 1 of 200 seriously injured soldiers developed ARF, while during the Vietnam conflict it occurred in only 1 of 600, although twice as many seriously injured patients survived to be treated. Patients treated during the Vietnamese conflict had a shorter period of evacuation and more adequate fluid volume replacement with very infrequent hypotension as compared with those injured in Korea. The most significant factor in the production of acute renal failure in the Vietnamese series appeared to be the severity of the wounds, and the presence of gastrointestinal trauma or peritonitis or both.[25,42]

MORTALITY

The survival of patients admitted to a dialysis unit for the treatment of postsurgical or posttraumatic ARF has not improved significantly over the past ten years in most dialysis centers. An exception to this is the report of Kleinknecht and coworkers, who reviewed their extensive experience in 1972.[22] They indicated a reduction of overall mortality with the use of prophylactic hemodialysis; deaths were reduced from 42 to 29 per cent, with significant lowering of the mortality from uremic causes. In this series, fatalities were reduced from 54 to 38 per cent in postsurgery patients, and from 55 to 33 per cent in posttrauma patients. Extension of this experience by the same authors, however, has shown somewhat poorer results, with the mortality rate now running at 42 per cent in surgical cases and 38 per cent in medical cases.[21] Most authors believe that the persistently high mortality rate is due to a change in the patient population needing dialytic therapy. In general, the milder cases have been prevented, and the patients with established renal failure are progressively older and have more serious illnesses or injuries.[21]

Overwhelming sepsis remains the most common factor in the death of patients with ARF following surgery or trauma.[7,21] In Kleinknecht's large series, sepsis was present in 40 per cent of all cases and was responsible for one-third of all fatalities. Origin of sepsis was most often in the abdomen or pelvis. Stott and coworkers[39] found sepsis present in 37 per cent; Brown and coworkers felt that it was a major cause of death in 31 per cent, but that at least 72 per cent had septicemia during the course of the illness. In Brown's series the commonest cause of overwhelming sepsis was pulmonary infection.

Gastrointestinal hemorrhage remains an important cause of death, and in Kleinknecht's series this occurred in 40 per cent of patients. Fatalities due to hemorrhage accounted for 30 per cent of the deaths. Prophylactic dialysis reduced the incidence of severe gastrointestinal hemorrhage, and this reduction was the main cause of improved survival with such a regimen. Other series have shown that gastrointestinal hemorrhage occurs in some 20 to 40 per cent of patients. In many of these patients, operation is required for control of bleeding, with an associated increase in mortality.

Deaths early in the course of ARF, within the first few days, were usually ascribed to the underlying conditions that caused the renal failure, i.e., hemorrhage or septic shock, respiratory or cardiac failure, cancer, intracranial hemorrhage, and so on. Dialysis was unable to influence the fatal course in this group of patients. With appropriate early and intensive dialysis, however, deaths due to the uremic complications of overhydration, acidosis, and hyperkalemia have become rare.

ETIOLOGY AND PATHOPHYSIOLOGY

In spite of intensive and highly sophisticated studies of the causes of ARF in patients with previously adequate renal function, the precise pathophysiologic mechanisms producing the disorder have not yet been clarified. Most theories implicate vasomotor alterations with reduction of cortical blood flow, or tubular obstruction due to toxic-anoxic damage of tubular cells with "passive backflow," or combinations of both.

Marked increase in renal cortical vascular resistance with decrease in cortical blood flow has been found in animals with induced renal failure,[9] and in human patients suffering from ARF.[18, 33] The increase in cortical vascular resistance appears to be in the afferent arteriole, with reduction of glomerular filtration pressure and a cessation of filtration. The renin-angiotensin system has been implicated in this vasomotor abnormality. Renin release is influenced both by vascular pressure and tension and by tubular sodium concentration, and thus could be implicated in either the vascular tone or tubular damage theories.[10, 11] If, indeed, the renin-angiotensin mechanism is active in the production of ARF of the vascular type, it presumably operates within the kidney interstitium rather than via the circulation, since experiments using infusions of renin-angiotensin inhibitors or passive antirenin immunization have not protected animals from ARF.[19, 31] It would seem that the vascular factor alone is not the entire cause of ARF, because the use of adrenergic blockade in animals[13] and in humans[17, 34] has not reversed the abnormality.

Ischemic damage with swelling of cells lining capillaries and tubules has been suggested as the cause of tubular blockage and as the reason vasodilator drugs fail to effect reopening of precapillary arterioles in established ARF.[23] The inability to restore normal circulation through the cortex after transient periods of vascular obstruction ("no-reflow") appears to be based on this type of endothelial cell damage. Most authorities agree that in addition to the vasomotor changes, some type of cellular damage occurs when the low-flow state is perpetuated. Flores and coworkers have shown endothelial cell swelling in the ischemic rat kidney and have demonstrated some improvement after treatment with nonabsorbable hypertonic solute, namely mannitol and dextran, in these animals.[16] Evidence to date thus indicates that ARF results from a combination of vasomotor alterations with decreased cortical blood flow, and tubular and capillary cell damage from ischemia, toxins, or other agents[15] (Table 1).

Table 1. CAUSES OF ACUTE RENAL FAILURE

Hypoperfusion
  Volume deficit
  Pump failure
  Excessive renal vasoconstriction
    Drugs
    Sympathetic stimulation
  Diffuse clotting in capillary beds (DIC)
Toxins
  Pigment
    Myoglobin
    Hemoglobin
  Mismatched transfusion
  Contast media
  Volume expanders (low-molecular dextran)
  Anesthesia (Penthrane)
  Antibiotics
    Coly-Mycin
    Gentamicin
    Polymyxin
    Kanamycin
    Amphotericin
  Solvents
    Carbon tetrachloride
    Phenol
  Heavy metals
    Arsenic
    Bismuth
    Cadmium
    Chromium
    Gold
    Mercury
    Uranium
  Peptide fragments
  Bacterial cells
    Endotoxin
    Extoxin

METABOLIC EFFECTS OF ARF

The long-term survival of patients with chronic renal failure when maintained on appropriate chronic dialysis regimens indicates that dialytic therapy can maintain reasonable body metabolism in the absence of serious intercurrent stress. Patients who develop ARF following renal transplantation fare far better than do patients who develop ARF following other types of surgery or trauma. In Kjellstrand's series, 95 per cent of 61 patients survived posttransplant ARF, whereas only 31 per cent of 85 patients survived postsurgical ARF.[20] In the survivors, renal function returned to adequate levels, with no discernible differences between the two groups of patients. Mortality in the postsurgery and posttrauma group, therefore, is primarily related to the underlying condition, and is worsened by metabolic derangements that usually are not fatal in the less stressed patient. In addition, the special care given transplant recipients, especially those measures taken to prevent infection, may play a role.

Studies of patients on chronic dialysis have indicated defects in protein metabolism; a deficiency in absorption of tryptophan; inefficient enzymatic breakdown of phenylalanine and tyrosine; and the possibility that protein synthesis is altered in uremic patients so that histidine may become an essential amino acid. Levels of certain dialyzable vitamins may be insufficient, with ascorbic acid being particularly sensitive in this regard. Red blood cell regeneration appears to be depressed, and there is some evidence of decreased red blood cell survival. Nerve function is altered, both in the central nervous system and in peripheral nerves. Electroencephalogram tracings show an increase in slow waves, less than 7 cycles per second, associated with altered consciousness, and the decrease in peripheral nerve transmission appears to coincide with decreased transketolase activity. The endoplasmic reticulum of the liver appears to be altered in animals, with structural changes appearing in light microscopic and ultrastructral sections, and functional depression results in a decrease in the rate of metabolism of certain drugs. Search for the precise "uremic toxin" producing these changes has not clarified the picture significantly, although guanidinosuccinic acid has been shown to be elevated in the plasma and urine and to be a toxic compound.

Clinically important metabolic alterations are an increased bleeding tendency, gastrointestinal ulceration, an increased susceptibility to infection, and failure of wound healing. Alterations in some of the steps of the clotting process, both in platelet aggregation and in Hageman factor, have been detected in some patients, but these findings remain to be confirmed. Defects in cell division in the intestinal mucosa have been shown in experimental animals, suggesting that failure of cell regeneration may contribute to gastrointestinal ulceration as well as to the failure of wound healing. Studies to determine the exact mechanism of loss of resistance to infection have been inconclusive to date.

PROPHYLAXIS

Because of the continuing mortality in patients who develop ARF following surgery and trauma, prevention of this complication is of the utmost importance. Animal studies have demonstrated that ARF occurs more readily in situations where renin levels are elevated; i.e., hypovolemia, dehydration, salt depletion, and low cardiac output states. Precipitating factors in humans appear to be low-flow states; tissue damage due to crush injury, burns, extensive trauma, or extensive surgical dissection; sepsis, predominantly intra-abdominal and pulmonary; massive transfusion; cardiopulmonary bypass; and liver dysfunction.

Optimization of the physiologic condition of every patient should be accomplished prior to operation, and the adequacy of cardiac output, red cell mass, circulating volume, and extracellular fluid composition is especially important in the type of patient described as at high risk for ARF. Preoperative evaluation of renal function should be done whenever time permits, especially in elderly patients. The performance of an endogenous creatinine clearance is a simple maneuver, requiring only a timed urine collection and a blood and urine sample, and gives a baseline for filtration function prior to stress.

Measurement of "clearance" is used as an indicator of glomerular filtration rate, using a substance filtered by the glomerulus that is neither excreted nor resorbed by the tubule. Creatinine is such a substance, and is normally present in the blood of all persons. Plasma creatinine is measured in mg/100 ml (P_{Cr}), urine creatinine is measured in mg (U_{Cr}), and the volume of urine produced per minute (V) is calculated by collecting a urine specimen over a timed period, usually 12 to 24 hours in a stable patient. The following formula gives the creatinine clearance in ml (of plasma cleared) per minute (glomerular filtration rate or GFR)

$$C_{Cr} = \frac{U_{Cr} \cdot V}{P_{Cr}}$$

The effectiveness of drug-induced diuresis in the normally hydrated patient in preventing ischemic renal injury has been shown by the use of both ethacrynic acid or furosemide[37] and mannitol.[29] The use of such diuresis intraoperatively or soon after trauma in patients in whom renal failure is suspected appears to be an important maneuver, especially if molecular fragments from damaged tissues are released into the blood stream and filtered into the urine.

DETECTION

There appears to be a stage in the development of ARF during which the vasomotor/tubular damage lesion can perhaps be halted or partially reversed by intensive therapy. It is therefore of utmost importance to detect the incipient stage of ARF and to institute appropriate therapy as soon as possible. A fall in urine output to below 0.5 ml/kg/hr should cause one to be on the alert, and any further decrease below this level, sustained for more than one hour, indicates that careful investigation of the patient is in order. Immediate examination of the urine should be made. The finding on microscopic study of tubular casts, tubular cell casts, granular casts, or red blood cell casts indicates renal tissue damage.[24] Decrease in the urine to plasma ratios for osmolality (<1.1), urea (<10), or creatinine (<2.5) indicates tubular cell damage with loss of concentrating power[12, 32] A urinary sodium concentration of over 30 to 40 mEq/liter indicates failure of normal sodium resorption. Patients with a high urine to plasma osmolality ratio and a low urinary sodium (10 mEq/liter) will usually diurese upon restoration of normal fluid volume and hemodynamics.

It must be kept in mind that some patients may develop ARF of the nonoliguric type without passing through an oliguric phase. In such patients a decrease in urine output does not occur, and the clinician must be alert enough in the case of high-risk patients to do the appropriate determinations on blood and urine. Measurement of serum creatinine, of urine to plasma ratios of osmolality, urea, or creatine, or preferably the performance of a creatinine clearance will detect the renal damage.

Restoration of the normal physiologic condition of body fluids, circulating volume, cardiac output, and chemical composition should be rapidly achieved in every patient. If oliguria is severe, however, or if toxic molecules are present, diuretic therapy should be started prior to the achievement of the normal physiologic condition, with the understanding that maximum improvement of the general state of the patient must be achieved concomitantly.

Furosemide has been used extensively as a test for incipient renal failure.[2] Reduction of intrarenal vascular resistance has been demonstrated following administration of furosemide both in animals[26] and in humans.[38] This increased blood flow, together with increase in tubular fluid flow and dilution of tubular solute, should theoretically reduce the ischemic/toxic damage to the lining cells of renal tubules and capillaries.

Suggestions as to diuretic therapy range from the initial use of a single 12.5 gm dose of mannitol, to the use of a single 200 mg dose of furosemide, to the use of a program of increasing doses of furosemide, up to 2000 mg/24 hours. Mannitol should be used cautiously beyond an initial dose, since if filtration is not occurring the osmotically active molecules will remain in the plasma, with increase in plasma volume. Central venous or pulmonary artery pressure should be closely monitored if cardiac reserve is limited. Mannitol should help to decrease swelling of damaged tubular and capillary lining cells. Furosemide can be used by doubling the intravenous dose every two hours, starting with 50 mg, but caution must be exercised in the rate of administration. Deafness, sometimes permanent, may result from the too rapid intravenous injection of large doses, and the continuous intravenous drip of 100 mg/hr should be used to infuse the large doses.

The therapeutic use of large doses of furosemide in patients suffering from established ARF has produced variable results. Many series have shown that the use of high-dosage furosemide therapy (up to 2000 mg/day), especially if begun early in the course of ARF, has produced a diuresis in a significant number of patients. Most of these patients are thus converted from oliguric to nonoliguric ARF, which makes subsequent management easier owing to improved water and potassium excretion. Muth feels that furosemide diuresis does not add to the therapeutic result in acute renal failure.[28] Cantarovich and coworkers, however, in a prospective study of 105 patients treated alternately with high-dosage furosemide (2000 mg/day) and daily dialysis, versus no furosemide and daily dialysis, found that the patients receiving furosemide showed a higher incidence of early diuresis (71.7 per cent versus 47.3 per cent) and a shorter anuric period (7 days versus 14 days), and required fewer dialyses (4.6 versus 9.2). However, both groups attained a normal serum creatinine level at the same time post-ARF, and the mortality in the two groups was exactly the same.[8] It would appear that early, high-dosage furosemide diuresis is important in therapy, but that the improvements to be expected are limited to an increase in the rate of early diuresis, and perhaps to a decrease in the number of dialyses required.

THERAPY

The two major improvements in the therapy of ARF over the past decade have been the acceptance of the concept of prophylactic dialysis, and an understanding of the need for adequate nutritional support. Teschan in 1955 found that the causes of death in his patients were hyperkalemia, rapidly developing clinical uremia, weight loss and emaciation, edema, progressive infection, impaired healing of wounds, and a bleeding tendency.[41] Early, active dialysis essentially prevents death from hyperkalemia, rapidly developing uremia, and edema; and appropriate nutritional support prevents the development of weight loss and emaciation. Sepsis, impaired wound healing, and gastrointestinal bleeding now remain as the most significant causes of mortality. In 1960, Scribner and coworkers[36] and Teschan and coworkers[40] clearly demonstrated that the use of prophylactic dialysis to maintain a nearly normal physiologic state gave superior results when compared with crisis dialysis begun only when fatal complications were imminent. Berlyne and coworkers in 1967 showed the importance of adequate calories, proteins, and essential amino acids in improvement of the general condition of the patient,[6] and Abel and coworkers demonstrated that intravenous alimentation containing essential amino acids and calories improved the metabolic state and decreased serum levels of magnesium, phosphate, and potassium, presumably owing to intracellular ionic shifts. Such therapy also stabilized blood urea nitrogen levels.[1]

Therefore, the basic principles of treatment for patients with established ARF are: Early intensive dialysis to maintain the blood urea nitrogen below 100 mg/100 ml and ideally below 50 mg/100 ml; adequate caloric and protein intake of 3500 to 4000 calories per day with 80 to 150 grams of protein; and active and vigorous therapy for the underlying surgical/traumatic/septic state.

With proper control by repeated cultures, antibiotics should be used in doses appropriately adjusted to sustain high therapeutic levels. The administration of any drug to a patient in established renal failure must be done carefully with a thorough understanding of the changes in drug metabolism and excretion resulting from renal lesion. Although various formulas have been devised based on a measurement of the creatinine clearance, by far the safest course is to measure actual drug levels in the plasma whenever possible. This is important not only to prevent overdosage, but also to assure that adequate levels are achieved. If the analytic capabilities are not available to measure actual drug levels frequently, the next safest method is to use tables that have been created based on the half-life of the particular drug related to the degree of renal impairment in the patient. These tables have been published by Bennett and coworkers[3-5] and by Neu.[30]

There are two methods which can be used to alter drug dosage to fit the clinical state. Usually the initial loading dose of the drug remains the same as in the normal state, since tissue saturation requires that the same amount of drug be administered. There is then the choice of administering the usual dose at extended intervals, or reducing the dose to be administered at regular intervals. Most clinicians find it easier to maintain drug levels with the usual dose administered at extended intervals. The drug administration tables give this information. If the tables are not available, one can approximate this method by multiplying the usual dose interval by the ratio of creatinine clearance of the normal divided by that of the patient. Thus, a patient with a creatinine clearance of 20 ml/minute would have a formula of 100 over 20, or five times the normal drug administration interval for maintenance, e.g., every 40 hours if the normal is every 8 hours. It has been stressed that some drugs bind to albumin, with higher levels of free drug resulting in the hypoalbuminemic patient to any given dose (oxacillin), and that some drugs bind to red cells with a higher drug level resulting in anemic patients (gentamicin). These factors, plus the influence of liver function and the possibility of cross reactions with other medications, make the use of drug administration tables much safer than attempting to calculate the dose from a formula. Also, many drugs are dialyzable, and this factor must be considered.[35] Needed surgical intervention must be early and complete, as hesitation leads to rapid deterioration. Vigorous search for foci of infection is essential.

Gastrointestinal bleeding must be prevented if at all possible, and although this complication is less frequent with the use of prophylactic dialysis, it still carries a high mortality when it occurs. Measurement of coagulation factors should be made frequently, and abnormalities corrected by administration of appropriate blood fractions. Antacid therapy by mouth or tube appears to be beneficial. If gastrointestinal bleeding does occur, blood replacement must be adequate, early endoscopy should be performed for diagnosis, and surgical intervention should be undertaken before deterioration of the patient's condition occurs. This is usually necessary when replacement of six units of blood has been required and bleeding is continuing. The operation for stress ulceration of the stomach must be extensive gastrectomy, as all lesser procedures are followed by an unacceptable rate of recurrent bleeding with markedly increased mortality.

Dialytic therapy is usually carried out by hemodialysis; in order to infuse appropriate amounts of fluids for nutritional supplement and to maintain blood urea nitrogen levels within an acceptable range in the hypercatabolic patient, this should be done daily, or at least on alternate days. Peritoneal dialysis can be used and is preferred by some centers, but must be maintained continuously, with a one to two liter per hour exchange, and catheter reinsertion after three to seven days to prevent infection. Peritoneal dialysis is preferable in patients with unstable hemodynamics. Oral intake of required nutrients is to be preferred whenever possible, but in most cases the patients are too ill to take adequate food by mouth or the surgical condition precludes normal alimentation. In such cases, intravenous alimentation should be used. Intravenous vitamin preparations should also be given, especially additional vitamin C. Appropriate support for other body systems should be supplied. The patient must be weighed daily, and fluid and electrolyte levels must be controlled by frequent blood sampling.

Even with intensive and sophisticated treatment, mortality in the patient with postsurgical renal failure remains the same as that experienced a decade ago. Patients with posttraumatic renal failure fare somewhat better, presumably because of their generally younger age, and patients with obstetrical renal failure survive in 85 to 95 per cent of cases. In the postsurgical group, mortality appears to be associated with advanced age. The increasing number of patients who die from uncontrollable sepsis, either from abdominal or pulmonary origin, is perhaps a reflection of the survival of these patients to reach a dialysis unit. Gastrointestinal hemorrhage appears to be decreasing with improved maintenance of the normal state by intensive dialysis. The present state of affairs in postsurgical ARF is well summed up by John P. Merrill, who stated in 1973, "Finally it must be remembered that the high mortality in acute renal failure results not from 'uremia' but from complications of trauma or surgery which were the predisposing causes in the first place."[27]

REFERENCES

1. Abel, R. M., Abbott, W. M., and Fischer, J. E.: Intravenous essential L-amino acids and hypertonic dextrose in patients with acute renal failure: effects on serum potassium, phosphate, and magnesium. Am. J. Surg., *123*:632, 1972.
2. Baek, S. M., Brown, R. S., and Shoemaker, W. C.: Early prediction of acute renal failure and recovery. II. Renal function response to furosemide. Ann. Surg., *178*:605, 1973.
3. Bennett, W. M., Singer, I., and Coggins, C. J.: Guide to drug usage in adult patients with impaired renal function. J.A.M.A., *223*:991, 1973.
4. Bennett, W. M., Singer, I., and Coggins, C. J.: A guide to drug therapy in renal failure. J.A.M.A., *230*:1544, 1974.
5. Bennett, W. M., Singer, I., Golper, T., Feig, P., and Coggins, C. J.: Guidelines for drug therapy in renal failure. Ann. Int. Med., *86*:754, 1977.
6. Berlyne, G. M., Bazzard, F. J., Booth, E. M., Janabi, K., and Shaw, A. B.: The dietary treatment of acute renal failure. Q. J. Med., *36*:59, 1967.
7. Brown, C. B., Cameron, J. S., Ogg, C. S., Bewick, M., and Stott, R. B.: Established acute renal failure following surgical operations. *In* Friedman, E. A., and Eliahou, H. E. (Eds.): Proceedings, Acute Renal Failure Conference. Washington, D.C., Department of Health, Education, and Welfare Publication No. (NIH) 74–608, May 1973.
8. Cantarovich, F., Galli, C., Benedetti, L., Chena, C., Castro, L., Correa, C., Perezloredo, J., Fernandez, J. C., Locatelli, A., and Tizado, J.: High dose furosemide in established acute renal failure. Br. Med. J., *4*:449, 1973.
9. Chedru, M., Baethke, R., and Oken, D.: Renal cortical blood flow and glomerular filtration in myohemoglobinuric acute renal failure. Kidney Int., *1*:232, 1972.
10. Cooke, C. R., Brown, T. C., Zacherle, B. J., and Walker, W. G.: The effect of altered sodium concentration in the distal nephron segments on renin release. J. Clin. Invest., *49*:1630, 1970.

11. Davis, J. O.: Control of renin release. Hosp. Pract., April 1974, p. 55.

12. Eliahou, H. E., and Bata, A.: The diagnosis of acute renal failure. Nephron, 2:287, 1965.

13. Eliahou, H. E., Brodman, R. R., and Friedman, E. A.: Adrenergic blockers in ischemic acute renal failure in the rat. *In* Friedman, A. E., and Eliahou, H. E. (Eds.): Proceedings, Acute Renal Failure Conference. Washington, D.C., Department of Health, Education, and Welfare Publication No. (NIH) 74–608, May 1973.

14. Eliahou, H. E., Modan, B., Leslau, V., Bar-Noach, N., Tchiya, P., and Modan, M.: Acute renal failure In the community: an epidemiological study. *In* Friedman, E. A., and Eliahou, H. E. (Eds.): Proceedings, Acute Renal Failure Conference. Department of Health, Education and Welfare Publication No. (NIH) 74–608, May 1973.

15. Flamenbaum, W.: Pathophysiology of acute renal failure. Arch. Intern. Med., 131:911, 1973.

16. Flores, J., DiBona, D. R., Beck, C. H., et al.: The role of cell swelling in ischemic renal damage and the protective effect of hypertonic solute. J. Clin. Invest., 51:118, 1972.

17. Fung, H., and Thomson, A. E.: Renal vascular responses to acetylcholine and phenoxybenzamine in acute renal failure in the dog and in man. Fifth International Congress of Nephrology. Abstracts, 359. Mexico, October 1972.

18. Hollenberg, N. K., Sandor, T., Conroy, M., Adams, D. F., Solomon, H. S., Adams, H. L. and Merrill, J. P.: Xenon transit through the oliguric human kidney: analysis by maximum likelihood. Kidney Int., 3:177, 1973.

19. Jackson, J. D., Macgregor, J., Brown, J. J., Lever, A. F., and Robertson, I. S.: The effect of angiotensin II antisera and synthetic inhibitors of the renin-angiotensin system on glycerol-induced acute renal failure in the rat. *In* Proceedings, Acute Renal Failure Conference. Friedman, E. A., and Eliahou, H. E. (Eds.): Department of Health, Education and Welfare Publication No. (NIH) 74–608, May 1973.

20. Kjellstrand, C. M., Simmons, R. L., Shideman, J. R., Buselmeier, T. J., von Hartitzsch, B., and Najarian, J. S.: Acute tubular necrosis after renal transplantation: pathogenesis, prognosis and comparison to surgical disease acute tubular necrosis. *In* Friedman, E. A., and Eliahou, H. E. (Eds.) Proceedings, Acute Renal Failure Conference. Washington, D.C., Department of Health, Education and Welfare Publication No. (NIH) 74–608, May 1973.

21. Kleinknecht, D., and Ganeval, D.: Preventive hemodialysis in acute renal failure: its effect on mortality and morbidity. *In* Proceedings, Acute Renal Failure Conference. Friedman, E. A., and Eliahou, H. E. (Eds.): Washington, D.C., Department of Health, Education and Welfare Publication No. (NIH) 74–608, May 1973.

22. Kleinknecht, D., Jungers, P., Chanard, J., Barbanel C., and Ganeval, D.: Uremic and non-uremic complications in acute renal failure: evaluation of early and frequent dialysis on prognosis. Kidney Int., 1:190, 1972.

23. Leaf, A.: Cell swelling and renal ischemia. *In* Friedman, A. E., and Eliahou, H. E. (Eds.): Proceedings, Acute Renal Failure Conference. Washington, D.C., Department of Health, Education and Welfare No. (NIH) 74–608, May 1973.

24. Levinsky, N. G.: The interpretation of proteinuria and the urinary sediment. D.M., March 1967, p. 30.

25. Lordon, R. E., and Burton, J. R.: Post-traumatic renal failure in military personnel in Southeast Asia. Experience at Clars USAF Hospital, Republic of the Philippines. Am. J. Med., 53:137, 1972.

26. Ludens, J., Hook, J. B., Brody, M. J., and Williamson, H. E.: Enhancement of renal blood flow by furosemide. J. Pharmacol. Exp. Ther., 103:456, 1968.

27. Merrill, J. P.: Newer aspects of acute renal failure. *In* Proceedings, Acute Renal Failure Conference. Washington, D.C., Friedman, E. A., and Eliahou, H. E. (Eds.): Department of Health, Education, and Welfare Publication No. (NIH) 74–608, May 1973.

28. Muth, R. G.: Furosemide in acute renal failure. *In* Proceedings, Acute Renal Failure Conference. Washington, D.C., Friedman, E. A., and Eliahou, H. E. (Eds.): Department of Health, Education, and Welfare Publication No. (NIH) 74–608, May 1973.

29. Najarian, J. S., Gulyassy, P. P., Stoney, R. J., Duffy, G., and Braunstein, P.: Protection of the donor kidney during homotransplantation. Ann. Surg., 164:398, 1966.

30. Neu, H. C.: Guidelines to antibiotic therapy in renal failure. Med. Times, 101:47, 1973.

31. Oken, D. E.: The renin-angiotensin axis in vasomotor nephropathy—fact and fancy. *In* Proceedings, Acute Renal Failure Conference. Friedman, A. E., and Eliahou, H. E. (Eds.): Washington, D.C., Department of Health, Education and Welfare Publication No. (NIH) 74–608, May 1973.

32. Orecklin, J. R., and Brosman, S. A.: Current concepts in the diagnosis of acute renal failure. J. Urol., *107*:892, 1972.
33. Pedersen, F., and Ladefoged, J.: Renal hemodynamics in acute renal failure in man measured by intra-arterial injection. Scand J. Urol. Nephrol., *7*:187, 1973.
34. Reubi, F. C., Vorburger, C., and Tuckman, J.: Renal distribution volumes of indocyamine green (^{51}Cr) EDTA, and ^{24}Na in man during acute renal failure after shock. Implications for the pathogenesis of anuria. J. Clin. Invest., *52*:223, 1973.
35. Schreiner, G. E., and Teehan, B. P.: Dialysis of poisons and drugs—annual review. Trans. Am. Soc. Artif. Intern. Organs, *18*:563, 1972.
36. Scribner, B. H., Magid, G. J., and Burnell, J. M.: Prophylactic hemodialysis iin the management of acute renal failure. Clin. Res., *8*:136, 1960.
37. Stahl, W. M., and Stone, A. M.: Prophylactic diuresis with ethacrynic acid for prevention of postoperative renal failure. Ann. Surg., *172*:361, 1970.
38. Stone, A. M., and Stahl, W. M.: Effect of ethacrynic acid and furosemide on renal function in hypovolemia. Ann. Surg., *174*:1, 1971.
39. Stott, R. B., Cameron, J. S., Ogg, C. S., and Bewick, M.: Why the persistently high mortality in acute renal failure? Lancet, *2*:75, 1972.
40. Teschan, P. E., Baxter, C. R., O'Brien, T. F., Freyhof, J. N., and Hall, W. H.: Prophylactic hemodialysis in the treatment of acute renal failure. Ann. Intern. Med., *53*:992, 1960.
41. Teschan, P. E., Post, R. S., Smith, L. H., Jr., Abernathy, R. S., Davis, J. H., Gray, D. M., Howard, J. M., Johnson, K. E., Klopp, E., Mundy, R. L., O'Meara, M. P., and Rush, B. F., Jr.: Post-traumatic renal insufficiency in military casualties. I. Clinical characteristics. Am. J. Med., *18*:172, 1955.
42. Whelton, A.: Post-traumatic acute renal failure in Vietnam: a milestone in progress. Conn. Med., *38*:7, 1974.

CHAPTER 20

THE BURN PATIENT IN THE INTENSIVE CARE UNIT

BASIL A. PRUITT, JR., M.D.

GARY W. WELCH, M.D.

An extensive burn exerts deleterious effects on every organ system and is one of the most severe injuries that one can sustain. Since burns of more than 40 per cent of the total body surface are associated with 30 per cent or greater mortality, all patients with such injuries are properly considered high-risk patients. Postburn pathophysiologic changes may be life-threatening, not only by virtue of the magnitude of the disturbance but also by virtue of the rapidity of the changes which occur. The physiologic sequelae of thermal injury persist from the time of injury until definitive closure of the wound is achieved, and the burn patient may require intensive care throughout this entire period measured in weeks and, at times, in months.

In the immediate postburn period, cardiopulmonary resuscitation is the principal aspect of burn care, with ventilation supported as necessary and fluids administered to maintain vital organ function without overloading the patient or needlessly accentuating edema formation. Following resuscitation, wound care is the central issue of burn treatment. Topical therapy, daily wound surveillance with biopsy monitoring as needed, application of biologic dressings, and extensive autografting are often best carried out with the patient in an intensive care facility to ensure optimum results. Lastly, burn patients with life-threatening complications involving the pulmonary system, gastrointestinal tract, or hematologic or vascular systems most often re-enter the intensive care unit (ICU), where the necessary intensive care and monitoring can be best provided (Table 1).

Each adult patient with greater than 30 per cent total body surface burns and children exceeding 10 kg in weight whose burns match or exceed their

Table 1. MONITORING EQUIPMENT FOR BURN UNIT ICU

Equipment for ICU

Blood gas analyzer
Accurate scale for body weight
Blood volume measuring device
Cardiac output computer
Oxygen analyzer
Carbon dioxide analyzer
Wright respirometer
Inspiratory force meter
Metabolic scale
Ultrasonic flowmeter (Doppler)
Portable x-ray equipment
Fiberoptic bronchoscopes
Fiberoptic gastroduodenoscopes

Equipment for Individual Patients

Foley catheter with urine collection device
Electrocardiograph
Pressure transducers
  Arterial
  Venous for CVP, PAP and/or PCWP
Rectal temperature device
Biopsy instruments
Blood, wound, and secretion culture media and equipment
Urinalysis "tapes"

body weight expressed in kilograms should be treated in the intensive care unit during the resuscitation period. Additionally, patients with high-voltage electric injury or inhalation injury, postresuscitation patients with life-threatening complications such as pneumonia or acute gastrointestinal ulceration with perforation or significant bleeding, or patients with burn wound infections are best cared for in the ICU.

During calendar year 1974, 161 or 66 per cent of 244 burn patients admitted to the U.S. Army Institute of Surgical Research were treated in our intensive care unit. These patients ranged in age from 11 months to 84 years, with 14.3 per cent in the pediatric age group, 21.2 per cent above 45 years of age, and 64.6 per cent in the 15 to 45 year age group. The extent of burns in these patients ranged from 14 to 100 per cent of the total body surface, with the average extent of third-degree burn in those 139 patients with third-degree burn being 31 per cent of the total body surface.

One hundred fifty-six of these patients were admitted directly to the ICU and 5 additional patients, initially cared for on the general ward, were later admitted to the ICU because of a worsening of their clinical condition. Seventy-two of these patients never improved sufficiently to leave the ICU and remained there during their entire hospital course of up to 75 days prior to death. The other 89 left the ICU at times ranging from a few hours to several days after admission, with their transfer to the general ward occurring on the fifth postburn day on the average. Thirty-one of these latter patients were returned to the ICU for a second period of care, which averaged 12 days in duration, with 13 expiring during their second ICU admission. Of the 18 who left the ICU a second time, eight were returned to the ICU for yet a third time for an average of 16 days of care. Five of these patients expired and three improved sufficiently to be returned to the ward. Two of these latter patients survived but the third was returned to the ICU for a fourth time, where he expired after a combined total of 97 ICU days.

The burn intensive care unit should be a physically separate, identifiable section of a burn unit or center. A minumum of 200 square feet per patient bed should be provided, and all patient beds should be visible from a central nursing station.[13] Sufficient space should be maintained between individual patients so the bedclothes or equipment being used for the care of one patient do not come in contact with other patients. Provision must be made for the daily cleansing of the wounds, either with the patient in bed or by transporting him to a hydrotherapy facility.

Air-borne contamination is of relatively minor importance compared with the direct transfer of microorganisms from patient to patient, usually by attending personnel. To minimize exogenous contamination of the burn patient, masks and gowns should be available at the entrance to the ICU and should be donned by all personnel entering the unit. A supply of sterile gloves should be placed near the bedside of each patient. When it is necessary to touch the burn patient, the hands must be gloved and subsequently washed before attending another patient. During wound care or other procedures, the involved personnel should wear disposable, impermeable aprons to prevent soilage and contamination of the front of their clothing, which could then spread microorganisms to the next patient they attend (Fig. 1). Similarly, visitors should be instructed not to touch the burn wound or the equipment being used for the patients they are visiting and to avoid any contact with the bedding, equipment, or person of any other patient.

The use of a portion of a general hospital intensive care unit for burn patients will usually require physical or procedural modification of that ICU. In order to maintain the standards of care for nonburn patients while meeting the special needs of the burn patient, the latter may need to be placed in an individual room or in a burn care area created by temporarily "walling off" a section of the ICU as an infection control measure. Additionally, locating the burn patient near a sink will facilitate the necessary hygiene on the part of the staff caring for the burn patient in such a "makeshift" situation.

The effectiveness of laminar flow environments per se in controlling burn wound infection, espoused by many, remains unconfirmed, and conventional nonrecirculating air conditioning with 7 to 12 changes per hour appears adequate for the burn ICU. The temperature of the ICU should be maintained at a level representing a compromise between comfort for the patient and comfort for the staff, usually in the neighborhood of 27 to 28°C. In such an environment, comfort of the nude burn patient can be improved by the use of heat lamps or other heat sources (Fig. 2). Maintenance of a relatively warm microenvironment not only will increase patient comfort but

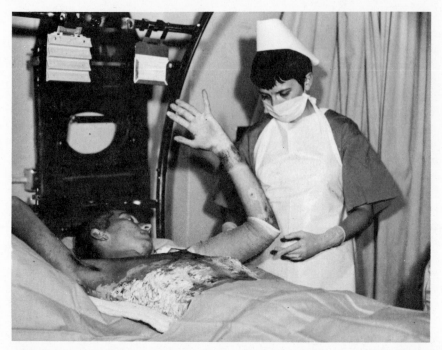

Figure 1. Attending personnel should wear disposable plastic aprons and gloves, as shown here, while carrying out wound care to prevent soilage of uniform and subsequent contamination of other patients. Note Sulfamylon burn cream on burns of right chest extending onto back and abdomen and use of Circ-O-Lectric bed, which permits turning of patient every three hours to prevent maceration of burned posterior surface.

will decrease modestly (approximately 10 per cent) the metabolic rate of patients with greater than 50 per cent burns.[42] The heating devices used for this purpose should be frequently monitored to ensure that the thermal energy supplied will not burn the patient and that the devices are adequately grounded to prevent electric shock injury to either patient or staff.

The burn patient requires frequent cleansing as a component of wound care. This is usually carried out in a hydrotherapy "tank" located on the burn ward, but can and should be done in the ICU for unstable or critically ill patients who will not tolerate movement to such a facility. Initial cleansing and debridement should be deferred until resuscitation has been instituted and cardiopulmonary stability is achieved, after which the patient can be moved to the hydrotherapy room or, depending upon his condition, cleansed in bed using any of several detergents. On a daily basis the topical wound care agent should be atraumatically removed, and the wound as well as unburned skin gently cleansed and thoroughly examined by the attending surgeon. Thereafter, the topical chemotherapeutic agent being used is reapplied with a sterile spatula or, preferably, with a sterile gloved hand.[31]

The frequency of inhalation injury and other pulmonary complications in burn patients necessitates obtaining chest roentgenographs at least daily during the first two weeks postburn and later in the postburn course, as indicated by the patient's condition. Associated injuries, such as fractures or blunt abdominal trauma, may require that other roentgenologic studies be obtained as well. Portable roentgenographic equipment must be available for the ICU to obtain these studies in critically ill patients who cannot be moved to the radiology department. The radiology department personnel must coordinate their procedures with the ICU staff in order not to interfere with other aspects of the burn patient's care and must be trained to observe appropriate hygienic precautions, such as incasing the x-ray cassettes in surgically clean linen when placing them in contact with the burn patient.

Housekeeping and equipment cleansing in the burn ICU are carried out as in other hospital areas. Outdoor carpeting has been used and reported as quite satisfactory in at least one burn ICU, but padded, seamless vinyl flooring is more commonly used because of its durability and ease of cleansing. On a regularly scheduled basis, ideally daily, the floor should be wet-vacuumed, using either a phenolic or, if the local water is "hard" and would cause plaque buildup, a quaternary ammonium detergent disinfectant. The walls of the ICU should be washed with the same type of solution. Beds and bedside furniture should be cleansed with a phenolic detergent disinfectant

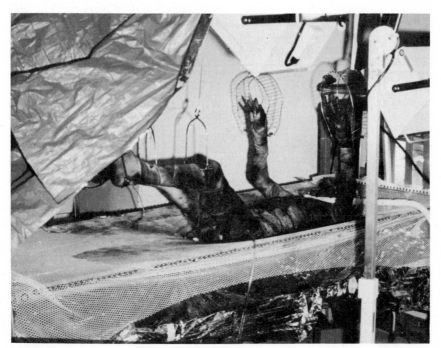

Figure 2. Extensively burned patient following excision and "mesh" grafting with skeletal suspension applied to all four limbs to prevent dislodgement of grafts by limb motion. Note the nylon mesh suspended from a modified Bradford frame, which prevents maceration of posterior truncal burn in this patient who must remain supine. The heat lamps and "space-blanket" shown here create a "microenvironment" of comfort and minimize heat loss.

when the patient leaves the ICU, or more often if soilage necessitates. Medical equipment should also be cleansed in similar fashion after each patient use with individual disposable delivery tubing sets used for any ventilatory device. The ICU ventilation system delivery filters should be changed or cleansed regularly and the air conditioning vents vacuumed weekly to remove dust and minimize air-borne debris. The filters and vents should be cultured periodically to detect microbial colonization, which has been reported in such equipment when condensation of water occurred.

FLUID REPLACEMENT AND MANAGEMENT

Fluid replacement is required to minimize blood volume deficits and to maintain organ flow in the immediate postburn period. The resuscitation should be begun as soon as possible with fluids administered through a secure pathway, preferably an intravenous cannula placed through un-burned skin in an upper extremity. Several formulas have been proposed for estimating fluid needs in the first 24 hours postburn, and all have been reported to be clinically effective (Table 2).[3,6,21,22] The attending physician should, therefore, utilize that formula with which he is most experienced and most comfortable, and modify the amount of fluid administered according to the individual patient's response. Loss of fluid from the vascular compart-ment due to increased vascular permeability is proportional to burn size and is clinically manifested by edema formation. In patients with burns of more than 30 per cent of the total body surface, fluid needs are further increased because of increased capillary permeability in unburned tissues. Since the capillary "leak" is greatest in the first few hours postburn, the rate of fluid administration must be correspondingly highest during that period. One gen-erally plans upon administering one-half of the fluid volume estimated for the first 24 hours during the first eight hours postburn, and the other half during the remaining 16 hours.

Table 2.   FORMULAS FOR ESTIMATING FLUID NEEDS IN
FIRST 24 HOURS POSTBURN

Evans's Formula: (1 ml colloid + 1 ml electrolyte)/kg/% burn   2000 ml 5% dextrose in water
Brooke Formula: (0.5 ml colloid + 1.5 ml electrolyte)/kg/% burn   2000 ml 5% dextrose in water
Lactated Ringer's (Moyer): Volume sufficient to maintain urine and   general condition of patient
Baxter's Formula: 4 ml lactated Ringer's/kg/% burn
Hypertonic Electrolyte Solution (250 mEq/liter): Volume sufficient to   maintain urine output at 30 ml/hr

Body-Weight Burn Budget of F. D. Moore:
    Colloid: 7.5% of body weight
    Electrolyte: 0.5 N saline, 1200 ml
                Ringer's lactate, 1000–4000 ml
    5% dextrose in water: 1500–5000 ml

Resuscitation volumes can be estimated by any of several published formulas detailed in Table 2. Studies at the U.S. Army Institute of Surgical Research have shown in a group of burn patients with extensive burns (average 65 per cent of the total body surface) that Brooke formula resuscitation permits a blood volume decrease of approximately 20 per cent but defends against further loss. Both blood and plasma volume decreased during the first 24 hours while the patient received resuscitation fluids, but returned toward normal during the second 24 hours postburn. Between 48 and 72 hours postburn, plasma volume had returned to normal in that group of burn patients and became supranormal in individual members of the group.[37]

Examination of the transcapillary dynamics in those patients revealed that in the first 24 hours postburn, infusion of colloid-containing fluids resulted in no greater intravascular volume restitution than an equal volume of electrolyte solution, suggesting that colloid-containing fluids administered during the first postburn day are in essence expensive salt water. During the second 24 hours postburn capillary integrity returns toward normal, so that plasma volume is augmented at all infusion rates with slight spontaneous increase observed even at a zero infusion rate. Studies by others have indicated that colloid-containing fluids are more effective for volume restoration in this period and that the use of colloids in the second 24 hours postburn minimizes both volume and salt loading in the burn patient.[6]

Fluid needs for the second 24 hours postburn are, therefore, generally between one-half and three-quarters of the volume required in the first 24 hours. Salt-containing infusions can usually be reduced and even omitted during the second 24 hours postburn to minimize salt loading. Colloid-containing solutions can be infused to repair persistent volume deficits, and glucose in water administered to meet metabolic and evaporative water losses. The preferred colloid is a heat-treated plasma product, free of hepatitis risk, or albumin diluted to "normal" plasma concentrations with an appropriate volume of saline or dextrose in water prior to infusion. At planned intervals during the second 24 hours, the fluid infusion rate should be reduced and, if urine flow remains at satisfactory levels, maintained thereafter at the slower rate. Accurate intake and output records and daily weights are essential for proper fluid management of the burn patient, not only in the immediate postburn period but, as noted below, throughout his hospital course. Frequently titration of fluid infusion to urinary output not only ensures adequate resuscitation but limits excessive fluid loading after vascular refilling has been achieved.

Based on clinical and laboratory studies, our present resuscitation regimen for the uncomplicated burn patient consists of only lactated Ringer's solution for the first 24 hours, with the volume need estimated as 2 ml/kg/per cent burn and the administered volume increased or decreased according to the individual patient's response. The majority of patients respond well to this regimen, and the actual volume required by adult burn patients seldom exceeds 2.5 ml/kg/per cent burn unless initiation of resuscitation has been delayed. During the second 24 hours, salt infusions are terminated and plasmanate is administered to minimize the volume needed to replace any persistent plasma volume deficit. Dextrose in water is also administered during the second 24 hours to satisfy metabolic and evaporative water losses while minimizing salt loading.

During resuscitation and even later in pediatric age group burn patients, salt-free fluid should be administered with caution and is best given either in small amounts interspersed with other fluids or mixed with salt-containing fluids to minimize the extent and rapidity of changes in serum sodium concentration. The most common cause of seizures in burned children at our Institute has been hyponatremia. Treatment of hyponatremia in the burn patient in virtually every case consists of limitation of fluid loading, administration of a rapid acting diuretic, such as Lasix, and anticonvulsant therapy, if necessary.[20]

Although destruction of red cells occurs owing to the thermal injury per se, the hematocrit rises in the first 24 hours postburn. This increased hematocrit is unresponsive to fluid therapy and renders the hematocrit an unreliable resuscitation guide. Except for patients with significant preinjury anemia or blood loss from associated injuries, whole blood is not given as part of the resuscitation fluids, since its administration would only further elevate an increased hematocrit and adversely affect flow in the microcirculation. Red cell loss during the first four to five days postburn proceeds at the rate of approximately nine per cent per day (some investigators have reported even greater losses during the first two postburn weeks.)[17,37] From the third postburn day onward, the hematocrit should be maintained between 30 and 35 per cent by infusions of packed red cells or, if secondary loss of whole blood occurs, by whole blood infusions. Despite marked elevation of erythropoietin levels, the need for periodic transfusion to replace wound and surgical losses persists until the burn wound is closed.[24]

The adequacy of resuscitation is monitored by determining the hourly urinary output and by frequent assessment of the patient's general condition (level of anxiety, restlessness, and the like) and vital signs. An hourly urinary output of 30 to 50 ml/hour in the adult burn patient and proportionately less in the pediatric burn patient is considered adequate and indicative of satisfactory fluid replacement. In the uncomplicated burn patient, the rate of fluid administration should be adjusted to achieve the above urinary outputs. Although urinary output may not precisely mirror renal blood flow and cardiac output, it is the most readily available and clinically useful guide to satisfactory volume replacement in the burn patient. Exceptions to this occur in patients with congestive heart failure and in patients who have previously received a diuretic and are undergoing an osmotic diuresis from any of several causes. The former can be identified by intravascular pressure measurements discussed below, and the latter by history and/or urinary glucose and urea measurement.

As a general rule, oliguria in the first 48 hours postburn indicates under-resuscitation, not renal failure, and calls for more rapid fluid administration, not the administration of a diuretic. Diuretics are useful and, in fact, indicated for prophylaxis against renal failure in four categories of burn patients, three of which are characterized by heavy concentrations of hemochromagens in the urine, i.e., patients with high-voltage electric injury, patients with associated soft tissue damage such as crush injury, and patients with white phosphorus burns in whom hemolysis has occurred secondary to inappropriate copper sulfate treatment. The other group in which diuretics are indicated includes patients with extensive burns who have received their estimated fluid needs plus additional fluids and who remain oliguric. The need for diuretics is otherwise infrequent, and renal failure is uncommon in adequately resuscitated burn patients as indicated by its occurrence in only 64 of 1,889 admissions to our Institute over a six-year period. In 7 of these patients, the renal failure was of the high output variety; of the remaining 57, all but 12 cases occurred secondary to terminal hypotension usually associated with overwhelming sepsis.

An indwelling urethral catheter should be placed upon admission in all patients with burns of more than 20 per cent of the body surface. The catheter should be taped to the abdominal skin to prevent pressure necrosis of the urethra, and the urinary drainage system should be of the closed type to minimize exogenous contamination. Antibiotic ointment should be applied to the urethral meatus daily, and urine cultures obtained by aspetic needle aspiration of the catheter. The catheter should be removed as soon as hemodynamic stability is achieved and the patient's state of consciousness ensures adequate voiding, usually by the fourth to fifth postburn day.

In the previously mentioned group of patients who were studied in detail during the resuscitation period, cardiac output was initially depressed but promptly rose to predicted levels by 18 hours postburn during a period of continued although modest blood and plasma volume decrease.[37] This finding indicated that patients receiving timely Brooke formula resuscitation do not sustain burn shock and suggests that blood and plasma volume measurements are probably not as sensitive an index of resuscitation effectiveness as cardiac output. During the second 24 hours postburn, cardiac output in the resuscitated burn patient rises to supranormal levels, where it remains in the absence of complications until the wound is healed or grafted.

If blood volume measurements are made in the immediate postburn period, the increased capillary permeability will permit the "leakage" of radioactively tagged albumin, resulting in the calculation of a greater than actual intravascular volume. The blood or plasma volume thus calculated provides one with an estimate of minimum deficit with the actual deficit of variably greater magnitude. Measurements of blood volume using radioactively tagged red cells may also be biased on the high side by trapping of such cells in injured vessels and intravascular cellular aggregates during the period of early postburn hypercoagulability. Despite the limitations of volume measurements during the period of increased capillary permeability, the measured volume does estimate minimum deficit and can serve as a rough guide to volume replacement needs.

The vast majority of burn patients do not require monitoring by the use of intravascular cannulae, but such may be helpful in the regulation of fluid therapy in burn patients of either extreme of age, in those with significant preexisting cardiopulmonary disease, in those with extensive burns unresponsive to fluid therapy, or in those who have been hypotensive because of a delay in initiating resuscitation. The limitations of the central venous pressure as an accurate reflection of myocardial function have led to the more frequent use of pulmonary artery and pulmonary capillary wedge pressure measurements for monitoring the state of the pulmonary circulation and adequacy of left heart function. Accurate, aseptic placement of such cannulae is essential, and the increased risk of infection in the burn patient necessitates that they be removed as soon as possible, at least within 72 hours after placement. If a Swan-Ganz catheter is used, the catheter must be gently inserted and the balloon deflated after each measurement of pulmonary capillary wedge pressure to minimize the occurrence of pulmonary parenchymal injury, reported to be as high as 7.2 per cent by some groups.[10] Laboratory studies at our Institute have shown that both pulmonary and peripheral vascular resistance increase immediately postburn, with the increase in pulmonary vascular resistance disproportionately high and persistent, suggesting that pulmonary capillary wedge pressure is a more reliable guide to myocardial function in the early postburn period.[4]

Electrocardiographic monitoring is required in those burn patients who have sustained high-voltage electric injury, in those with a history of cardiac disease, especially prior infarction, and in the elderly and other patients who respond poorly to resuscitation. Acute myocardial infarction was diagnosed in 11 burn patients, and old myocardial infarcts in two burn patients who expired during a recent 21-month period at our Institute. The extent of burn in those patients ranged from 13 to 81 per cent, with a mean size of 53 per cent of the total body surface, and the ages ranged from 19 to 75 years, with five under 40 years of age. Seven of the 10 acute myocardial infarctions that could be dated occurred within the first five postburn days. Chest pain was an inconstant, unreliable feature, and three patients had no symptoms of myocardial infarction. Diagnostic electrocardiographic changes were observed in only four patients, but significant arrhythmias indicating myocardial irritability were observed in eight patients. In addition to digitalis therapy and vasopressors and ventilatory support, pacemakers were implanted in two patients and antiarrhythmia medication administered to six. The seriousness of this complication is indicated by the universal mortality of those patients with a clinically diagnosed acute myocardial infarction.[2]

Following resuscitation, the burn patient is predisposed to the development of hypernatremia. The burn wound, having lost its water vapor barrier, acts like a free water surface, permitting prodigious evaporative water losses in proportion to the size of the burn. Additionally, renin and aldosterone secretion are elevated and the salt load administered during resuscitation is avidly retained. Consequently, the most common electrolyte abnormality in the postresuscitation period is hypernatremia due, in the vast majority of cases, to inadequate replacement of evaporative water loss.[40] The evaporative water loss of the burn patient can be predicted by the formula:

$$\text{Evaporative water loss in milliliters per hour} = (25 + \text{extent of burn on body surface}) \times \text{body surface area in square meters.}$$

The adequacy of hydration and of fluid replacement therapy can be assessed by changes in body weight, serum sodium concentration, and serum osmolality, all of which should be measured daily. The second most common cause of hypernatremia is dehydration secondary to an osmotic diuresis. In burn patients, particularly those receiving high carbohydrate and high protein feedings, glucosuria or azotemia, frequently accentuated in the septic patient, may be the cause of diuresis. Both blood and urine glucose and urea levels must be measured daily and the diet adjusted if significant elevation of blood glucose or urea or urinary spillage of glucose occurs.

PERIPHERAL CIRCULATION

The formation of edema beneath a tight, inelastic, circumferential eschar on a limb or the chest may impair limb blood flow or chest wall motion, respectively. Elevation of tissue pressure above venous pressure will cause secondary extravasation of fluid into the burned limb and further increase tissue pressure until arterial flow ceases. Adequacy of distal limb blood supply must be assessed hourly or more often during the first 48 hours in patients with circumferential third-degree or deep second-degree burns. Clinical signs of vascular impairment include cyanosis, impairment of capillary refilling, and progressive neurologic change, especially paresthesias, with the latter being the most accurate of the clinical signs.[33] Studies at our Institute have shown the Doppler ultrasonic flowmeter to be more accurate than clinical signs in determining the need for escharotomy. Use of the flowmeter permitted detection of arterial flow in the posterior tibial artery or distal palmar artery in 50 per cent of limbs judged on the basis of clinical signs to need escharotomy (Fig. 3). Elevation of the involved limb with active exercise to increase venous return five minutes out of every hour was associated with maintenance of blood flow in circumferentially burned limbs and significantly reduced the need for escharotomy.[26] In the intensive care unit the attending personnel must ensure elevation of circumferentially burned limbs and directly supervise the scheduled hourly active motion of such limbs, encouraging the patient to move the part despite discomfort and the physical limitations imposed by edema formation.

If distal pulses are absent on examination or fade even with elevation and exercise, escharotomy should be performed with incision in the midlateral and/or midmedial line of the involved limb throughout the length of the constricting eschar (Fig. 4). This procedure can be carried out on the ward,

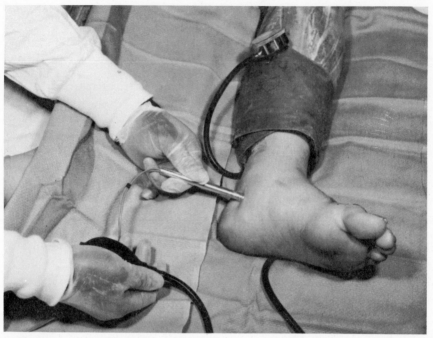

Figure 3.   Use of the ultrasonic flowmeter to detect flow in the distal palmar arch or, as shown here, in the posterior tibial artery is the most sensitive guide to the need for escharotomy in the circumferentially burned limb.

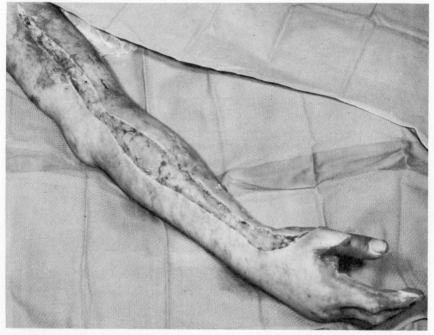

Figure 4.   Escharotomy incisions should extend for the entire length of the circumferential limb burn and, as shown here, must extend across involved joints.

since anesthesia is not required (the third-degree burn is insensate) and blood loss is minimal if the incision is carried only through the eschar and the superficial fascia. This will permit separation of the eschar with release of tissue pressure and not transect patent vessels in viable subcutaneous tissue. Escharotomy may be insufficient to restore blood flow in three categories of patients: (1) patients with high-voltage electric injury, (2) patients with associated fractures or soft tissue injury, and (3) patients with deep thermal injury directly involving muscle, in all of whom edema occurs beneath the investing fascia. In these patients, fasciotomy with incision of the investing fascia will be required to restore flow to distal unburned tissues. The latter procedure should be carried out in the operating room where appropriate anesthesia can be employed and proper aseptic precautions taken.

Edema formation beneath a circumferential upper truncal burn may limit the respiratory excursion of the thoracic cage and be manifested by rapid, shallow respirations, anxiety, and arterial hypoxia. In such cases, escharotomy along the anterior axillary line bilaterally will permit greater respiratory excursion, decrease anxiety, and improve ventilatory exchange and blood oxygenation. If the eschar extends onto the anterior abdominal wall, subcostal escharotomies connecting those in the anterior axillary line will further "release" the thoracic cage. In rare cases, penile and anterior cervical escharotomies have been employed for the release of tissue pressure and vascular occlusion in the penis and neck, respectively.

PULMONARY CONSIDERATIONS IN THE BURN ICU

The extensively burned patient is liable to all the pulmonary complications of any seriously ill surgical patient, including pulmonary edema during the diuretic phase, atelectasis, and pneumonia (either air-borne or hematogenous), during virtually the entirety of his hospital course.[34] In addition, inhalation injury (a chemical tracheobronchitis resulting from inhalation of smoke and products of incomplete combustion), limitation of chest wall excursion by eschar, and accentuation of postinjury hyperventilation by topical agents are problems peculiar to the burn patient which require special consideration. A total of 88 of the 161 burn patients treated in our ICU in 1974 had an endotracheal tube in place at some time during their ICU stay, and 35 of these patients required a tracheostomy for prolonged access to the lower tracheobronchial tree. A total of 99 of these patients (61.5 per cent) required mechanical ventilatory assistance while in the ICU, indicating a frequent need for careful, sophisticated pulmonary monitoring and care in burn unit ICUs.

Assessment of ventilatory adequacy can be made in the vast majority of patients on the basis of blood gas levels, blood pH, vital capacity, V_D/V_T, $D(A-a)o_2$ gradient and inspiratory force, which can all be determined by means of blood gas and pH measurements and pulmonary function tests which can be performed at the bedside. Blood gas measuring equipment should be indigenous to the burn ICU, or such equipment should be available in a responsive 24-hour-a-day central laboratory.

Ventilatory support may be needed in the burn patient immediately after a high-voltage electric injury because of respiratory arrest. This need is usually of brief duration and ends when spontaneous respiration is restored following cardiopulmonary resuscitation in such patients. In electric injury patients with cerebral or brain stem involvement, the need may persist or recur and frequent monitoring as described below must be carried out.

Clinical signs of inhalation injury include hoarseness, wheezing, coughing, and production of carbonaceous sputum, with the latter being the most reliable.[12] Although these signs may be present on admission, patients with severe inhalation injury may have a misleadingly benign early clinical course, and the signs first appear several days after injury (average time of onset is the second postburn day). Recent studies at our Institute have shown that the use of ^{133}xenon lung scans using 10 microcuries of ^{133}xenon injected into a peripheral vein permits the early diagnosis of inhalation injury with an 86 per cent accuracy. Direct examination of the tracheobronchial tree using the fiberoptic bronchoscope and the use of pulmonary function tests increase the accuracy of diagnosis to 96 per cent. The ^{133}xenon lung scans were performed in 84 of the total of 161 burn patients treated in our ICU in 1974, and fiberoptic bronchoscopic examination was carried out in 70. The diagnosis of inhalation injury was confirmed in 45 of these patients and the findings were suggestive but equivocal in an additional 10, i.e., a total of 34 per cent of the entire group required special care directed to their pulmonary status while in the ICU.

The ^{133}xenon lung scan should be performed as soon after hemodynamic stabilization has been achieved as is possible and in all events prior to the fourth postburn day, when the rate and depth of respiration characteristically begin to increase and the resulting hyperventilation may produce a falsely negative test. Inhalation injury is considered to be present if there is retention of the radioactive gas beyond 90 seconds postinjection, or if unequal radiation density is noted in the lung fields. Falsely positive tests may occur in patients with preexisting obstructive pulmonary disease (e.g., chronic bronchitis in a heavy smoker). A repeat ^{133}xenon lung scan following 24 to 48 hours of intensive inhalation therapy in patients with preexisting lung disease will usually show significant decrease or absence of ^{133}xenon retention if inhalation injury is not actually present.[27]

Identification of inhalation injury of the larger airways and the supraglottic region can be made by direct fiberoptic bronchoscopic examination of the tracheobronchial tree. Topical anesthesia should be employed as necessary to perform the bronchoscopic examination in an atraumatic manner and endobronchial cultures obtained to facilitate selection of antibiotics should pneumonia subsequently develop in the injured lungs. The bronchoscope can be passed either per os or per nares, depending upon the status of the individual patient. The endobronchial changes indicative of inhalation injury include edema, erythema, ulceration, and carbon particle deposition.[16] If edema of the vocal chords or of the supraglottic airway is identified, nebulized racemic epinephrine (1 ml in 8 ml of sterile water) should be administered with intermittent positive pressure breathing as often as every 15 minutes, until clinical evidence of airway compromise abates. Intubation of the airway as an elective procedure is indicated if the nebulized epinephrine is ineffective or if, at the time of bronchoscopic examination, complete obstruction of the airway appears imminent.

In patients with negative [133]xenon lung scans, large airway inflammatory changes can be present and their identification, using the bronchoscope, enables one to institute appropriate therapy, including frequent toilet, to clear the airways of necrotic debris and maintain their patency. Since falsely negative examinations have occurred in burn patients who underwent bronchoscopy while hypotensive, direct examination of the tracheobronchial tree should be performed only in adequately resuscitated, stable patients. To identify pneumothorax as a complication of bronchoscopy, a chest roentgenogram should be obtained following such procedures.

Pulmonary function tests are the most sensitive means of identifying inhalation injury and have an accuracy of 91 per cent. Recent studies at our Institute have shown significant changes in Po_2, airway resistance, nitrogen washout, slope, and ventilation perfusion gradient to occur in burn patients with inhalation injury. Contrary to reports by others, Pco_2, pH, and compliance were unchanged in those patients with inhalation injury. The most discriminating tests appear to be the maximum expiratory flow volume curve (MEFV) and flow rates measured at 25, 50, and 75 per cent of vital capacity. Peak flow is depressed and the shape of the MEFV curve altered in patients with inhalation injury. With resolution of the inflammatory process, serial flow-volume curves measured over a period of several days will show a return of peak flow toward normal and the curve to assume a more normal configuration. Conversely, persistently diminished or decreasing peak flow rates indicate progression of the inflammatory changes and further compromise of the airways. Additionally, the effectiveness of therapeutic agents, such as Isuprel, can be assessed by noting the improvement in peak flow rates following administration of the agent.

Use of any two of these three diagnostic modalities virtually eliminates falsely negative assessment for inhalation injury.[1] Although some falsely positive assessments will occur with two diagnostic modalities, every patient requiring treatment will be identified so that treatment can be begun prior to clinical progression. The treatment of inhalation injury depends upon the severity of the disease process. In patients with mild disease the provision of warm, humidified oxygen, encouragement of coughing, and intermittent positive pressure breathing therapy will often suffice. More severe involvement may necessitate use of bronchodilators and mechanical clearing of debris from the tracheobronchial tree through the bronchoscope with the frequency of bronchoscopy determined by the amount of debris and the patient's ability to clear his airway spontaneously. Progressive hypoxemia will require the use of mechanical ventilatory support, and unrelenting bronchospasm may respond to corticosteroid therapy. Massive dose steroid therapy should be reserved for patients with severe pulmonary insufficiency because of the enhancement by these agents of the risk of infection and acute ulceration of the gastrointestinal tract. A broad spectrum antibiotic is administered at the first sign of pneumonia, with the antibiotics changed, if necessary, when the results of endotracheal cultures are available.

The characteristic ventilatory response to burn injury per se is hyperventilation resulting from an increase in both rate and depth of respiration. Minute volume increases in the immediate postburn period, with a further increase in general proportional to burn size in patients with greater than 40 per cent total body surface area burns beginning on the third to fifth day and peaking at levels of 20 to 25 liters per minute on the eighth to tenth postburn day. A slow return to the usual postburn level of two to three times normal occurs thereafter with subsequent lysis to normal levels. In the absence of inhalation injury, lung resistance is normal as is the lung clearance index, with the latter indicating uniform distribution of inspired air. As anticipated, arterial carbon dioxide tensions are commonly low and the blood pH is slightly alkaline in the hyperventilating burn patient. Although still within normal limits, arterial oxygen tensions commonly reach their lowest levels at the peak of the postburn hyperventilation period.[23]

In contrast to the normality of gas exchange indices, the mechanical properties were disturbed in the lungs of a group of burn patients recently studied at our Institute. Static lung compliance was depressed, with the greatest depression noted in patients with most extensive burns, and they showed a proportional decrease in dynamic compliance. The absence of a further fall in dynamic compliance as rate of breathing increased indicated that severe alteration of the small airways was not a principal cause of the hyperventilation. The decrease in compliance was associated with a modest increase in pressure-volume work of breathing, but fully half of the measurements of this index of pulmonary function in 35 study patients fell within the upper limits of normal for our laboratory. Of interest is the apparent temporal relationship of maximum hyperventilation, decrease in lung compliance, lowest arterial oxygen tension, and fullness of the circulation due to edema resorption in the latter part of the first postburn week. It is our clinical impression that diminution of the hyperventilation has occurred in some patients following restriction of fluid intake and diuretic therapy.

This postburn hyperventilation can be accentuated, particularly during the edema resorption period, by the use of Sulfamylon topical therapy for the burn wound. As noted above, the findings of earlier studies were consistent with fluid overload and pulmonary edema, and that process may have accounted for the exaggerated minute ventilation (approaching 70 liters per minute in some patients) and the respiratory insufficiency noted in the studies of Morris and Spitzer. More recent studies from which patients with any indication of pulmonary edema have been excluded have shown the application of Sulfamylon burn cream to patients previously treated with another agent to be associated with a 50 per cent rise in minute ventilation, tidal volume, and ventilatory equivalent.[29] This was accompanied by an increase in respiratory rate and the V_D/V_T ratio, an increase in arterial oxygen tension, and a fall in base excess. This latter study suggests that the basic cause of postburn hyperventilation is the increased metabolic demand of the burn patient and, additionally, that a portion of the hyperventilation is "wasted ventilation."

Prolonged postburn hyperventilation per se may cause some of the observed changes in pulmonary function, including increased pulmonary vascular resistance, decreased compliance, ventilation perfusion abnormalities, and increased work of breathing, which can all be further accentuated by pneumonia or pulmonary edema. The accentuation of postburn hyperventilation by Sulfamylon burn cream, therefore, appears relatively modest and the recent studies indicate that minute ventilation exceeding 25 liters per minute, even in patients treated with Sulfamylon burn cream, should prompt search for and correction of an underlying disease such as sepsis or fluid overload.

The respiratory alkalosis and lowered serum bicarbonate levels characteristic of postburn hyperventilation will predispose the burn patient who develops a secondary pulmonary complication, such as pneumonia, to a rapid shift from alkalosis to acidosis. In such patients, retention of carbon dioxide can occur with the absolute values still within normal limits and result in a fall in pH because of a change in the bicarbonate/carbon dioxide ratio. For this reason, frequent, at least daily, blood gas and blood pH measurements and chest roentgenograms are necessary to monitor the acid-base status of the burn patient with significant hyperventilation who develops secondary pulmonary complications. Persistent minute ventilation of 25 liters or more per minute, an increase in arterial carbon dioxide content, and the development of acidosis are indications for discontinuing Sulfamylon topical therapy and substituting another topical agent that does not inhibit carbonic anhydrase. If the acidosis is severe, buffering may also be necessary.

In addition to the problems specific to the burn patient, pulmonary complications common to all patients can occur and be the cause of respiratory insufficiency in patients with burns. The diagnosis of pulmonary insufficiency and the criteria for the need of mechanical ventilatory assistance and for the application of positive and expiratory pressure are the same for burn patients as for any other patient, with the exception of the V_D/V_T ratio in patients treated with Sulfamylon burn cream in whom that ratio frequently exceeds 0.5 because of the inhibition of carbonic anhydrase associated with the use of that agent.

A pulmonary function flow sheet should be maintained at the bedside for each patient requiring mechanical ventilation. Measurements of the pulmonary function indices noted above should be obtained and recorded on a scheduled basis with the frequency determined by the degree of pulmonary insufficiency. Pulmonary care and support devices should be adjusted as indicated by the patient's condition and the test values obtained.

Endotracheal intubation is performed for the same reasons in the burn patient as in other surgical patients, not simply because the head and neck are burned. The indications for intubation in the burn patient include acute upper airway edema, associated chest wall injury such as a flail chest, inability to handle secretions or vomitus and, as noted previously, severe inhalation injury. If mechanical ventilation is to be employed, the endotracheal tube should have a sponge or prestretched balloon type cuff to minimize tracheal trauma. Ideally, a nasotracheal tube should be employed initially, with a tracheostomy performed later if prolonged access to the tracheobronchial tree is necessary. Whichever tube is used, it should be removed as soon as possible to minimize the trauma caused by such devices, and careful hygiene should be observed during endobronchial aspiration procedures to minimize exogenous contamination. Humidification of ventilator-supplied air should be provided either by a humidifier in which the water is heated or by a nebulizer which is adequately disinfected between uses and in which the reservoir is replenished in an aseptic manner. The tubing leading from the ventilator to any seriously ill patient should be replaced by new, disposable tubing or by adequately sterilized previously used tubing on a daily basis.

WOUND CARE

Following resuscitation, burn patient treatment centers on wound care. The eschar per se is an excellent culture medium because of the presence of warm, moist, avascular, necrotic tissue. Since it is essentially impossible to prevent microbial colonization, topical chemotherapy is necessary to control and limit bacterial proliferation and prevent invasive burn wound sepsis. Several topical agents of documented effectiveness are available for burn wound care, in the form of either solutions applied as soaks or creams applied directly to the burn wound (Table 3).[15,25,31] Although topical therapy regimens may be varied according to individual patient needs, creams are usually applied with the sterile-gloved hand or a sterile spatula to all burn wounds once a day, with the cream renewed 12 hours later to those areas from which it has been abraded by the bedclothes. Silver nitrate soaks, 0.5 per cent, are changed every 8 to 12 hours and saturated with the solution every 2 hours to prevent wound desiccation.

The prolonged immobility of the burn patient with an intensive burn combined with the loss of tissue over bony prominences and the bacterial colonization of the burn wound predispose such patients to the development of decubiti. The burn wound, unless treated by soaks, should be kept as dry as possible by alternately exposing the anterior and posterior surfaces. This can best be achieved by nursing the burn patient in a Circ-O-

Table 3. Topical Antimicrobials for the Burn Wound

Agent	Type of Wound Care	Diffusable	Principal Limitations
Sulfamylon cream	Open	Yes	Pain on application Hypersensitivity reaction Accentuation of hyperventilation
0.5% silver nitrate solution	Soaks	No	Electrolyte disturbances Discoloration
Silver sulfadiazine cream	Open or dressed	Minimal	Hypersensitivity Bone marrow depression Insensitivity of some gram-negative organisms

Lectric bed and turning the patient every 3 hours following resuscitation (Fig. 1). The armrest attachments of those beds can be modified to facilitate elevation of burned arms and hands, which is especially important in the immediate postburn period. Armrest modification also permits more comfortable positioning of the arms when such patients are lying prone. Stryker or Foster frames can also be used for treatment of patients with burns on both the anterior and posterior surfaces. During the resuscitation period of all patients with burns of more than 20 per cent of the body surface, we have found recovery room–type beds with side rails and removable headboards useful in terms of ease of positioning and access to all areas of the patient. Following resuscitation, patients with burns on only one surface of the body or less than 20 per cent of the total body surface can be satisfactorily cared for in virtually any hospital bed. Burn patients with posterior surface burns and fractures requiring skeletal traction can best be nursed on a coarse-mesh nylon net attached to a modified Bradford frame (Fig. 2). Such a device prevents maceration of the posterior surfaces of such patients who cannot be turned. The air-fluidized bed is useful for nursing patients with extensive burns who have sustained a significant weight loss and have developed a decubitus ulcer or are at risk of doing so. Additionally, the air-fluidized bed prevents maceration of posterior surface donor sites in the patient on whom skin grafts have been placed and are exposed on the anterior surface.[28]

Since none of the available topical agents sterilize the burn wound, the microbial flora of the burn may escape from control and invasive burn wound sepsis of bacterial, fungal, and even viral etiology develop. Because of this possibility, the entirety of the burns of every patient must be examined daily for the clinical signs of invasive burn wound sepsis (Table 4). Should these signs be identified in any area of the burn, that area of the burn should be biopsied with the specimens divided for quantitative culture and microscopic examinations.[35] If invasive burn wound sepsis is confirmed by histologic criteria (Table 5), wound care must be altered. If the involved area is limited in extent, excision or even amputation should be considered. If a nonabsorbable topical agent is being used, it should be stopped and Sulfamy-

Table 4. CLINICAL SIGNS OF INVASIVE BURN WOUND INFECTION

Appearance of focal dark-brown or black discoloration of wound

Degeneration and "neoeschar" formation of granulation tissue

Hemorrhagic discoloration of unburned subcutaneous tissue

Unexpectedly rapid eschar separation

Advancing violaceous wound margin

Metastatic lesions in unburned skin

Vesicular lesions in second-degree burn (Herpes infection)

---

lon burn cream therapy instituted. For Pseudomonas invasive burn wound sepsis, daily subeschar injections of carbenicillin, 10 gm in 150 ml of saline, have been found helpful in arresting invasive sepsis when used in combination with systemic antibiotics to which the organism is sensitive.[7]

The burn wound should be cleansed daily if topical creams are being used so that wound inspection can be carried out. At that time, debridement of loose eschar to the point of bleeding or pain and unroofing of any subeschar collections of liquefied fat or purulent material should be accomplished. Following this procedure, the topical agent should be reapplied to intact eschar and a biologic dressing (xenograft or allograft skin) applied to any sizable (1 per cent of the total body surface or more) area free of eschar and necrotic tissue. Alternatively, small areas of open wound (in the aggregate less than 20 per cent of the total body surface) can be treated with 5 per cent Sulfamylon acetate solution soaks until all nonviable dermal debris has been removed and granulation tissue has appeared over the wound bed.[9]

Biologic dressings can and should be used as temporary wound covers to continue microbial control after the bulk of the eschar has been separated.[31] The ICU personnel should be well versed in the technique of applying cutaneous allograft or xenograft and the indications for the removal of such tissue. Biologic dressings are preferably left exposed unless applied to circumferentially burned limbs or an area in contact with the bedclothes, in

Table 5. HISTOLOGIC CRITERIA OF INVASIVE BURN WOUND INFECTION

Presence of microorganisms in unburned tissue

Marked inflammatory reaction in viable tissue at margin of burn

Microbial proliferation in subeschar space

Small vessel thrombosis in unburned tissue with ischemic necrosis

Intracellular virions in healed or healing second-degree burn.

---

which cases they are held in place by occlusive dressings. Exposed grafts are examined every four hours for the presence of subgraft suppuration, which is evacuated by incising the graft and extruding purulent material by rolling a cottontip applicator over the graft, or by removing the entire graft if there is diffuse subgraft suppuration and no graft adherence. A persistent elevation of temperature or other signs of systemic sepsis following application of biologic dressings in the presence of nonadherence of the grafts is indication for removal of the biologic dressing and resumption of topical therapy and daily debridement for further preparation of the wound.

As with any patient with recently applied grafts, the burn patient with the physiologic dressings must be moved with care and spontaneous motion limited for the first two to three days postgrafting. Grafted extremities should be slightly elevated and not permitted to assume a dependent position. When allografts show good adherence to the wound, one can be assured of a good "take" of autograft skin. Autografts are cared for in the same manner as biologic dressings in terms of cautious, passive movement of the patient, evacuation of subgraft purulent collections, elevation of autografted limbs, and limitation of spontaneous motion. Sheets of split-thickness skin graft are usually left exposed if not in contact with the bedclothes, but "meshed" autograft skin is commonly dressed with a layer of fine-mesh gauze next to the grafts and beneath gauze sponges kept moist with 5 per cent Sulfamylon acetate solution to limit bacterial proliferation in the interstices of such grafts. In cases where one is concerned about the state of a "mesh" grafted wound, the outer layers of the dressing can be removed and the graft "inspected" with the fine-mesh gauze in place in order not to unnecessarily disturb the grafts. The most common cause of skin graft failure on a properly prepared burn wound is motion, and it may be necessary to utilize skeletal traction to adequately immobilize the limbs of an uncontrollably restless patient (Fig. 2). The skin entrance sites of skeletal traction pins or wires should be kept clean and free of crusts. It is our practice to apply a gauze sponge moistened and kept moist with skin disinfectant to the skin-metal junction. Aside from limited osteolysis of cortical bone around the pin tracts, we have seldom encountered significant osteomyelitis associated with the use of such devices in the burn patient.

LIFE–THREATENING COMPLICATIONS

Sepsis remains as the most common life-threatening complication of burn patients in spite of the marked decrease in burn wound sepsis brought about by effective topical therapy. This is most commonly pneumonia, either air-borne or hematogenous, closely followed in incidence by suppurative thrombophlebitis. Air-borne pneumonia, which occurs earlier in the postburn period and occurs with greater frequency in association with inhalation injury, is less commonly fatal than hematogenous pneumonia, but is more often the principal cause of death. Assiduous aseptic tracheal toilet in the early postburn period, prevention of aspiration, and specific antibiotic therapy minimize the morbidity and mortality of this form of pneumonia. The appearance of focal pulmonary infiltrates late in the postburn course is suggestive of hematogenous spread of organisms from invasive burn wound sepsis, intraluminal suppuration in a previously cannulated vein, occult perforation of a viscus (most commonly, perforation of an acute gastric or duodenal ulcer), or an inapparent soft tissue abscess. All of these sites must be considered and ruled out in the burn patient with pneumonia or persistently positive blood culture and no other obvious source of infection.[32]

Suppurative thrombophlebitis can occur in any previously cannulated vein in the burn patient, although the frequency of the disease is directly related to the duration of cannula residence within the vein. Since less than one-half of burn patients with this disease will have any local signs of phlebitis, it is necessary to examine each previously cannulated vein by opening the cut-down site, removing residual ligatures from the vein, and digitally "milking" the vein in both directions toward the venotomy site. Extrusion of pus confirms the diagnosis, and the entirety of the involved vein should be excised. If intravenous cannulae were placed subcutaneously or nothing is expressed from the aforementioned venotomy site, the vein should be surgically explored at the estimated level of the previously resident catheter tip. Again, the presence of gross pus or identification of infection microscopically in extracted clot confirms the diagnosis of suppurative thrombophlebitis.[38]

Even high-flow central veins are not immune to this septic process, although it is less common in such veins.[39] Frequently, removal of a central venous cannula and treatment with systemic antibiotics are rewarded by clearing of a positive blood culture. Pulmonary embolization of infected clot is considered an indication for anticoagulant therapy in these patients. Persistently positive blood cultures in the presence of adequate blood levels of effective antibiotics in patients with central vein thrombophlebitis is a grave prognostic sign, although success has been reported following direct surgical or Fogarty catheter extraction of infected central vein thrombi in such patients.

Persistence of staphylococcal-positive blood cultures in the absence of another source of sepsis is an ominous suggestion of acute bacterial endocarditis.[5] In the recent past, the organisms causing such infections in our burn center have been resistant to methicillin, and vancomycin has proved to be the most effective agent. It is important that any antibiotic given to such patients be given in doses adequate to achieve effective "trough" levels. Failure to clear the blood culture with antibiotics in patients in whom peripheral sources of sepsis are absent is strongly suggestive of microbe-containing cardiac vegetations. The development of cardiac insufficiency in such patients may necessitate valve excision with insertion of a prosthetic valve, but salvage of such patients has been vanishingly small.

Massive adrenal hemorrhage is another complication related to infection in patients with extensive burns. In our experience, the first clinical sign has been cardiovascular instability, manifested by postural hypotension and cyanotic mottling of the skin. The clinical findings have otherwise been inconsistent except for upper abdominal pain of a somewhat diffuse character unassociated with specific abdominal signs. Laboratory findings in the patient in whom this diagnosis was made during life were remarkable for the rapid change from avid sodium retention at the apparent time of hemorrhage to urinary "salt-wasting" thereafter. Reciprocal changes in urinary potassium levels have also been observed, as has the occurrence of eosinophilia. Treatment consisting of steroid replacement therapy, general supportive therapy, and identification and treatment of any focus of infection has been universally disappointing.[14]

Hemorrhage from or perforation of an acute ulcer of the upper gastrointestinal tract is another life-threatening complication of thermal injury which is burn size–related. Studies by Czaja and coworkers have described the natural history of postburn changes of the gastric and duodenal mucosa and documented the occurrence of mucosal change as early as five hours postburn in over 80 per cent of patients with burns of 30 per cent or more of the total body surface (84 per cent had gastritis and 76 per cent duodenitis).[11] These changes are not associated with increased acid production, increased mucosal hydrogen ion permeability, sepsis, microvascular fibrin thrombi, or changes in mucus production or quality. In the majority of the patients, these mucosal lesions healed uneventfully; but in 26 per cent of patients with mucosal change, primarily those with sepsis or other complications, the lesions progressed to frank ulceration, some by the fifth postburn day, and in slightly more than 12 per cent, clinically significant bleeding occurred. Operative intervention for the treatment of bleeding or perforation was required in only two of this recently studied group of patients. Recently, those same investigators have identified increased gastric acid production in those burn patients with progressive mucosal disease and an increased hydrogen ion back diffusion, which appears to be a reflection of the severity of mucosal change.[19]

More recent studies carried out at our Institute indicate that prophylactic administration of antacids reduces the incidence of clinically significant complications of Curling's ulcer.[18] The antacid solution (a magnesium and aluminum hydroxide mixture is preferred) is instilled through a nasogastric tube in an amount sufficient to maintain an intragastric pH of 7.0. The gastric contents are aspirated hourly, with the amount of antacid instilled at that time adjusted according to the pH of the aspirate. Antacid therapy may predispose the burn patient to constipation, and monitoring of bowel movements to avoid impaction is an important aspect of ICU burn care.

The nasogastric aspirate and the stools should be closely observed for the presence of blood, and bleeding is an indication for endoscopic examination of the stomach and duodenum to assess the extent of mucosal disease and identify the source of hemorrhage. Ice water lavage should be instituted if significant bleeding is verified, and if the bleeding is massive or prolonged, operative intervention is required. Monitoring of the bleeding patient entails assessment of vital signs every 15 minutes and of the hematocrit every four hours. The strong association of sepsis as a predisposing factor to frank ulceration and hemorrhage demands a search for a focus of infection and its control if identified.

Perforation, massive hemorrhage with unresponsive hypotension, a need for more than six units of blood in 12 hours, and persistence of less severe hemorrhage for more than 24 hours are indications for operative intervention. Preexisting complications such as pneumonia, burns of the abdominal wall per se, and the presence of invariably contaminated burn wounds elsewhere on the body make one reluctant to intervene surgically, but prolonged delay only further prejudices the operative outcome in these patients. In the case of children, replacement of more than 60 per cent of the estimated blood volume has been associated with a fatal outcome, and when blood replacement volume approaches this level, operative therapy should be undertaken.[8]

Although our experience with nonresectional therapy has been limited, it has been discouraging because of rebleeding and perforation. We feel that the goal of surgical therapy is the removal of the ulcer, with antrectomy and vagotomy being the procedure of choice.[36] If the lesion is situated in a more cephalad position, a more extensive resection should be carried out. Twenty of 53 patients requiring surgery for the treatment of complications of Curling's ulcer have survived surgery and their burns. An additional seven patients survived surgery and resumed oral alimentation only to succumb to another complication of their burn injury, and these patients are considered potential survivors. When the latter group are added to the actual survivors, they represent a potential salvage rate of 51 per cent for operated patients as compared with an overall 23 per cent salvage for all burn patients with Curling's ulcer treated at our Institute.

The frequency of postoperative wound infections in these patients is so high as to necessitate use of retention sutures for abdominal closure in all these patients without suture of the skin edges and physiologic closure of the wound by means of viable cutaneous allografts. Postoperative complications are frequent and commonly related to conditions existing prior to operation, such as postoperative exacerbation of preexisting pneumonia and other septic processes. Intensive postoperative care is essential for these patients to prevent further deterioration and achieve maximum survival.

NUTRITIONAL CARE IN THE BURN ICU

The pronounced hypermetabolism of the burn patient can be only slightly ameliorated by manipulation of the environment, but its effects upon body mass and energy reserves can be minimized by provision of adequate amounts of calories and nitrogen.[30] The calorie and nitrogen needs for individual burn patients have been determined by indirect calorimetry and balance studies, which indicate that calorie and nitrogen equilibrium can be achieved in the majority of patients with burns of 30 to 60 per cent of the body surface by the administration of 2,000 to 2,200 calories per square meter of body surface per day and 15 gms of nitrogen.[41] These needs may be modified by coexistent injuries or complications, preburn dietary habits, and the patient's age.

Oral alimentation is preferred over all other routes, but spontaneous postburn food intake appears to be fixed at preburn levels, which will not satisfy the elevated needs of the patient. Calorie and nitrogen balance can be approached only by giving the burn patient around-the-clock feedings of any of several high-calorie, protein-containing liquid supplements which provide approximately one calorie per milliliter. Facial burns, oropharyngeal thrush, obtundation, or ileus as a manifestation of sepsis may limit oral alimentation, and if the patient has lost or is anticipated to lose more than 10 per cent of his preburn body weight, parenteral nutrition will, in general, be necessary.

Parenteral alimentation of the burn patient employs the solutions utilized for the nutrition of other surgical patients. The techniques of administration and monitoring are also the same as for other patients, including the use of carefully regulated infusion pumps to administer the hypertonic fluid at a constant rate throughout the entire day. The magnitude of evaporative water loss in the burn patient necessitates that sufficient "salt-free" water be added to the nutrient solutions to replace such losses, with the total amount of administered fluid adjusted as indicated by the indices of adequate hydration. Since potassium requirements are commonly elevated in the burn patient, as may be the phosphorus requirements, these minerals should be added to the nutrient solutions as necessary for the individual patient.

Sepsis is of particular concern in the burn patient receiving hyperalimentation, and the frequency of bacteremia and septicemia and the high density of skin microorganisms necessitates changing of the intravenous alimentation catheter site at least every three days on a regularly scheduled basis. The frequency of sepsis in the burn patient necessitates more frequent monitoring of serum and urine glucose levels than in other patients. Intolerance to a previously tolerated glucose load in the burn patient receiving intravenous alimentation has been closely associated with the development of sepsis and should prompt a thorough search for such a process with concomitant adjustment of the nutrient load.

REFERENCES

1. Agee, R. N., Long, J. M., III, Hunt, J. L., Petroff, P. A., Lull, R. J., Mason, A. D., Jr., and Pruitt, B. A., Jr.: Use of [133]xenon in early diagnosis of inhalation injury. J. Trauma, *16*:218, 1976.
2. Andes, W. A., and Hunt, J. J.: Myocardial infarction in the thermally injured patient. Proceedings Sixth Annual Meeting American Burn Assoc., Abstract 35, 1974.
3. Artz, C. P., and Soroff, H. S.: Modern concepts in the treatment of burns. J.A.M.A., *159*:411, 1955.
4. Asch, M. J., Feldman, R. J., Walker, H. L., et al.: Systemic and pulmonary hemodynamic changes accompanying thermal injury. Ann. Surg., *178*:218, 1973.

5. Baskin, T. W., Rosenthal, A., and Pruitt, B. A., Jr.: Acute bacterial endocarditis: a silent source of sepsis in the burn patient. Ann. Surg. (in press).
6. Baxter, C. R.: Fluid volume and electrolyte changes of the early postburn period. Clin. Plast. Surg., *1*:693, 1974.
7. Baxter, C. R., Curreri, P. W., and Marvin, J. A.: The control of burn wound sepsis by the use of quantitative bacteriologic studies and subeschar clysis with antibiotics. Surg. Clin. North Am., *53*:1509, 1973.
8. Bruck, H. M., and Pruitt, B. A., Jr.: Curling's ulcer in children: a 12-year review of 63 cases. J. Trauma, *12*:490, 1972.
9. Curreri, P. W., Shuck, J. M., Lindberg, R. B., and Pruitt, B. A., Jr.: Treatment of burn wounds with five per cent aqueous Sulfamylon and occlusive dressings. Surg. Forum, *20*:506, 1969.
10. Curry, C. R., and Quie, P. G.: Fungal septicemia in patients receiving parenteral hyperalimentation. N. Engl. J. Med., *285*:1221, 1971.
11. Czaja, A. J., McAlhany, J. C., and Pruitt, B. A., Jr.: Acute gastroduodenal disease after thermal injury: an endoscopic evaluation of incidence and natural history. N. Engl. J. Med., *291*:925, 1974.
12. DiVincenti, F. C., Pruitt, B. A., Jr., and Reckler, J. M.: Inhalation injuries. J. Trauma, *11*:109, 1971.
13. Downs, J. J.: Guidelines for organization of critical care units. The Committee on Guidelines of the Society for Critical Care Medicine, May 1971.
14. Foley, F. D., Pruitt, B. A., Jr., and Moncrief, J. A.: Adrenal hemorrhage and necrosis in seriously burned patients. J. Trauma, *7*:863, 1967.
15. Fox, C. L., Jr., Rappole, B. W., and Stanford, W.: Control of Pseudomonas infection in burns by silver sulfadiazine. Surg. Gynecol. Obstet., *128*:1021, 1969.
16. Hunt, J. L., Agee, R. N., and Pruitt, B. A., Jr.: Fiberoptic bronchoscopy in acute inhalation injury. J. Trauma, *15*:641, 1975.
17. Loebl, E. C., Baxter, C. R., and Curreri, P. W.: The mechanism of erythrocyte destruction in the early postburn period. Ann. Surg., *178*:681, 1973.
18. McAlhany, J. C., Jr., Czaja, A. J., and Pruitt, B. A., Jr.: Antacid control of complications from acute gastroduodenal disease after burns. J. Trauma (in press).
19. McAlhany, J. C., Czaja, A. J., Villarreal, Y., Mason, A. D., Jr., and Pruitt, B. A., Jr.: The gastric mucosal barrier in thermally injured patients: correlation with gastroduodenal endoscopy. Surg. Forum, *25*:414, 1974.
20. McManus, W. F., Hunt, J. L., and Pruitt, B. A., Jr.: Postburn convulsive disorders in children. J. Trauma, *14*:396, 1974.
21. Monafo, W. W.: The treatment of burn shock by the intravenous and oral administration of hypertonic lactated saline solution. J. Trauma, *10*:575, 1970.
22. Moore, F. D.: Body weight burn budget. Basic fluid therapy for the early burn. Surg. Clin. North Am., *50*:1249, 1970.
23. Morris, A. H., and Spitzer, K. W.: Pulmonary pathophysiologic changes following thermal injury in burned soldiers. U.S. Army Inst. Surg. Res., Ann. Res. Prog. Rept., 30 June 1972, BAMC, Ft. Sam Houston, Texas, Sect. 49.
24. Mortensen, F. R., and Eurenius, K.: Erythrokinetics and ferrokinetics after thermal injury in the rat. Surg. Gynecol. Obstet., *138*:713, 1974.
25. Moyer, C. A., Brentano, L., Gravens, D. L., et al.: Treatment of large human burns with 0.5 per cent silver nitrate solution. Arch. Surg., *90*:812, 1965.
26. Moylan, J. A., Jr., Inge, W. W., Jr., and Pruitt, B. A., Jr.: Circulatory changes following circumferential extremity burns evaluated by the ultrasonic flowmeter: an analysis of 60 thermally injured limbs. J. Trauma, *11*:763, 1971.
27. Moylan, J. A., Wilmore, D. W., Mouton, D. E., and Pruitt, B. A., Jr.: Early diagnosis of inhalation injury using [133]xenon lung scan. Ann. Surg., *176*:477, 1972.
28. Newsome, T. W., Johns, L. A., and Pruitt, B. A.: Use of an air-fluidized bed in the care of patients with extensive burns. Am. J. Surg., *124*:52, 1972.
29. Petroff, P. A., Hander, W. E., and Mason, A. D., Jr.: Ventilatory patterns following burn injury and effect of Sulfamylon. J. Trauma, *15*:650, 1975.
30. Pruitt, B. A., Jr.: Postburn hypermetabolism and nutrition of the burn patient. In Manual of Surgical Nutrition. Philadelphia, W. B. Saunders Company, 1975, pp. 396–412.
31. Pruitt, B. A., Jr., and Curreri, P. W.: The burn wound and its care. Arch. Surg., *103*:461, 1971.

32. Pruitt, B. A., Jr., DiVincenti, F. C., Mason, A. D., Jr., et al.: The occurrence and significance of pneumonia and other pulmonary complications in burn patients: comparison of conventional and topical treatments. J. Trauma, *10*:519, 1970.

33. Pruitt, B. A., Dowling, J. A., and Moncrief, J. A.: Escharotomy in early burn care. Arch. Surg., *96*:502, 1968.

34. Pruitt, B. A., Jr., Erickson, D. R., and Morris, A.: Progressive pulmonary insufficiency and other pulmonary complications of thermal injury. J. Trauma, *15*:369, 1975.

35. Pruitt, B. A., Jr., and Foley, F. D.: The use of biopsies in burn patient care. Surgery, *73*:887, 1973.

36. Pruitt, B. A., Jr., Foley, F. D., and Moncrief, J. A.: Curling's ulcer: a clinicopathologic study of 323 cases. Ann. Surg., *172*:523, 1970.

37. Pruitt, B. A., Jr., Mason, A. D., and Moncrief, J. A.: Hemodynamic changes in the early postburn patient. The influence of fluid administration and of a vasodilator (Hydralazine). J. Trauma, *11*:36, 1971.

38. Pruitt, B. A., Jr., Stein, J. M., Foley, F. D., et al.: Intravenous therapy in burn patients: suppurative thrombophlebitis and other life-threatening complications. Arch. Surg., *100*:399, 1970.

39. Warden, G. D., Wilmore, D. W., and Pruitt, B. A., Jr.: Central venous thrombosis: a hazard of medical progress. J. Trauma, *13*:620, 1973.

40. Warden, G. D., Wilmore, D. W., Rogers, P. W., et al.: Hypernatremic states in hypermetabolic burn patients. Arch. Surg., *106*:420, 1973.

41. Wilmore, D. W.: Nutrition and metabolism following thermal injury. Clin. Plast. Surg., *1*:603, 1974.

42. Wilmore, D. W., Mason, A. D., Johnson, D. W., and Pruitt, B. A.: Effect of ambient temperature on heat production and heat loss in burn patients. J. Appl. Physiol., *38*:593, 1975.

CHAPTER 21

THERAPEUTIC CONFLICTS IN THE INTENSIVE CARE UNIT

SAMUEL F. POWERS, M.D.

Patients who are admitted to an intensive care unit may pose problems in management that are infrequently encountered on the general hospital ward. Admission to the medical or surgical services is almost invariably for a single disease, such as pneumonia or acute appendicitis. Once the diagnosis has been established, the therapy is usually self-evident. On the other hand, patients who are admitted to the intensive care unit may be suffering from multiple injuries or diseases involving multiple organ systems. Although the specific treatment for any single organ system is reasonably clear-cut, the management of the entire patient may involve several methods of treatment that appear to be mutually contraindicated. The intensive care physician, above all others, must guard against the tunnel vision of the medical specialists and consider the entire patient, including both the physical and emotional states. Emotional distress associated with severe illness is more frequent in the intensive care unit than on other services in the hospital. An example of therapeutic conflict is seen in the middle-aged male patient who has been under severe emotional stress due to loss of his job and is involved in a single car accident. On admission to the intensive care unit, he is found to have a fractured femur and to be hypotensive and mentally agitated. The actual sequence of events might have been profound mental strain leading to a myocardial infarction that occurred while driving for a job interview, leading in turn to the single car accident and a fractured femur. Placing this patient in an open intensive care ward will be bad for his mental state and probably bad for his myocardial infarction; on the other hand, however, it is desirable because of the need for close monitoring of his hemodynamic status. The administration of intravenous fluids may be required to support his peripheral circulation because of blood loss associated with the fracture, but at the same time the administration of such fluids is contraindicated if he is suffering from hypotension secondary to myocardial damage. Successful

326

management of this patient will depend upon the skillful resolution of each of these conflicts at the appropriate time so that the entire patient— myocardium, peripheral circulation, and psyche—is adequately supported.

Therapeutic conflicts in the intensive care unit can be divided into four general categories:

1. Ethical conflicts—the decision of whether a patient should be admitted to the intensive care unit, whether any treatment should be instituted, and if instituted, when and under what circumstances it should be terminated. These considerations are discussed in detail in the chapter titled Ethical and Legal Considerations in the Intensive Care Unit, and will not be discussed further in this section.

2. Conflicts between the risks of invasive diagnostic and therapeutic techniques and the expected benefits to be achieved from such invasive methods.

3. Conflicts resulting from the need for emergency management of an acute problem utilizing a therapeutic modality that may be hazardous because of the presence of preexisting disease.

4. Conflicts that arise because the therapy which is necessary for treating one organ system may damage another. A corollary to this problem is that the organ system which demands therapeutic priority over others will change from day to day and sometimes from hour to hour.

CONFLICTS BETWEEN THE RISK OF INVASIVE THERAPEUTIC MANEUVERS AND PROBABLE BENEFITS

Patients who are admitted to the intensive care unit are generally at a high risk for serious complication or death, so that the tolerance for diagnostic and therapeutic error is reduced almost to a vanishing point. Clinical syndromes appear suddenly and progress to irreversibility with startling rapidity. The time-honored practice of sequential clinical observation followed by tentative therapeutic trials is a luxury denied to the physician in the intensive care unit. The use of the balloon tip flow-directed catheter in the usual patient on the general medical ward suffering from congestive heart failure could not be countenanced, since the risk involved would far outweigh the probable therapeutic benefit. On the other hand, the use of this device in the patient with a combined myocardial infarction and fractured femur as described previously is mandatory. Here, the risk of the procedure is small compared with the essential information that can be immediately obtained. Delay in management to permit sequential observations of the electrocardiogram would undoubtedly provide the correct diagnosis, but this would appear only in the clinical summary of the autopsy report. Other devices that may be useful in the care of patients in the intensive care unit but that are associated with finite risk include an arterial cannula, a urethral catheter, and an endotracheal tube. Each of these may serve to introduce infection into the patient and should not be lightly undertaken. Systemic sepsis is now the number one cause of death of patients admitted to intensive care units.

A conflict in therapy is typified by the problem of tracheostomy in patients with extensive burns. The recognition of an airway burn is an indication for prolonged airway support. Under most circumstances, a tracheostomy would be the indicated therapy. A conflict arises because tracheostomy involves an elective incision. Burn patients are infected, and an open wound will serve as a portal of entry for pathogenic organisms. The performance of a tracheostomy in any seriously injured patient poses an additional conflict whenever prolonged nutritional support by means of intravenous hyperalimentation is expected. The site of election for introduction of the hyperalimentation catheter is the subclavian vein adjacent to the incision for tracheostomy. Infection in the tracheostomy wound may spread along the course of the hyperalimentation catheter into the circulation. Faced with these conflicts, the decision to avoid tracheostomy and accept the risk of subglottic stenosis and vocal cord damage associated with an endotracheal tube must be accepted.

Hyperalimentation lines have an extremely high risk of introducing infection or of having the catheter serve as a nidus for perpetuating sepsis. The duration of expected therapy and the type of fluid infused increase the risk of bacterial contamination. Patients with systemic sepsis are more likely to develop colonization of the hyperalimentation catheter, but they may be the patients who are most in need of nutritional support. A satisfactory compromise for this conflict is to insert hyperalimentation catheters that are changed from one side to the other at least twice a week. With all possible precautions, there is still a significant risk that must be accepted because of the greater benefits that may accrue.

The insertion of urethral catheters and intra-arterial lines poses a significant risk for both local and systemic infection. Neither invasion should be undertaken without due consideration of the possible consequences inherent in these techniques. In the early postinjury period, a urethral catheter and a radial artery cannula can provide lifesaving information. Once stabilization has taken place, the additional information to be obtained is relatively trivial, while the risk of infection increases with time.

The use of prophylactic ventilatory support in the immediate postinjury or portsurgical period poses additional therapeutic conflicts. Certain patients who have sustained multiple long bone fractures, pulmonary contusions, or severe crushing injuries are at significantly increased risk for development of the respiratory distress syndrome. Current evidence suggests that prophylaxis of this disorder is more effective than treatment once it has developed. A decision must be made as to whether the benefits of prophylactic respiratory support for a period of 24 to 48 hours result in a lesser risk to the patient than does the invasion by an endotracheal tube and respirator. There is no simple answer to these questions, and the final decision must be based on long experience with the treatment of the severely injured and seriously ill.

THERAPEUTIC CONFLICTS DUE TO THE PRESENCE OF THE PREEXISTING DISEASE

Cardiac disorders are the most important preexisting diseases to pose difficult and unusual therapeutic conflicts. The cardinal rule for management of cardiac patients is the avoidance of excessive intravenous fluids, particularly those containing sodium. The seriously injured or septic patient may require large quantities of precisely this type of solution for the maintenance of hemodynamic support. Diuretic therapy is the cornerstone of the management of congestive heart failure, but if applied to the hypovolemic injured patient, it can result in peripheral circulatory failure, decrease in myocardial blood flow, and worsening of the cardiac disorder. The patient with preexisting myocardial disease who sustains severe injury or undergoes a complicated operative procedure demands the most careful management if he is to survive. Every myocardium has a series of optimum conditions for its operation. These include the filling pressure of the left ventricle, which will provide adequate stroke work and assure that oxygen delivery to the myocardium can be maintained. Insertion of a balloon tip flow-directed catheter into the pulmonary artery permits the measurement of pulmonary wedge pressure and an estimation of the filling pressure of the left ventricle. Cardiac output, pulse rate, and mean arterial pressure provide the necessary information to estimate stroke work and, in conjunction with the pulmonary wedge pressure, to construct a Starling curve for this individual patient's myocardium. Sophisticated analyses of this type were once confined to the animal laboratory, but are now a clinical reality in modern intensive care units. Optimal oxygen delivery to the myocardium depends not only on the provision of the proper fluid volume to fill the left ventricle, but also on a reasonably normal concentration of hemoglobin and adequate oxygen saturation. Even here, a therapeutic conflict arises. Adequate oxygenation of arterial blood in critically ill patients may involve the use of a ventilator and may require positive and end-expiratory pressure (PEEP). Recent studies have shown that high levels of PEEP may result in decreased stroke work or, in some patients, left ventricular myocardial failure. The solution to this conflict requires frequent determination of stroke work, pulmonary wedge pressure, large vessel hematocrit, and oxygen saturation. Therapeutic maneuvers that result in improvement in one parameter with deterioration in others must be evaluated in terms of cardiac function and also in terms of peripheral organ perfusion.

Other examples of conflicts between therapy for the acute problem with its deleterious effects on preexisting disease include the use of certain antimicrobial agents in patients with known renal damage. The decision of whether to use an antibiotic agent that may be specific against an invasive organism but that is known to be nephrotoxic is a frequent occurrence. Whether to use gentamicin in patients with gram-negative sepsis and associated renal failure is an unfortunately frequent dilemma.

THERAPEUTIC CONFLICTS CONCERNING THE SUPPORT OF DIFFERENT ORGAN SYSTEMS AT DIFFERENT POINTS IN TIME

Attempts to improve myocardial function may cause deterioration of ventilation. Therapeutic attempts to maintain renal function and prevent subsequent tubular necrosis may threaten myocardial reserve. Emergency blood replacement with unmatched blood may improve oxygen-carrying capacity but result in a severe coagulopathy. The only possible solution to the dilemma of multiple organ dysfunction is to develop a table of priorities based on those efforts that are necessary for the immediate maintenance of life followed by those that are necessary to prevent isolated organ failure. Immediate resuscitative efforts demand adequate replacement of all lost and translocated fluid volume. All other therapeutic interventions must be subservient to this prime consideration. There is an optimal quantity and composition of fluid replacement for each individual clinical situation. The difficulty is in matching the clinical situation to the fluid requirement. Shires, in a classic study, demonstrated that the very severely injured whose expected mortality with standard replacement therapy was in the range of 80 per cent might require very large supplemental infusions of a balanced electrolyte solution. Conversely, those patients who have sustained moderate trauma for which the expected mortality is low and particularly where coexistent cardiac disease is present should receive little, if any, supplemental electrolyte solution. A frequent therapeutic conflict is whether volume replacement should be carried out with an electrolyte solution or a colloid such as albumin. The proper answer depends on many factors, including the elapsed time following the onset of illness or injury and the presence or absence of respiratory distress. Recent evidence suggests that in the early postinjury period, colloid solutions may be well tolerated, whereas at a subsequent phase of this illness when capillary endothelial damage has developed, the use of albumin solution may be contraindicated. The answer to the dilemma depends upon the type of illness or injury, the presence of preexisting disease, and the elapsed time from the onset of the disorder.

The use of a ventilator with positive end-expiratory pressure frequently poses a therapeutic conflict because its use may result in a decrease in cardiac output. This will be particularly severe in patients who are volume depleted. Patients with pulmonary contusions are likely to obtain improved pulmonary function if ventilator support with positive end-expiratory pressure is initiated as soon as possible. The dilemma arises because these patients generally have associated injuries, which result in a depleted vascular volume. The use of positive end-expiratory pressure may produce serious reductions in peripheral profusion with myocardial, renal, and hepatic failure. The solution to this particular dilemma is to make certain that left atrial pressure, as determined from a pulmonary wedge catheter, is restored to the range of 8 to 12 mm Hg before the end-expiratory pressure is increased.

Prophylaxis of acute tubular necrosis is the single most important therapeutic maneuver for acute renal failure. Once acute renal failure has developed, the mortality is high, whereas prophylaxis of this disorder can generally be accomplished. Fluid resuscitation is the keystone for prevention of acute tubular necrosis, which may involve the use of an osmotic or a loop diuretic in the hope of preventing acute renal failure. If the diuretic is administered at a time when the oliguria is secondary to volume depletion, then the resulting diuresis will cause a further volume depletion and may be the cause of acute renal failure rather than its hoped for prevention. The solution to this therapeutic dilemma is to avoid the use of diuretic agents until the adequacy of volume repletion has been established by means of measurements of pulmonary wedge pressure or left ventricular stroke work. It follows from this that the first priority is intravenous volume repletion, with concern about specific organ failure taking a slightly delayed position. The delay, however, should be measured in minutes rather than hours or days.

The final group of therapeutic conflicts is concerned with in toto patient management. A problem that has received insufficient attention is the conflict between the psychiatric implications of the intensive care unit with its 24-hour per day lighting, continuous activity, and coldly impersonal nature versus the physical benefit to be obtained from these surroundings. Patients in intensive care units easily become disoriented to place and time and may develop hallucinations and delusions. Transfer of such a patient into a hospital environment that more closely approximates his home surroundings, including the introduction of favorite personal belongings into the sick room, may provide therapeutic benefits that outweigh the physical facilities of the intensive care unit for monitoring the patient's somatic disorders.

A therapeutic management dilemma occurs in patients with multiple fractures for which the preferred method of management may be the use of skeletal traction when the patient is suffering from respiratory complications. The ability to turn the patient from side to side is a prime requisite of good pulmonary management, and this cannot be accomplished when the patient is being maintained in traction. Internal fixation should be used in these circumstances, since management of the overall patient will be improved, with only a slight increased risk from the alternate method of fracture management.

A special therapeutic conflict arises when a seriously ill patient who is clinically deteriorating may require a surgical procedure to correct one of the causes of an organ failure. Specific examples include the debridement and radical amputation of necrotic areas in patients with acute tubular necrosis, the drainage of infected tissue in a patient with evidence of systemic sepsis, and in certain instances, the performance of an emergency hysterectomy in a patient suffering from septic shock secondary to uterine infection. In each case, the performance of a surgical procedure poses a risk in a desperately ill patient, but the surgical procedure may offer the only hope for survival. A good rule of thumb is that the more seriously ill the patient, the more urgent is the surgical correction of a potentially treatable acute process.

In summary, the intensive care physician must be aware of the changing clinical priorities of the patient and be prepared to change therapeutic emphasis from one organ system to another. Willingness to compromise a method of treatment that may be ideal for the management of one diseased organ in order to improve the function of another more immediately critical organ is the keystone of successful management of the patient with multiple organ dysfunction.

Index